Neuroimmunomodulation

From Fundamental Biology to Therapy

ANNALS OF THE NEW YORK ACADEMY OF SCIENCES
Volume 1153

Neuroimmunomodulation
From Fundamental Biology to Therapy

Edited by
WILSON SAVINO, PRISCILLA OLIVEIRA SILVA, AND HUGO BESEDOVSKY

Published by Blackwell Publishing on behalf of the New York Academy of Sciences
Boston, Massachusetts
2009

Library of Congress Cataloging-in-Publication Data

Neuroimmodulation: from fundamental biology to therapy/edited by Wilson Savino, Priscilla Oliveira Silva, and Hugo Besedovsky.

    p. ; cm. – (Annals of the New York Academy of Sciences, ISSN 0077-8923; v. 1153)

    Result of a conference entitled the VII Congress of the International Society for Neuroimmunomodulation (ISNIM), held Apr. 14-27, 2008 in Rio de Janeiro, Brazil.

    Includes bibliographical references and index.

    ISBN 978-1-57331-746-7

    1. Neuroimmunology–Congresses. 2. Immune response–Regulation–Congresses. I. Savino, W. (Wilson) II. Besedovsky, Hugo O. III. Silva, Priscilla Oliveira. IV. International Society for Neuroimmunomodulation. Congress (7th: 2008: Rio de Janeiro, Brazil) V. Series: Annals of the New York Academy of Sciences; v. 1153. [DNLM: 1. Neuroimmunomodulation–physiology–Congresses. 2. Brain–immunology–Congresses. 3. Brain–physiopathology–Congresses. 4. Inflammation–immunology–Congresses. W1 AN626YL v.1153 2009/QW 504 N4937 2009]

    QP356.47.N4695 2009
    616.07'9–dc22

                                   2009001804

The *Annals of the New York Academy of Sciences* (ISSN: 0077-8923 [print]; ISSN: 1749-6632 [online]) is published 32 times a year on behalf of the New York Academy of Sciences by Wiley Subscription Services, Inc., a Wiley Company, 111 River Street, Hoboken, NJ 07030-5774.

MAILING: The *Annals* is mailed standard rate. POSTMASTER: Send all address changes to *ANNALS OF THE NEW YORK ACADEMY OF SCIENCES*, Journal Customer Services, John Wiley & Sons Inc., 350 Main Street, Malden, MA 02148-5020.

Journal Customer Services: For ordering information, claims, and any inquiry concerning your subscription, please go to interscience.wiley.com/support or contact your nearest office:

Americas: Email: cs-journals@wiley.com; Tel: +1 781 388 8598 or 1 800 835 6770 (Toll free in the USA & Canada).
Europe, Middle East and Asia: Email: cs-journals@wiley.com; Tel: +44 (0) 1865 778315
Asia Pacific: Email: cs-journals@wiley.com; Tel: +65 6511 8000
Information for Subscribers: The *Annals* is published in 32 issues per year. Subscription prices for 2008 are:
Print & Online: US$4862 (US), US$5296 (Rest of World), €3432 (Europe), £2702 (UK). Prices are exclusive of tax. Australian GST, Canadian GST and European VAT will be applied at the appropriate rates. For more information on current tax rates, please go to www3.interscience.wiley.com/aboutus/journal_ordering_and_payment.html#Tax. The price includes online access to the current and all online

back files to January 1, 1997, where available. For other pricing options, including access information and terms and conditions, please visit www.interscience.wiley.com/journal-info.

Delivery Terms and Legal Title: Prices include delivery of print publications to the recipient's address. Delivery terms are Delivered Duty Unpaid (DDU); the recipient is responsible for paying any import duty or taxes. Legal title passes to the customer on despatch by our distributors.

Membership information: Members may order copies of *Annals* volumes directly from the Academy by visiting www.nyas.org/annals, emailing membership@nyas.org, faxing +1 212 298 3650, or calling 1 800 843 6927 (toll free in the USA), or +1 212 298 8640. For more information on becoming a member of the New York Academy of Sciences, please visit www.nyas.org/membership. Claims and inquiries on member orders should be directed to the Academy at email: membership@nyas.org or Tel: 1 800 843 6927 (toll free in the USA) or +1 212 298 8640.

Printed in the USA.

The *Annals* is available to subscribers online at Wiley InterScience and the New York Academy of Sciences Web site. Visit www.interscience.wiley.com to search the articles and register for table of contents e-mail alerts.

ISSN: 0077-8923 (print); 1749-6632 (online)
ISBN-10: 1-57331-746-2; ISBN-13: 978-1-57331-746-7

A catalogue record for this title is available from the British Library.

ANNALS OF THE NEW YORK ACADEMY OF SCIENCES

Volume 1153

Neuroimmunomodulation: From Fundamental Biology to Therapy

Editors

WILSON SAVINO, PRISCILLA OLIVEIRA SILVA, AND HUGO BESEDOVSKY

This volume is the result of a conference entitled the **VII Congress of the International Society for Neuroimmunomodulation (ISNIM)**, held April 14–27, 2008 in Rio de Janeiro, Brazil.

CONTENTS

Part III. Behavioral Effects on Neuroimmunomodulation

Part IV. Stress, Inflammation, and Disease

Contents

Preface

The network of bidirectional interactions between the neuroendocrine and immune systems, essential "circuits" required for the homeostatic regulation of the organism, is now well defined. Accordingly, any imbalance in these physiological circuits can trigger or modulate a number of diseases; conversely, a number of diseases can affect these same circuits. This volume of the *Annals of the New York Academy of Sciences* presents papers devoted to the field of neuroimmunomodulation, comprising a large and integrative spectrum of the most recent advances in the subject, including physiological and pathological aspects of immunoneuroendocrine interactions, as well as neuroimmunomodulation-based therapy.

Articles are grouped together in sub-themes that include signaling pathways used in immunoneuroendocrine interactions; cytokine networks acting in the nervous and endocrine tissues; neuroimmunomodulation-related behavioral effects; and stress, inflammation, and disease (including autoimmune and infectious diseases). Each contribution to the volume was presented at the VII Congress of the International Society of Neuroimmunomodulation (ISNIM), held April 14–27, 2008 in Rio de Janeiro, Brazil, where more than three hundred researchers and students gathered to discuss topics in neuroimmunomodulation. We thank all the contributors to the proceedings herein, for their dedication and support, and hope that readers will find this volume of the *Annals* to be an excellent and thorough update of the neuroimmunomodulation field.

Wilson Savino
Oswaldo Cruz Foundation, Rio de Janeiro, Brazil

Priscilla Oliveira Silva
Oswaldo Cruz Foundation and Biology Institute
Fluminense Federal University, Brazil

Hugo Besedovsky
Institute for Physiology and Pathophysiology
Marburg, Germany

Neuroimmunomodulation: Ann. N.Y. Acad. Sci. 1153: xi (2009).
doi: 10.1111/j.1749-6632.2009.04479.x © 2009 New York Academy of Sciences.

Growth Hormone Modulates Migration of Developing T Cells

Mireille Dardenne,[a] Salete Smaniotto,[b] Valéria de Mello-Coelho,[c] Déa Maria Serra Villa-Verde,[d] and Wilson Savino[d]

[a]*Université Paris Descartes, Centre National de la Recherche Scientifique, Paris, France*

[b]*Laboratory of Immunohistology, Institute of Biological and Health Sciences, Federal University of Alagoas, Maceió, Brazil*

[c]*Laboratory of Immunophysiology, Institute of Biomedical Sciences, Federal University of Rio de Janeiro, Rio de Janeiro, Brazil*

[d]*Laboratory on Thymus Research, Oswaldo Cruz Institute, Oswaldo Cruz Foundation, Rio de Janeiro, Brazil*

In the context of the cross-talk between the neuroendocrine and immune systems, it is well known that growth hormone (GH) exerts physiological effects in central as well as peripheral compartments of the immune system. GH modulates a variety of thymic functions. For example, GH upregulates proliferation of thymocytes and thymic epithelial cells. Accordingly, GH-transgenic mice, as well as animals and humans treated with exogenous GH, exhibit an enhanced cellularity in the thymus organ. GH also stimulates the secretion of thymic hormones, cytokines, and chemokines by the thymic microenvironment as well as the production of extracellular matrix proteins. These effects lead to an increase in thymocyte migratory responses and intrathymic traffic of developing T cells, including the export of thymocytes from the thymus organ, as ascertained by experimental studies with intrathymic injection of GH in normal mice and with GH-transgenic animals. Because GH promotes a replenishment of the thymus and an increase of thymocyte export, it has been applied as a potential adjuvant therapeutic agent in the treatment of immunodeficiencies associated with thymic atrophy.

Key words: GH; IGF-1; thymic epithelium; thymocyte migration

Introduction

In the context of the cross-talk between the neuroendocrine and immune systems, it is well known that growth hormone (GH) exerts physiological effects in central as well as peripheral compartments of the immune system.[1–3] In respect to the thymus, we and others have shown that GH enhances the production of the thymic hormone thymulin by thymic epithelial cells (TEC) as well as the expression of extracellular matrix (ECM) ligands and receptors by these cells of the microenvironment.[1] GH also enhances thymopoiesis, as seen by the higher numbers of thymocytes in GH-transgenic mice compared to age-matched normal littermates.[4] This is in keeping with the data obtained with GH-injected mice, which presented 10–15% more cells in the synthesis + G2 mitosis (S + G2M) phases compared to denatured GH-injected animals.[5]

Importantly, in addition to the thymopoietic role in the thymus, GH also modulates thymocyte migration, and such effect will be the focus of the present review.

Address for correspondence: Mireille Dardenne, Paris Descartes University, CNRS UMR-8147, Hôpital Necker, 161, rue de Sèvres, 75015, Paris, France. Voice: 33 1 44 49 53 91; fax: 33 1 44 49 06 76. mireille.dardenne@inserm.fr

Neuroimmunomodulation: Ann. N.Y. Acad. Sci. 1153: 1–5 (2009).
doi: 10.1111/j.1749-6632.2008.03977.x © 2009 New York Academy of Sciences.

GH Enhances the Entrance of Bone Marrow-derived Precursors into the Thymus

Although few studies addressed the issue of a neuroendocrine control of T cell precursors into the thymus, it was demonstrated[6] that GH increases human T cell engraftment into the thymus of severe combined immunodeficiency-syndrome mice. This influence is mediated, at least partially, by adhesion molecules because it can be abrogated with antibodies directed against β1- or β2-integrin chains.[6] These data are in keeping with the findings showing that the entrance of bone marrow-derived progenitors into the thymus organ is partly mediated by the vascular cell adhesion molecule-1/fibronectin receptor, the integrin receptor α4β1 or CD49d/CD29.[7]

Thymocyte Traffic in Thymic Nurse Cells is Upregulated by GH

Thymic nurse cells (TNCs) are lymphoepithelial structures formed by one epithelial cell that harbors many developing thymocytes, which apparently physiologically traffic through this particular niche.[1] Because thymocyte traffic in the context of TNCs is mediated by ECM,[8] and given the fact that GH is able to enhance ECM production by TEC, we investigated whether GH could modulate intra-TNC thymocyte traffic. We found that, compared with control TNCs, GH significantly accelerated thymocyte release from TNCs and enhanced the entrance of thymocytes to reconstitute new lymphoepithelial complexes. This could be abrogated by antibodies recognizing laminin, fibronectin, or their corresponding receptors. More recently, we noticed that the production of laminin by TNCs derived from GH-transgenic mice is increased compared to wild-type control mice. Accordingly, thymocyte release from TNCs was also faster in GH-transgenic animals.[4] Taken together, these data clearly indicate that GH acceler-

ates the intra-TNC cell traffic and that ECM-mediated interactions are involved in such an effect.

Growth Hormone Stimulates Thymocyte Migration by a Combined Effect of Extracellular Matrix and Chemokines

The effects of GH upon thymocyte migration were further approached *ex vivo* by using *transwell* migration chambers.[9] We evaluated the effects of intrathymic high GH levels in two distinct models: intrathymic injection of GH in BALB/c mice and GH-transgenic mice. We showed that thymocyte adhesion to laminin is higher in GH-treated and in GH-transgenic animals compared with control mice. An enhancing effect was also observed in relation to the numbers of migrating cells in laminin-coated transwells.[4] Considering that intrathymic deposition of laminin is also enhanced *in vivo* upon GH stimulation, it is likely that hyper-responsive thymocytes, encountering higher amounts of laminin, further accelerate their traffic within the thymus organ.

GH also modulates other interactions related to thymocyte migration. In fact, thymocyte migratory response triggered by the chemokine CXCL12 is higher in GH-transgenic and GH-treated mice compared with control animals.[4] Such a GH-dependent increase in thymocyte migration is even more important when both laminin and CXCL12 were applied in the transwell chambers.

Thymocyte migration appears to result from various molecular interactions as if cells migrate under a multivectorial system of interactions involving various ligand/receptor pairs.[10] In this respect, it is possible that GH modulates the expression of other cell migration-related molecules that play a role in the generation of a resulting migration vector. This issue is completely open to further investigation.

Growth Hormone Modulates Thymocyte Export

Thymocyte export is a major event in the physiology of the thymus organ, allowing mature thymocyte to daily contribute to the maintenance of the peripheral T cell pool. One direct strategy to evaluate the exit of cells from the thymus is the evaluation of recent thymic emigrants (RTEs). It is well established that intrathymic injection of fluorescein isothiocyanate (FITC) randomly labels thymocyte cell membranes, which allows us to detect in the periphery of the immune system those cells (now labeled by FITC) that have recently been exported from the thymus.[9,11] When normal mice were intrathymically injected with GH in combination with FITC, there was an increase in the percentage of CD4+FITC+ cells in the lymph nodes. Similar data were obtained when FITC was injected alone within the thymus of GH-transgenic animals.[4,5]

These data match data from previous reports showing an increase in human RTEs in the blood of acquired immunodeficiency syndrome (AIDS) patients who received GH in conjunction with specific anti-retroviral therapy.[12,13] Additionally, we had previously found that adult AIDS patients bear a severe thymic atrophy,[14] whereas other researchers showed a decrease in GH production.[15] Also, HIV-positive children bearing a GH deficiency exhibited diminished thymus volume and reduced blood CD4+ T cells compared to HIV-bearing children that did not present GH deficiency.[16]

By contrast, in a rather reverse situation, acromegalic patients show an increase in the relative numbers of CD4+ T lymphocytes in the blood compared to age-matched healthy individuals.[17]

Is There an Autocrine/Paracrine Circuitry in the Thymus Involving Local GH and IGF-1 Production?

In addition to the endocrine effects of GH upon the thymus, we should consider the possibility of an autocrine/paracrine GH-dependent pathway. In this respect, the expression of GH receptors on thymocytes and microenvironmental cells has been demonstrated by various methods. Moreover, GH itself is produced by thymocytes and TECs.[1] Thus, in addition to the classical endocrine role of GH upon the thymus, it is conceivable that a GH-mediated autocrine/paracrine circuit exists within the thymus organ.

In addition, a number of data clearly show that GH effects in the thymus are mediated by insulin-like growth factor-1 (IGF-1). We found that the effects of GH upon the thymic epithelium could not only be seen by the use of IGF-1 but could also be abrogated by anti-IGF-1 or anti-IGF-1 receptor antibodies, as ascertained by thymic hormone production and expression of ECM ligands and receptors.[18,19] Moreover, GH enhances the expression of IGF-1 and IGF-1 receptor by cultured thymic epithelium,[20] which is in keeping with the fact that GH-transgenic mice have high levels of circulating IGF-1.[21]

Furthermore, administration of IGF-1 together with bone marrow cells resulted in an increase in thymus cellularity compared with transfer of bone marrow cells alone, and IGF-1 potentiated the colonization of fetal thymus organ cultures with T cell precursors,[22] indicating that IGF-1 by itself enhances the entrance of cell precursors into the thymus.

GH-based Therapy to Recover Thymopoietic Function

GH and related molecules (IGF-1 and ghrelin) have been applied to abrogate or to revert thymic involution. It was initially demonstrated that injections of GH-producing cells in old rats resulted in significant recovery of their age-related thymic atrophy.[23] As mentioned above, GH therapy was attempted in AIDS patients because early research had already shown that AIDS promotes a severe thymic atrophy.[14] Thymopoiesis as well as the numbers of CD4+ T

RTEs were increased in middle-aged AIDS patients that received anti-retroviral therapy plus GH.[13] This is in keeping with the fact that in young adult mice receiving intrathymic GH injections and young and aging GH-transgenic mice the size of the thymus increased and revealed higher numbers of CD4+ RTEs in spleen and subcutaneous lymph nodes compared to corresponding controls.[4,5]

These findings lead to the notion that GH can also affect the total numbers and the patterns of lymphocyte migration in peripheral compartments of the immune system. In this respect, we recently studied *ex vivo* migration patterns of lymphocytes derived from spleen and lymph nodes of GH-transgenic mice. We showed that ECM and chemokine-driven peripheral T cell migration is also enhanced in those animals overexpressing GH.[24]

Interestingly, enhancement of thymopoieisis in aging animals was also achieved with the use of IGF-1[25] as well as ghrelin, a potent GH secretagogue.[26]

Concluding Remarks

It is now largely accepted that GH exerts a pleiotropic role upon the thymus. In addition to enhancing proliferation of thymic cells, this hormone upregulates cytokine production by the thymic microenvironment and increases the ECM/chemokine-driven intrathymic T cell traffic as well as thymocyte export. Because GH enhances thymus replenishment and increases intrathymic T cell traffic, ultimately modulating thymocyte export, it should really be envisioned as a potential adjuvant therapeutic agent in the treatment of immunodeficiencies associated with thymic atrophy. The data discussed above, concerning GH treatment in AIDS patients, is a clear-cut example of how beneficial GH can be for individuals suffering severe immunodeficiency.

Acknowledgments

This work was developed at the Centre National de la Recherche Scientifique (CNRS)-Fiocruz Associated Laboratory of Immunology and Immunopathology. It was partially funded with grants by CNRS/Fiocruz French/Brazilian conjoint program, CNRS, Fiocruz, Conselho Nacional de Desenvolvimento Cientifico e Tecnologica (CNPq), and Capes (Brazil).

Conflicts of Interest

The authors declare no conflicts of interest.

References

1. Savino, W. & M. Dardenne. 2000. Neuroendocrine control of the thymus. *Endocrine Rev.* **21:** 412–443.
2. Meazza, C., S. Pagani, P. Travaglino, *et al.* 2004. Effect of growth hormone (GH) on the immune system. *Pediatr. Endocrinol. Rev.* **3:** 490–495.
3. Sumita, K., N. Hattori & C. Ninagaki. 2005. Effects of growth hormone on the differentiation of mouse B-lymphoid precursors. *J. Pharmacol. Sci.* **97:** 408–416.
4. Smaniotto, S., V. Mello-Coelho, D.M.S. Villa-Verde, *et al.* 2005. Growth hormone modulates thymocyte development in vivo through a combined action of laminin and CXCL12. *Endocrinoloy* **146:** 3005–3017.
5. Smaniotto, S., M.M. Ribeiro-Carvalho, M. Dardenne, *et al.* 2004. Growth hormone stimulates the selective trafficking of thymic CD4+CD8− emigrants to peripheral lymphoid organs. *Neuroimmunomodulation* **11:** 299–306.
6. Taub, D.D., G. Tsarfary, A.R. Lloyd, *et al.* 1994. Growth hormone promotes human T cell adhesion and migration to both human and murine matrix proteins in vitro and directly promotes xenogeneic engraftment. *J. Clin. Invest.* **94:** 293–300.
7. Scimone, M.L., I. Aifantis, I. Apostolou, *et al.* 2006. A multistep adhesion cascade for lymphoid progenitor cell homing to the thymus. *Proc. Natl. Acad. Sci. USA* **103:** 7006–7011.
8. Villa-Verde, D.M., J.M. Lagrota-Candido, M.A. Vannier-Santos, *et al.* 1994. Extracellular matric components of the mouse thymus microenvironment. IV. Modulation of thymic nurse cells by extracellular matrix ligands and receptors. *Eur. J. Immunol.* **24:** 659–664.
9. Savino, W., D.A. Mendes-da-Cruz, J.S. Silva, *et al.* 2002. Intrathymic T cell migration: a combinational interplay of extracellular matrix and chemokines? *Trends Immunol.* **23:** 305–313.

10. Mendes-da-Cruz, D.A., S. Smaniotto, A.C. Keller, *et al.* 2008. Multivectorial abnormal cell migration in the NOD mouse thymus. *J. Immunol.* **180:** 4639–4647.

11. Savino, W., D.A. Mendes-da-Cruz, S. Smaniotto, *et al.* 2004. Control of thymocyte migration: an interplay of distinct cellular interactions. *J. Leuk. Biol.* **75:** 951–961.

12. Napolitano, L.A., J.C. Lo, M.B. Gotway, *et al.* 2002. Increased thymic mass and circulating naïve CD4 T cells in HIV-1-infected adults treated with growth hormone. *AIDS* **16:** 1103–1111.

13. Napolitano, L.A., D. Schmidt, M.B. Gotway, *et al.* 2008. Growth hormone enhances thymic function in hiv-1-infected adults. *J. Clin. Invest.* **118:** 1085–1098.

14. Savino, W., M. Dardenne, C. Marche, *et al.* 1986. Thymic epithelium in aids. An immunohistologic study. *Am. J. Pathol.* **122:** 302–307.

15. Barbey-Morel, C., K. McDonnell & C.B. Pert. 2002. Peptide T bolus normalizes the growth hormone secretion pattern in two children with AIDS. *Peptides* **23:** 2279–2281.

16. Vigano, A., M. Saresella, D. Trabattoni, *et al.* 2004. Growth hormone in T-lymphocyte thymic and post-thymic development: a study in HIV-infected children. *J. Pediatrics* **145:** 542–548.

17. Colao, A., D. Ferone, P. Marzullo, *et al.* 2002. Lymphocyte subset pattern in acromegaly. *J. Endocrinol. Invest.* **25:** 125–128.

18. Timsit, J., W. Savino, B. Safieh, *et al.* 1992. Growth hormone and insulin-like growth-factor I stimulate hormonal function and proliferation of thymic epithelial cells. *J. Clin. Endocrinol. Metab.* **75:** 183–188.

19. Mello-Coelho, V., D.M.S. Villa Verde, M. Dardenne, *et al.* 1997. Pituitary hormones modulate by extracellular matrix-mediated interactions between thymocyte and thymic epithelial cells. *J. Neuroimmunol.* **76:** 39–49.

20. de Mello Coelho, V., D.M. Villa-Verde, D.A. Farias-de-Oliveira, *et al.* 2002. JM, Dardenne M, Savino W: Functional insulin-like growth factor-1/insulin-like growth factor-1 receptor-mediated circuit in human and murine thymic epithelial cells. *Neuroendocrinology* **75:** 139–150.

21. Sotelo, A.I., A. Bartke, J.J. Kopchick, *et al.* 1998. Growth hormone (GH) receptors, binding proteins and IGF-I concentrations in the serum of transgenic mice expressing bovine GH agonist or antagonist. *J. Endocrinol.* **158:** 53–59.

22. Montecino-Rodrigues, E., R.G. Clarck, L. Power-Braxton, *et al.* 1997. Primary B cell development is impaired in mice with defects of the pituitary/thyroid axis. *J. Immunol.* **159:** 2712–2719.

23. Kelley, K.W., S. Brief, H.J. Westly, *et al.* 1986. GH3 pituitary adenoma cells can reverse thymic aging in rats. *Proc. Natl. Acad. Sci. USA* **83:** 5663–5667.

24. Smaniotto, S., D.A. Mendes-da-Cruz, C.E. Carvalho-Pinto, *et al.* 2006. Combined role of extracellular matrix and chemokines on peripheral lymphocyte migration in growth hormone transgenic mice. *Neuroimmunomodulation* **13:** 214.

25. Beschorner, W.E., J. Divic, H. Pulido, *et al.* 1991. Enhancement of thymic recovery after cyclosporine by recombinant human growth hormone and insulin-like growth factor 1. *Transplantation* **52:** 879–884.

26. Dixit, V.D., H. Yang, Y. Sun, *et al.* 2007. Ghrelin promotes thymopoiesis during aging. *J. Clin. Invest.* **117:** 2778–2790.

Intracellular Molecular Signaling

Basis for Specificity to Glucocorticoid Anti-inflammatory Actions

Ana C. Liberman,[a,b] Jimena Druker,[a,b] Fernando Aprile Garcia,[a] Florian Holsboer,[c] and Eduardo Arzt[a,b]

[a]*Laboratorio de Fisiología y Biología Molecular, Departamento de Fisiología y Biología Molecular y Celular, Facultad de Ciencias Exactas y Naturales, Universidad de Buenos Aires, Buenos Aires, Argentina*

[b]*Members of the Instituto de Fisología y Biologia Molecular y Neurociencias-Consejo Nacional de Investigaciones Científicas y Técnicas*

[c]*Max-Planck Institute of Psychiatry, Munich, Germany*

The molecular interaction between hormonal and cytokine signals is crucial for providing specificity to their actions and represents a key step for understanding, at the molecular level, the ultimate response of physiological neuroendocrine-immune interactions. In this article we will describe new insights into the mechanisms underlying glucocorticoid-mediated anti-inflammatory action, focused on the regulation of immune–cytokine pathways. There are different levels of interaction between intracellular signals elicited by glucocorticoids and cytokines, with the final outcome being regulation of gene expression. One such interaction involves the molecular cross-talk between the activated glucocorticoid receptor (GR) and transcription factors implicated in the regulation of cytokine synthesis and function. This interaction results in the regulation of gene transcription, as we will illustrate with the helper T (Th)1 and Th2 transcription factors T-bet and GATA-3, respectively, implicated in the outcome of specific adaptive immune responses. A further level of mutual regulation is the posttranslational modification of GR by the ubiquitin–proteasome and sumoylation systems. These posttranslational modifications regulate GR activity and will be discussed for the small ubiquitin-related modifier (SUMO) pathway and its enhancer RWD RING finger-containing proteins, WD-repeat-containing proteins, and yeast DEAD (DEXD)-like helicases-containing sumoylation enhancer (RSUME). The impact of posttranslational modifications on inflammatory pathways, such as nuclear factor-$\kappa\beta$ and regulated cytokines, will also be discussed.

Key words: glucocorticoids; GATA-3; T-bet; SUMO; RSUME

Introduction

An important feature of the immune or inflammatory response is the marked increase in cytokine synthesis. Cytokines activate the hypothalamic–pituitary–adrenal system, causing an elevation of systemic glucocorticoid (GC) levels. GCs participate actively in the interaction between the neuroendocrine and the immune systems. The goal of this regulatory interplay is to maintain homeostasis of the whole body, avoiding excessive destruction and inflammation.[1] GCs inhibit cytokine gene expression and their actions on target cells; GCs act as immunosuppressive and anti-inflammatory agents that contain overreactions of the immune system as well as

Address for correspondence: Dr. Eduardo Arzt, Laboratorio Fisiología y Biología Molecular, FCEN-Universidad de Buenos Aires, Ciudad Universitaria, Pabellón II (C1428EHA), Buenos Aires, Argentina. Voice: 54-11-4576-3368; fax: 54-11-4576-3321. earzt@fbmc.fcen.uba.ar

Neuroimmunomodulation: Ann. N.Y. Acad. Sci. 1153: 6–13 (2009).
doi: 10.1111/j.1749-6632.2008.03958.x © 2009 New York Academy of Sciences.

autoaggressive responses in order to maintain body homeostasis. In this context, cytokines and hormones act as messengers that send systemic information to many cellular effectors. The final outcome of an adaptive response will depend on the satisfactory integration of this information at the intracellular level, which occurs through the molecular interaction between cytokines and steroid receptor signaling. In this article we will illustrate the integrative pathways with two examples: the helper T (Th)1/Th2 regulation by GCs and how specific intracellular pathways, such as posttranslational modifications, may fine-tune the immune and inflammatory responses.

Glucocorticoid Action

GCs are lipophilic compounds with the capability of diffusing through the cell membrane and binding their cytoplasmatic receptors. GCs exert their biological effects through binding to the GC receptor (GR), which is a transcription factor (TF) capable of regulating either positively or negatively the expression of target genes.[2-4] Upon interaction with GCs, the GR dissociates from the complex with heat shock proteins (hsp), hsp-associated proteins, and immunophilins and translocates to the nucleus.[2,3] In the nucleus the GR binds as homodimer to specific palindromic DNA consensus sequences, the glucocorticoid response elements (GREs). Genes positively regulated by GR have GREs in the promoter. This mechanism is named transactivation. The GR can also modulate gene responses by protein–protein interaction, which is commonly responsible for repression of transcription of target genes. This mechanism is called transrepression and involves the physical association between GR and other TFs, such as activating protein-1 (AP-1), nuclear factor-κβ (NF-κβ), and signal transducers and activators of transcription (STAT) family members implicated in signaling of inflammatory and immunoregulatory responses. New insights about their role in the regulation of Th cells will be described below.

Helper T1/Helper T2 Cells

After T cell receptor activation, naive Th cells differentiate into cells that contribute to eradicating extracellular or intracellular pathogens.[5,6] Th1 cells mediate cellular immunity defense against intracellular pathogens and Th2 cells participate in humoral and eosinophil/mast cell responses.[5,6] Th function is characterized by the specific pattern of cytokines they secrete.[5,6] Interferon-gamma (IFN-γ), tumor necrosis factor-beta (TNF-β), and interleukin-2 (IL-2) are secreted by Th1 cells and IL-4, IL-5, IL-10, and IL-13 are produced by Th2 lymphocytes. Mutual inhibitory regulation of Th1 and Th2 response exist; IFN-γ and IL-12 were shown to inhibit Th2 cytokine production and IL-4, IL-10, and IL-13 were shown to inhibit the Th1 responses,[7-9] thus avoiding the simultaneous activation of these two types of host defense and providing specificity to the immune response.

The committed Th cells express specific TFs: T-box expressed in T cells (T-bet) for Th1 and GATA-3 for Th2 differentiation.[10,11] T-bet and GATA-3 are known as master regulators of Th differentiation.[12,13] Ectopic expression of GATA-3 augments the production of Th2 cytokines, such as IL-4, IL-5, and IL-10.[14,15] At the same time GATA-3 inhibits Th1 polarization and cytokine production.[15] Likewise, ectopic expression of T-bet in T cells under different stages of Th2 differentiation is able to generate IFN-γ-producing Th1 cells and may also inhibit IL-4 and IL-5 Th2 cytokine production.[10]

T-bet is expressed only in Th1 cells and natural killer cells that produce IFN-γ,[10,12,16] a hallmark of Th1 cell-mediated immunity.[5,6] Ectopic expression of T-bet activates the *IFN-γ* gene and induces endogenous IFN-γ production, upregulation of IL-12 receptor β2 chain (IL-12Rβ2), and chromatin remodeling of IFN-γ alleles.[10,17,18] Mice lacking T-bet fail to develop Th1 cells and have reduced IFN-γ production.[12] Moreover, T-bet-deficient mice show normal lymphoid development

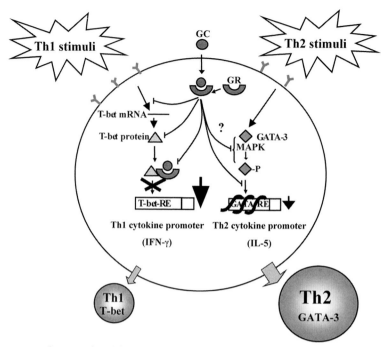

Figure 1. Helper T (Th)1/Th2 external stimuli induces T-bet or GATA-3 expression and protein synthesis. In turn, T-bet or GATA-3 induces Th1/Th2 gene expression. Glucocorticoids (GCs) inhibit T-bet mRNA and protein expression and strongly inhibit T-bet transcriptional activity by a transrepression mechanism involving the mutual interaction between the activated GC receptor (GR) and T-bet and inhibition of T-bet binding to DNA. GCs also inhibit GATA-3 activity by means of modification of chromatin structure and also could be modulating GATA-3 activation by kinase pathways. The differential stronger inhibition on T-bet compared to GATA-3 might induce a Th2 anti-inflammatory response. (Abbreviations: RE, DNA response element.)

but altered Th1 immune responses[19] and a corresponding increase in Th2 cytokines. T-bet is a target of posttranslational modifications by IL-2-inducible T cell kinase. This phosphorylation is necessary for the inhibition of Th2 cytokine expression but does not affect IFN-γ production and is exerted by the physical association between phosphorylated T-bet with GATA-3.[20] Thus, T-bet is a key TF that controls lineage commitment of Th cells by simultaneously activating Th1 genetic programs and by repressing the development of the opposing Th2 subset.[10]

GATA-3[21] is a member of the three Zn-finger domain-containing family proteins, which bind to a consensus site [(A/T)GATA (G/A)]. GATA-3 is selectively expressed in Th2 cells and is downregulated in Th1 cells.[11,14] Expression of a dominant-negative mutant of GATA-3 in mice leads to reduction in the levels of Th2 cytokines IL-4, IL-5, and IL-13[22] and, on the other hand, attenuates airway eosinophilia, mucus production, and IgE synthesis, all features of asthma and inflammation.[22] Posttranslational modifications, such as phosphorylation, also impacts GATA-3 TF activity. It has been shown that cAMP can induce GATA-3 phosphorylation via p38 mitogen-activated protein kinases and stimulate GATA-3 promoter activity (Fig. 1).[23] GATA-3 phosphorylation may be important for its interaction with other factors to promote Th2 cytokine gene expression or to make the chromatin environment accessible to other factors. Also, GATA-3 nuclear translocation is dependent on its phosphorylation and may also be an important step in the regulation of Th2 cytokine gene expression.[24]

Glucocorticoid Helper T-specific Anti-inflammatory Action

The Th1 and Th2 cytokine profiles are differently regulated by GC.[25] When T cells are exposed to GCs early during the activation phase, GCs promote a Th2 response that is evidenced by inhibition of the Th1 cytokines IL-2 and IFN-γ and stimulation of Th2 cytokines, such as IL-4 and IL-10.[26,27] GCs also inhibit IL-12 production.[27] However, in acute treatments GCs also inhibit IL-4[28,29] and IL-5 Th2 cytokines.[30] The *in vivo* Th2-preferred response caused by GCs could be explained by their modulatory action on key TF relative levels.[25,31,32] In addition, Th1 and Th2 cytokines may act together with GCs to regulate downstream specific TFs to determine the final outcome of the inflammatory and immune response.

Glucocorticoids Inhibit Helper T1 and Helper T2 Transcription Factors

The ability of GCs to inhibit inflammatory cellular immunity may be explained by the physical interaction between the activated GR and T-bet, which blocks the ability of T-bet to bind to DNA and to activate gene transcription[33] (Fig. 1). Consistent with its immunosuppressive action, GCs additionally inhibit T-bet both at mRNA and protein expression levels, revealing another layer of GR action on T-bet (Fig. 1).

IFN-γ is a central immunoregulatory cytokine responsible for several immunological effects, rendering its regulation important for protective cellular immunity.[5,6,34] Studies of the *IFN-γ* gene have shown that T-bet elements play an important role in the induction of transcription and production of this cytokine.[10,12,16–19] Transfection of EL-4 cells,

with T-bet expression vector and the entire IFN-γ locus, results in IFN-γ cytokine production.[10] GC inhibition of T-bet transcriptional activity impacts IFN-γ production and promoter activity,[33] thereby contributing to the understanding of the anti-inflammatory action of GCs by the specific inhibition of the Th1 cellular immune response (Fig. 1). These results indicate that T-bet might be useful as a GC target for pharmacological treatment of immune disorders. The understanding of T-bet regulation may ultimately help to improve Th2-inflammatory disease treatments by GCs.[35]

The interaction on the IL-5 promoter between GCs and nuclear factor of activated T cells,[36,37] AP-1, or NF-κβ,[30,37] the interaction between the GR and STAT-6,[38] and the inhibition of STAT-4 phosphorylation by dexamethasone[39] constitute some additional evidence about the underlying molecular mechanisms involved in the participation of GCs in Th responses.

IL-5 is a central immunoregulatory cytokine that plays an important role in the activation and survival of eosinophils. Also, IL-5 is involved in the development of a number of eosinophil-associated diseases, including bronchial asthma and airway inflammation. IL-5 is primarily synthesized by Th2 cells along with other Th2 cytokines, such as IL-4 and IL-13, that are also believed to participate in the pathogenesis of asthma. IL-5 synthesis is regulated at the level of gene transcription by a number of TFs, among them GATA-3. GATA-3 directly controls the expression of the *IL-5* gene[11,14,15,40] by binding and transactivation of elements on the −70 to −59 region. Inhibition of GATA-3 activity by GCs impacts *IL-5* gene expression.[37] It would be of much interest to elucidate the underlying molecular mechanisms involved in GC inhibition of GATA-3 activity, which may involve not only chromatin remodeling[37] but also inhibition of the kinase pathways involved in GATA-3 phosphorylation (Fig. 1). Identification of the exact molecular effect of GCs on GATA-3 Th2 cytokine production, such as IL-5, could allow the development of specific inhibitors that lack the extensive side effects of chronic use of GCs and could open new ways for the design of specific anti-inflammatory therapies.

The strong transrepressive inhibitory action of GCs on T-bet/Th1 cells[33] supports the notion that a differential mechanistic inhibition at the molecular level of T-bet and GATA-3 may be the way by which GCs induce Th2 differentiation (Fig. 1). A greater sensitivity to GC inhibition of T-bet with respect to GATA-3 could explain the Th2 induction exerted by GCs. Consistent with its immunosuppressive action, GCs inhibit both Th1 and Th2 master TFs but favor a Th2 development, which could be more evident in long-term treatments as already described.[41–44] Moreover, the effect of GCs is not only directly on Th cells but also on antigen-presenting cells (APC). Whole blood cell cultures treated with dexamethasone show an inhibition of IL-12 and no effect or even stimulation of IL-10 mRNA expression,[27,39] which may result in a decreased capacity of monocytes to induce IL-12 and an increased ability to induce IL-4 in T cells.[45] The presence of GCs at early stages of the immune response may create an imbalance not only on Th T-bet- and GATA-3-mediated cytokine release but also on APC cytokine production, thereby favoring a shift toward Th2 responses. T-bet-preferred inhibition by GCs provides the molecular basis to further understand the subtle regulation taking place during Th1/Th2 development.

Posttranslational Modifications Add Specificity to Glucocorticoid Interaction with Immune and Anti-inflammatory Transcription Factors

The interaction of GCs with TFs may be further modified by posttranslational modifications. Transcriptional activity of steroid receptors as well as several TFs involved in immune and inflammatory responses may be regulated by posttranslational modifications,

such as phosphorylation, acetylation, prenylation, and even by covalent attachment of polypeptides, such as ubiquitin and SUMO (small ubiquitin-related modifier).[4] The ubiquitin system induces the selective degradation of targeted proteins by the proteasome machinery.[46] On the other hand, SUMO modification regulates different cellular processes, including subcellular localization, transcription, chromatin structure, protein–protein interactions, and protein stability.[47–49] In some cases, SUMO and ubiquitin ligation compete for the same lysine residues on protein substrates; thus sumoylated proteins can avoid ubiquitin-mediated degradation, this being the case of the inhibitor of κβ (Iκβ).[50,51] Nuclear targets of many cytokine signaling pathways are sumoylated[52,53] as well as steroid receptors,[48,54,55] suggesting that SUMO modification could play a key role in modulating GC anti-inflammatory action. Accordingly, GR is modified by SUMO,[56,57] and this modification regulates the activity of the GR. Since GR function can be regulated by sumoylation, it might be possible that this mechanism leads to functional consequences on GR anti-inflammatory action. The RWD RING finger-containing proteins, WD-repeat-containing proteins, and yeast DEAD (DEXD)-like helicases-containing sumoylation enhancer (RSUME), a small RWD-containing protein, has a central role in the regulation of sumoylation by enhancing SUMO conjugation.[58] RSUME increases Iκβ sumoylation and stability. Moreover, immunoprecipitation experiments show a direct interaction between RSUME and Iκβ. In addition, RSUME inhibits TNF-α-induced κB-LUC (Luciferase) reporter activity, showing the functional consequence of Iκβ increased stability.[58] RSUME-enhanced sumoylation of Iκβ leads to the inhibition of NF-κB activity on two well-known inflammatory genes, *IL-8* and cyclooxygenase-2 (*Cox-2*) and therefore may also favor anti-inflammatory pathways (Fig. 2). Also, RSUME might have an additional activity on GR further modifying GC action. Understanding the impact of sumoylation and the

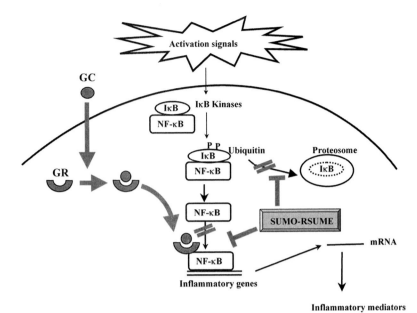

Figure 2. Nuclear factor (NF)-κβ activation involves the phosphorylation of inhibitor of κβ (Iκβ) by specific kinases and further ubiquitination and proteasome degradation. Then, free NF-κβ can bind κβ elements in the promoter regions of its target inflammatory genes. RWD RING finger-containing proteins, WD-repeat-containing proteins, and yeast DEAD (DEXD)-like helicases-containing sumoylation enhancer (RSUME)-enhanced sumoylation of Iκβ leads to an increase of Iκβ stability by avoiding ubiquitin-mediated degradation and therefore inhibits NF-κβ activity on target genes. GCs can inhibit NF-κβ activity by a transrepression mechanism involving the binding of the activated GR to NF-κβ. Also, the GR can be sumoylated, and this posttranslational modification may further modify its anti-inflammatory action. (Abbreviations: SUMO, small ubiquitin-related modifier.)

effect of its enhancer RSUME on inflammatory responses provides further insight in the regulatory network of immune–inflammatory signals.

Conclusions

GCs and cytokines interact at the molecular level on their target cells. This interaction is elicited by the activated downstream TFs that are at the same time further modified by posttranslational modifications, such as phosphorylation or sumoylation. Posttranslational modifications further impact TF signaling and gene expression. The final outcome of this complex network of interaction depends on the satisfactory integration of this information at the intracellular level, which finally generates an adequate im-

mune response helping to maintain homeostasis of the whole body and avoiding deleterious inflammatory or immunological effects.

Acknowledgments

This work was supported by grants from the University of Buenos Aires, the Argentine National Research Council (CONICET), and Agencia Nacional de Promoción Científica y Tecnológica-Argentina.

Conflicts of Interest

The authors declare no conflicts of interest.

References

1. Besedovsky, H.O. & A. del Rey. 1992. Immune-neuroendocrine circuits: integrative role of cytokines. *Front Neuroendocrinol.* **13:** 61–94.

2. De Bosscher, K., W. Vanden Berghe & G. Haegeman. 2003. The interplay between the glucocorticoid receptor and nuclear factor-kappaB or activator protein-1: molecular mechanisms for gene repression. *Endocr. Rev.* **24:** 488–522.

3. Ashwell, J.D., F.W. Lu & M.S. Vacchio. 2000. Glucocorticoids in T cell development and function. *Annu. Rev. Immunol.* **18:** 309–345.

4. Liberman, A.C. *et al.* 2007. Glucocorticoids in the regulation of transcription factors that control cytokine synthesis. *Cytokine Growth Factor Rev.* **18:** 45–56.

5. Abbas, A.K., K.M. Murphy & A. Sher. 1996. Functional diversity of helper T lymphocytes. *Nature* **383:** 787–793.

6. Mosmann, T.R. & R.L. Coffman. 1989. TH1 and TH2 cells: different patterns of lymphokine secretion lead to different functional properties. *Annu. Rev. Immunol.* **7:** 145–173.

7. Parronchi, P. *et al.* 1992. IL-4 and IFN (alpha and gamma) exert opposite regulatory effects on the development of cytolytic potential by Th1 or Th2 human T cell clones. *J. Immunol.* **149:** 2977–2983.

8. Oriss, T.B. *et al.* 1997. Crossregulation between T helper cell (Th)1 and Th2: inhibition of Th2 proliferation by IFN-gamma involves interference with IL-1. *J. Immunol.* **158:** 3666–3672.

9. Manetti, R. *et al.* 1993. Natural killer cell stimulatory factor (interleukin 12 [IL-12]) induces T helper type 1 (Th1)-specific immune responses and inhibits the development of IL-4-producing Th cells. *J. Exp. Med.* **177:** 1199–1204.

10. Szabo, S.J. *et al.* 2000. A novel transcription factor, T-bet, directs Th1 lineage commitment. *Cell* **100:** 655–669.

11. Zhang, D.H. *et al.* 1997. Transcription factor GATA-3 is differentially expressed in murine Th1 and Th2 cells and controls Th2-specific expression of the interleukin-5 gene. *J. Biol. Chem.* **272:** 21597–21603.

12. Szabo, S.J. *et al.* 2002. Distinct effects of T-bet in TH1 lineage commitment and IFN-gamma production in CD4 and CD8 T cells. *Science* **295:** 338–342.

13. Zhu, J. *et al.* 2004. Conditional deletion of Gata3 shows its essential function in T(H)1-T(H)2 responses. *Nat. Immunol.* **5:** 1157–1165.

14. Zheng, W. & R.A. Flavell. 1997. The transcription factor GATA-3 is necessary and sufficient for Th2 cytokine gene expression in CD4 T cells. *Cell* **89:** 587–596.

15. Ferber, I.A. *et al.* 1999. GATA-3 significantly downregulates IFN-gamma production from developing Th1 cells in addition to inducing IL-4 and IL-5 levels. *Clin. Immunol.* **91:** 134–144.

16. Robinson, D.S. & A. O'Garra. 2002. Further checkpoints in Th1 development. *Immunity* **16:** 755–758.

17. Mullen, A.C. *et al.* 2001. Role of T-bet in commitment of TH1 cells before IL-12-dependent selection. *Science* **292:** 1907–1910.

18. Afkarian, M. *et al.* 2002. T-bet is a STAT1-induced regulator of IL-12R expression in naive CD4+ T cells. *Nat. Immunol.* **3:** 549–557.

19. Neurath, M.F. *et al.* 2002. The transcription factor T-bet regulates mucosal T cell activation in experimental colitis and Crohn's disease. *J. Exp. Med.* **195:** 1129–1143.

20. Hwang, E.S. *et al.* 2005. T helper cell fate specified by kinase-mediated interaction of T-bet with GATA-3. *Science* **307:** 430–433.

21. Ho, I.C. *et al.* 1991. Human GATA-3: a lineage-restricted transcription factor that regulates the expression of the T cell receptor alpha gene. *Embo J.* **10:** 1187–1192.

22. Zhang, D.H. *et al.* 1999. Inhibition of allergic inflammation in a murine model of asthma by expression of a dominant-negative mutant of GATA-3. *Immunity* **11:** 473–482.

23. Chen, C.H. *et al.* 2000. Cyclic AMP activates p38 mitogen-activated protein kinase in Th2 cells: phosphorylation of GATA-3 and stimulation of Th2 cytokine gene expression. *J. Immunol.* **165:** 5597–5605.

24. Maneechotesuwan, K. *et al.* 2007. Regulation of Th2 cytokine genes by p38 MAPK-mediated phosphorylation of GATA-3. *J. Immunol.* **178:** 2491–2498.

25. Kovalovsky, D. *et al.* 2000. Molecular mechanisms and Th1/Th2 pathways in corticosteroid regulation of cytokine production. *J. Neuroimmunol.* **109:** 23–29.

26. Ramirez, F. *et al.* 1996. Glucocorticoids promote a TH2 cytokine response by CD4+ T cells in vitro. *J. Immunol.* **156:** 2406–2412.

27. Visser, J. *et al.* 1998. Differential regulation of interleukin-10 (IL-10) and IL-12 by glucocorticoids in vitro. *Blood* **91:** 4255–4264.

28. Wu, C.Y. *et al.* 1991. Glucocorticoids suppress the production of interleukin 4 by human lymphocytes. *Eur. J. Immunol.* **21:** 2645–2647.

29. Chen, R. *et al.* 2000. Glucocorticoids inhibit calcium- and calcineurin-dependent activation of the human IL-4 promoter. *J. Immunol.* **164:** 825–832.

30. Mori, A. *et al.* 1997. Two distinct pathways of interleukin-5 synthesis in allergen-specific human T-cell clones are suppressed by glucocorticoids. *Blood* **89:** 2891–2900.

31. Refojo, D. *et al.* 2003. Integrating systemic information at the molecular level: cross-talk between steroid receptors and cytokine signaling on different target cells. *Ann. N. Y. Acad. Sci.* **992:** 196–204.

32. Liberman, A.C., D. Refojo & E. Arzt. 2003. Cytokine signaling/transcription factor cross-talk in T

cell activation and Th1-Th2 differentiation. *Arch. Immunol. Ther. Exp. (Warsz.)* **51:** 351–365.

33. Liberman, A.C. *et al.* 2007. The activated glucocorticoid receptor inhibits the transcription factor T-bet by direct protein-protein interaction. *Faseb J.* **21:** 1177–1188.

34. Young, H.A. & K.J. Hardy. 1990. Interferon-gamma: producer cells, activation stimuli, and molecular genetic regulation. *Pharmacol. Ther.* **45:** 137–151.

35. Boumpas, D.T. *et al.* 1993. Glucocorticoid therapy for immune-mediated diseases: basic and clinical correlates. *Ann. Intern. Med.* **119:** 1198–1208.

36. Quan, A., M.N. McCall & W.A. Sewell. 2001. Dexamethasone inhibits the binding of nuclear factors to the IL-5 promoter in human CD4 T cells. *J. Allergy Clin. Immunol.* **108:** 340–348.

37. Jee, Y.K. *et al.* 2005. Repression of interleukin-5 transcription by the glucocorticoid receptor targets GATA3 signaling and involves histone deacetylase recruitment. *J. Biol. Chem.* **280:** 23243–23250.

38. Biola, A. *et al.* 2000. The glucocorticoid receptor and STAT6 physically and functionally interact in T-lymphocytes. *FEBS Lett.* **487:** 229–233.

39. Franchimont, D. *et al.* 2000. Inhibition of Th1 immune response by glucocorticoids: dexamethasone selectively inhibits IL-12-induced Stat4 phosphorylation in T lymphocytes. *J. Immunol.* **164:** 1768–1774.

40. Zhang, D.H., L. Yang & A. Ray. 1998. Differential responsiveness of the IL-5 and IL-4 genes to transcription factor GATA-3. *J. Immunol.* **161:** 3817–3821.

41. Miyaura, H. & M. Iwata. 2002. Direct and indirect inhibition of Th1 development by progesterone and glucocorticoids. *J. Immunol.* **168:** 1087–1094.

42. Ramirez, F. 1998. Glucocorticoids induce a Th2 response in vitro. *Dev. Immunol.* **6:** 233–243.

43. Daynes, R.A. & B.A. Araneo. 1989. Contrasting effects of glucocorticoids on the capacity of T cells to produce the growth factors interleukin 2 and interleukin 4. *Eur. J. Immunol.* **19:** 2319–2325.

44. Brinkmann, V. & C. Kristofic. 1995. Regulation by corticosteroids of Th1 and Th2 cytokine production in human CD4+ effector T cells generated from CD45RO- and CD45RO +subsets. *J. Immunol.* **155:** 3322–3328.

45. Blotta, M.H., R.H. DeKruyff & D.T. Umetsu. 1997. Corticosteroids inhibit IL-12 production in human monocytes and enhance their capacity to induce IL-4 synthesis in CD4 +lymphocytes. *J. Immunol.* **158:** 5589–5595.

46. Hershko, A. & A. Ciechanover. 1998. The ubiquitin system. *Annu. Rev. Biochem.* **67:** 425–479.

47. Melchior, F. 2000. SUMO–nonclassical ubiquitin. *Annu. Rev. Cell Dev. Biol.* **16:** 591–626.

48. Gill, G. 2004. SUMO and ubiquitin in the nucleus: different functions, similar mechanisms? *Genes Dev.* **18:** 2046–2059.

49. Hay, R.T. 2005. SUMO: a history of modification. *Mol. Cell* **18:** 1–12.

50. Desterro, J.M., M.S. Rodriguez & R.T. Hay. 1998. SUMO-1 modification of IkappaBalpha inhibits NF-kappaB activation. *Mol. Cell* **2:** 233–239.

51. Hay, R.T. *et al.* 1999. Control of NF-kappa B transcriptional activation by signal induced proteolysis of I kappa B alpha. *Philos. Trans. R. Soc. Lond. B. Biol. Sci.* **354:** 1601–1609.

52. Carbia-Nagashima, A. & E. Arzt. 2004. Intracellular proteins and mechanisms involved in the control of gp130/JAK/STAT cytokine signaling. *IUBMB Life* **56:** 83–88.

53. Bossis, G. *et al.* 2005. Down-regulation of c-Fos/c-Jun AP-1 dimer activity by sumoylation. *Mol. Cell Biol.* **25:** 6964–6979.

54. Tirard, M. *et al.* 2007. Sumoylation and proteasomal activity determine the transactivation properties of the mineralocorticoid receptor. *Mol. Cell Endocrinol.* **268:** 20–29.

55. Poukka, H. *et al.* 2000. Covalent modification of the androgen receptor by small ubiquitin-like modifier 1 (SUMO-1). *Proc. Natl. Acad. Sci. USA* **97:** 14145–14150.

56. Le Drean, Y. *et al.* 2002. Potentiation of glucocorticoid receptor transcriptional activity by sumoylation. *Endocrinology* **143:** 3482–3489.

57. Tian, S. *et al.* 2002. Small ubiquitin-related modifier-1 (SUMO-1) modification of the glucocorticoid receptor. *Biochem. J.* **367:** 907–911.

58. Carbia-Nagashima, A. *et al.* 2007. RSUME, a small RWD-containing protein, enhances SUMO conjugation and stabilizes HIF-1alpha during hypoxia. *Cell* **131:** 309–323.

Organizing the Thymus Gland

The Role of Eph and Ephrins

**Juan José Muñoz,[a] Javier García-Ceca,[a] David Alfaro,[a]
Marco Augusto Stimamiglio,[b] Teresa Cejalvo,[a] Eva Jiménez,[c]
and Agustín G. Zapata[a]**

[a]*Department of Cell Biology, Faculty of Biology, Complutense University, Madrid, Spain*

[b]*Laboratory of Thymus Research, Fundação Oswaldo Cruz, Rio de Janeiro, Brazil*

[c]*Department of Cell Biology, Faculty of Medicine, Complutense University, Madrid, Spain*

Eph receptors and their ligands, ephrins, are molecules involved in the morphogenesis of numerous tissues, including the central nervous system in which they play a key role in determining cell positioning and tissue domains containing or excluding nerve fibers. Because common features have been suggested to occur in the microenvironmental organization of brain and thymus, a highly compartmentalized organ central for T cell differentiation, we examined the expression and possible role of Eph/ephrins in the biology of the thymus gland. We reviewed numerous *in vivo* and *in vitro* results that confirm a role for Eph and ephrins in the maturation of the thymic epithelial cell (TEC) network and T cell differentiation. Their possible involvement in different steps of early thymus organogenesis, including thymus primordium branching, lymphoid colonization, and thymocyte–TEC interactions, that determine the organization of a mature three-dimensional thymic epithelial network is also analyzed.

Key words: **thymocytes; thymic epithelial cells; Eph; ephrins**

The thymus is a highly compartmentalized organ in which lymphoid progenitors mature under the influence of a specialized epithelial cell microenvironment, which has been compared with that present in the brain.[1] It is, therefore, possible to speculate that molecules important for brain development could also be involved in thymus organogenesis.

Among these molecules are the Eph, a family of tyrosine kinase receptors (16 members) known to participate in the topological organization of the developing central nervous system,[2] and their ligands, ephrins (nine members). Both groups of molecules are divided into two families, A and B, based on sequence similarities of the molecules and ligand binding preferences. In fact, it is a very promiscuous molecular system in which each Eph and ephrin binds different ligands. Accordingly, different combinations of Eph and ephrin signals result in different behavior of the interacting cells. Furthermore, both the receptors (Eph) and their ligands (ephrins) transmit signals (forward and reverse, respectively) to the molecule-expressing cell, making the system particularly complex. Eph/ephrins are involved in numerous cellular processes, including cell attachment/detachment, migration, positioning, shape, and chemotaxis, and also in more general biological phenomena, such as gene expression, apoptosis, cell proliferation, and cell differentiation.[3,4]

Over the past few years we have analyzed the expression and possible role played by Eph/ephrins in the biology of the thymus and T cell differentiation. We and other authors have demonstrated that most Eph and ephrins

Address for correspondence: Dr. Agustín G. Zapata, Department of Cell Biology, Faculty of Biology, Complutense University of Madrid, C/ José Antonio Nováis 2; Ciudad Universitaria, C.P. 28040, Madrid, Spain. Voice: +34 91 394 49 79; fax: +34 91 394 49 81. zapata@bio.ucm.es

Neuroimmunomodulation: Ann. N.Y. Acad. Sci. 1153: 14–19 (2009).
doi: 10.1111/j.1749-6632.2008.03965.x

CORTEX　　**MEDULLA**

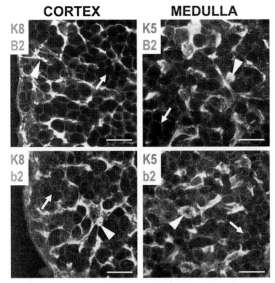

Figure 1. Expression of EphB receptors and ephrinB ligands in mouse thymus. Immunofluorescence detection of EphB2 (B2) and ephrinB2 (b2) on thymus cryosections from adult wild-type (WT) mice. EphB2 and ephrinB2 are expressed on both thymocytes (keratin-negative cells shown by arrows/green cells) and epithelial cells (arrowheads/yellow cells) of thymic cortex (K8+ cells) and medulla (K5+ cells). Scale bar: 10 μm. (In color in *Annals* online.)

are expressed in the thymus.[5–8] Furthermore, all thymocyte subsets, as well as both cortical and medullary thymic epithelial cells (TECs) from fetal and adult thymus, express Eph and ephrins, especially those of the B family. One thymic cell may, therefore, express several Eph and/or ephrins (Fig. 1).

Blockade of Eph/Ephrin Signaling Differentially Affects the Thymus

With respect to the possible functions of Eph/ephrins in the thymus, we first demonstrated that EphA-Fc fusion proteins blocked *in vitro* T cell differentiation, drastically reducing the numbers of thymocytes, especially those of the double positive (DP) (CD4+CD8+) cell compartment, in correlation with increased proportions of apoptotic cells. Furthermore, the lack of one or more Eph/ephrins A or B results in hypocellularity, increased numbers of apoptotic cells, and decreased proportions of cycling

cells *in vivo* but affects T cell differentiation differently.

Some authors have reported that the thymi of both EphB6−/− and EphB2−/− mice do not show special changes compared to those of wild-type (WT) mice.[9–11] However, ephrin B1, one of the main ligands of EphB2, has been claimed to be critical for T cell development,[12,13] and EphB6 overexpression results in the breakdown of the thymic cortex-medulla limits.[11] On the other hand, EphA4-deficient mice show a blockade of T cell maturation, exhibiting reduced proportions of DP thymocytes.[14] In this case, we demonstrated that the blockade of T cell development was dependent on the changes taking place in the nonlymphoid thymic microenvironment. Thus, mutant bone marrow lymphoid progenitors normally differentiate in severe combined immunodeficiency (SCID) thymus, but EphA4-deficient alymphoid thymic stroma grafted under the kidney capsule of WT mice and colonized by WT lymphoid progenitors supported defective T cell differentiation with decreased proportions of DP cells.[14] In fact, immunohistochemical analysis of the mutant thymi showed a profound collapse of the cortical thymic epithelial network.

EphB-deficient Mice Show Profound Alterations of the Maturation and Organization of Thymic Epithelial Cells

The lack of EphB2 and/or EphB3 only slightly affected T cell differentiation, resulting in just a slight accumulation of double negative (DN) (CD4−CD8−) cells but, importantly affected the thymic cell content and the TEC network (Fig. 2) (García-Ceca *et al.*, submitted manuscript) resulting in disorganization of the cortical epithelial network, increased numbers of K5+K8+ epithelial cells in the thymic cortex, and the presence of K5−K8− areas that correlated well with the presence of degenerated TECs but could also be a consequence of

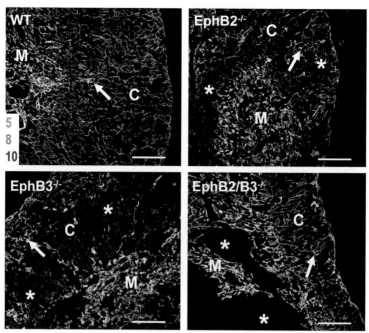

Figure 2. Immunofluorescence study of the thymus of adult WT and EphB-deficient mice. The immunofluorescence analysis was carried out combining specific markers for thymic epithelial cells (TECs) [keratin 5 (5), keratin 8 (8), mouse thymic stromal (MTS)10 (10)]. WT thymi consist of an outer cortex (C), showing largely a K5⁻K8⁺MTS10⁻ TEC population (red cells) and a few K5⁺K8⁺MTS10⁻ cells (arrow/yellow cells), and a central medulla (M) formed mainly by K5⁺K8⁻MTS10⁺ TEC cell population (blue cells). EphB-deficient thymi presented altered distribution and organization of these two compartments as well as important variations in their cell content, including among other features the existence of large K5⁻K8⁻ areas (asterisks) and increased numbers of cortical K5⁺K8⁺ cells (arrows/yellow cells). Scale bar: 100 μm. (In color in *Annals* online.)

downregulated keratin expression and/or altered thymocyte–TEC interactions.

Apart from these remarkable and common changes in the thymic epithelial phenotypes, the deficient thymi showed specific features for every mutant studied. These features began early in thymus ontogeny and became more severe at the end of fetal life and in the neonatal thymus (García-Ceca *et al.*, submitted manuscript), suggesting a role for these EphB in TEC maturation.

Imbalance of Eph/EphrinB Signaling Is Critical for T Cell Development

The balance between the different transmitted signals rather than the presence or ab-

sence of Eph and/or ephrins is determinant, as previously demonstrated in other systems,[4] for the final phenotype of tissues. Thus, despite the minimal effects observed in EphB-deficient mice on the thymocyte phenotype, important alterations occurred *in vivo* in chimeric thymi generated in SCID mice, expressing Eph and ephrinB as WT mice, that received either WT or EphB-deficient bone marrow lymphoid progenitors (Alfaro *et al.*, manuscript in preparation). SCID mice receiving EphB2⁻/⁻ lymphoid progenitors show a total blockade of T cell differentiation with an increased percentage of DN (CD4⁻CD8⁻) cells and a severe reduction in DP (CD4⁺CD8⁺) thymocytes. However, SCID thymi colonized by lymphoid progenitors expressing a EphB2 devoid of the cytoplasmic domain but containing an ectodomain capable of activating ephrinB signaling in ephrinB-expressing cells (EphB2-LacZ mice) supported a maturation of DN thymocytes in the DP cell compartment, although only a small proportion of single positive (SP) (both CD4$^+$CD8$^-$ and CD4$^-$CD8$^+$) cells are formed. Therefore, the absence of EphB2 determines the blockade of T cell maturation at the DN stage, while a signaling reversal, presumably generated by the interactions of EphB2-LacZ-expressing lymphoid progenitors with ephrinB-expressing TECs, allows the progression of DN cells to the DP cell compartment. However, this signal seems to be insufficient to permit progression of the DP thymocytes to the mature SP cell compartment. A forward signal seems to be necessary for the final maturation to SP thymocytes. The condition in the SCID mice injected with EphB3$^{-/-}$ lymphoid progenitors is intermediate with a significant but lesser reduction in the percentage of DP thymocytes. Transmitted signaling through EphB2, therefore, seems to be more important for the maturation of DN thymocytes than those mediated through EphB3. Accordingly, the differentiation of double EphB2/B3-deficient lymphoid progenitors in the SCID thymus exhibits a similar blockade to that observed for EphB2-deficient progenitors.

Together, these results support a role for Eph/ephrins in thymus morphogenesis, controlling cell survival, apoptosis, and cell proliferation and modulating gene expression in both developing thymocytes and TECs. As a result, Eph/ephrins seem to affect TEC development and, to a variable degree, T cell differentiation.

Role of Eph/Ephrins in Early Thymus Ontogeny

Over the last few years, increasing interest for the thymic epithelial stroma has allowed two steps to be recognized in the maturation of thymic epithelium primordium: an early lymphocyte-independent stage and a lymphoid-dependent differentiation after

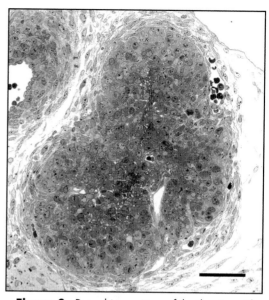

Figure 3. Branching pattern of the thymic epithelium during early development. Histological section of a 12.5-day-old fetal thymic lobe showing a central area (red) exhibiting a branching pattern that will determine the histological compartmentalization of the organ in later stages of development. Scale bar: 100 μm. (In color in *Annals* online.)

the lymphoid colonization of primordium.[15,16] The organization of mouse thymic primordium on day 10.5 post coitum is the result of the interaction of the third pharyngeal pouch endoderm with the neural crest-derived mesenchyme.[17] One day later, molecules of the Wnt family activate the transcription factor Foxn1, which induces the maturation of TEC progenitors.[18–20] Because very little is known about the histological, cellular, and molecular mechanism governing this first stage of thymus development and because the involvement of Eph/ephrins in the organogenesis of other tissues is clearly established, we have also analyzed the role of EphB in early thymus organogenesis.

At 11.5 days post coitum, when the thymic primordium is still joined to the pharyngeal cavity and most cells already express keratins K5 and K8, the branching of the thymic epithelium, which is folded repeatedly to histologically organize a gland, seems to begin. Thus, as early as 12.5 days post coitum it is possible to clearly distinguish a branching tree (Fig. 3) that exhibits an incipient $K5^+K8^{-/lo}$ medullary thymic epithelial phenotype in the central area, in the outer zone $K8^+$ cells, and in an enlarged area between the two that still contains numerous presumptive $K5^+K8^+$ epithelial cell progenitors. Accordingly, the commitment to the thymic cortex and medulla seems to be an early process intimately associated with an epithelial branching outgrowth pattern.

Comparative analysis of the thymic epithelial branching in EphB2-deficient mice demonstrates that this follows a general pattern similar to that found in WT mice but the epithelial branches of the mutants exhibit a more compact, almost collapsed, histological organization compared with that of WT mice, suggesting that EphB could also be involved in determining the branching pattern of thymic epithelial parenchyma.

For many years, lymphoid colonization of thymus has been extensively studied although the mechanisms involved are as yet unknown. In this line, we have studied by flow cytometry and confocal microscopy the colonization of dGuo-treated fetal thymic lobes by Lin$^-$ bone marrow cell progenitors from WT EphB2-deficient mice and EphB2-LacZ mice and showed that EphB2$^{-/-}$ but not EphB2-LacZ lymphoid progenitors colonize the alymphoid thymic lobes less efficiently; however, once lymphoid progenitors are inside the thymic parenchyma, the behavior of both EphB2-deficient cells and EphB2-LacZ-expressing thymocytes is similar. In both cases, the cells remain at the periphery rather than scattered at random throughout the parenchyma, as found in lobes receiving WT lymphoid progenitors.

These results demonstrate that different signals mediated through EphB are involved in colonization of the thymic primordium and the intrathymic migration of developing thymocytes; reverse signaling mediated through ephrinB-expressing thymic cells is sufficient to recover the capacity of lymphoid precursors to colonize the thymic lobes but not to control the migration of developing cells throughout the thymic parenchyma. We are currently analyzing the underlying mechanisms that govern this role of EphB2 in lymphocyte migration to and throughout the thymic parenchyma (Stimamiglio *et al.*, manuscript in preparation) on the basis of the relationship between this family of molecules and both integrins[21] and chemokines.[22]

Finally, once lymphoid progenitors have colonized the thymic primordium, thymocyte–TEC interactions become important for the development of both thymocytes and TECs. In order to evaluate the possible importance of Eph/ephrinB in this process, we tested the effects of ephrinB1-Fc (or IgG-Fc as a control) fusion proteins on the thymocyte–TEC interactions established in re-aggregates (RTOC) constituted by fetal thymic lobes and isolated DP thymocytes.[23] After 24 h, the control RTOC showed a compact organization in which thymocytes were closely associated to the TEC processes that formed a continuous epithelial network. On the contrary, in the RTOC to which ephrinB1-Fc proteins had been added, the epithelial cells appeared rounded without organized keratin filaments in the cell processes and were unable to interact with thymocytes. Accordingly, in the presence of ephrinB1-Fc, thymocytes and TECs are unable to organize a three-dimensional epithelial network housing the developing thymocytes.[8]

These results suggest that Eph/ephrin are key molecules for establishing links between histological organization, topological distribution, and phenotypical differentiation of TEC progenitors and thymocytes. Further studies must focus on confirming the role of Eph/ephrins in the earliest stages of thymus development and to determine both the specific Eph signals involved in every step of TEC maturation and the nature of the molecules associated with Eph/ephrins in the control of all these processes.

Acknowledgments

This work was supported by Grants BFU 2004-03132 and BFU 2007-65520 from the

Spanish Ministry of Education and Science, RD06/0010/0003 from Spanish Ministry of Health and Consumption, and S-BIO/0204/2006 and R74/91 05552/08 from the Regional Government of Madrid.

Conflicts of Interest

The authors declare no conflicts of interest.

References

1. Mentlein, R. & M.D. Kendall. 2000. The brain and thymus have much in common: a functional analysis of their microenvironments. *Immunol. Today* **21:** 133–140.

2. Goldshmit, Y., S. McLenachan & A. Turnley. 2006. Roles of Eph receptors and ephrins in the normal and damaged adult CNS. *Brain Res. Brain Res. Rev.* **52:** 327–345.

3. Pasquale, E.B. 2008. Eph-ephrin bidirectional signaling in physiology and disease. *Cell* **133:** 38–52.

4. Pasquale, E.B. 2005. Eph receptor signalling casts a wide net on cell behaviour. *Nat. Rev. Mol. Cell Biol.* **6:** 462–475.

5. Munoz, J.J. *et al.* 2002. Expression and function of the Eph A receptors and their ligands ephrins A in the rat thymus. *J. Immunol.* **169:** 177–184.

6. Vergara-Silva, A., K.L. Schaefer & L.J. Berg. 2002. Compartmentalized Eph receptor and ephrin expression in the thymus. *Mech. Dev.* **119**(Suppl 1): S225–229.

7. Wu, J. & H. Luo. 2005. Recent advances on T-cell regulation by receptor tyrosine kinases. *Curr. Opin. Hematol.* **12:** 292–297.

8. Alfaro, D. *et al.* 2008. Alterations in the thymocyte phenotype of EphB-deficient mice largely affect the double negative cell compartment. *Immunology* **125:**(1): 131–143.

9. Luo, H. *et al.* 2004. EphB6-null mutation results in compromised T cell function. *J. Clin. Invest.* **114:** 1762–1773.

10. Shimoyama, M. *et al.* 2002. Developmental expression of EphB6 in the thymus: lessons from EphB6 knockout mice. *Biochem. Biophys. Res. Commun.* **298:** 87–94.

11. Coles, M.C. *et al.* 2004. The role of Eph receptors and ephrins ligands in T-cell development in the thymus. 12th Int. Congress of Immunology and 4th Annual Conference of FOCIS, Montreal, Canada, July 18–23. Clin Invest Med56D.

12. Yu, G. *et al.* 2004. EphrinB1 is essential in T-cell-T-cell co-operation during T-cell activation. *J. Biol. Chem.* **279:** 55531–55539.

13. Yu, G. *et al.* 2006. Ephrin-B1 is critical in T-cell development. *J. Biol. Chem.* **281:** 10222–10229.

14. Munoz, J.J. *et al.* 2006. Thymic alterations in EphA4-deficient mice. *J. Immunol.* **177:** 804–813.

15. Manley, N.R. & C.C. Blackburn. 2003. A developmental look at thymus organogenesis: where do the non-hematopoietic cells in the thymus come from? *Curr. Opin. Immunol.* **15:** 225–232.

16. Rodewald, H.R. 2008. Thymus organogenesis. *Annu. Rev. Immunol.* **26:** 355–388.

17. Blackburn, C.C. & N.R. Manley. 2004. Developing a new paradigm for thymus organogenesis. *Nat. Rev. Immunol.* **4:** 278–289.

18. Blackburn, C.C. *et al.* 1996. The nu gene acts cell-autonomously and is required for differentiation of thymic epithelial progenitors. *Proc. Natl. Acad. Sci. USA* **93:** 5742–5746.

19. Balciunaite, G. *et al.* 2002. Wnt glycoproteins regulate the expression of FoxN1, the gene defective in nude mice. *Nat. Immunol.* **3:** 1102–1108.

20. Su, D.M. *et al.* 2003. A domain of Foxn1 required for crosstalk-dependent thymic epithelial cell differentiation. *Nat. Immunol.* **4:** 1128–1135.

21. Sharfe, N. *et al.* 2008. EphA and ephrin-A proteins regulate integrin-mediated T lymphocyte interactions. *Mol Immunol.* **45:** 1208–1220.

22. Sharfe, N. *et al.* 2002. Ephrin stimulation modulates T cell chemotaxis. *Eur. J. Immunol.* **32:** 3745–3755.

23. Alfaro, D. *et al.* 2007. EphrinB1-EphB signaling regulates thymocyte-epithelium interactions involved in functional T cell development. *Eur. J. Immunol.* **37:** 2596–2605.

Neuropilins, Semaphorins, and Their Role in Thymocyte Development

Daniella Arêas Mendes-da-Cruz,[a,b] **Yves Lepelletier,**[b]
Anne C. Brignier,[b] **Salete Smaniotto,**[c] **Amédée Renand,**[b]
Pierre Milpied,[b] **Mireille Dardenne,**[b] **Olivier Hermine,**[b,d,e]
and Wilson Savino[a,e]

[a]*Oswaldo Cruz Institute, Oswaldo Cruz Foundation, Rio de Janeiro, Brazil*

[b]*Paris Descartes University, Centre National de la Recherche Scientifique, Unité Mixte de Recherche 8147, Necker Hospital, Paris, France*

[c]*Institute of Biomedical and Health Sciences, Federal University of Alagoas, Maceió, Brazil*

[d]*Assistance Publique, Hôpitaux de Paris, Paris, France*

Some molecules described in the nervous system are also expressed in cells involved in the control of the immune response, suggesting they have a role as common mechanisms between neuroendocrine and immune systems. In this review, we focus on the expression and role of neuropilins (NPs) and their soluble ligands class 3 semaphorins in thymus physiology, particularly migration of developing thymocytes. We also discuss the concept of multivectorial thymocyte migration, including semaphorins, as a new individual cell migration vector.

Key words: semaphorins; neuropilins; thymus; thymocyte migration; thymocyte development

It is largely accepted that a variety of molecular interactions typically found in nervous tissue can be found in the immune system. In particular, the thymus is a primary site for T cell development in which various interactions mediated by neuroendocrine moieties have been defined.[1] Herein we will focus on the expression and role of neuropilins (NPs) and their soluble ligands semaphorins (SEMAs) in thymus physiology, particularly migration of developing thymocytes. Yet, before entering the discussion of recent data on this subject, we briefly provide some background data on thymus physiology and "neuroendocrine"-mediated intrathymic cellular interactions.

General Aspects of the Thymus

Thymocyte differentiation occurs as cells migrate within the thymic lobules. Thymocyte precursors enter the thymus by the corticomedullary region and subsequently migrate to the subcapsular region of the organ. Most of the immature thymocytes, including those bearing the phenotypes T cell receptor (TCR) TCR$^-$CD3$^-$CD4$^-$CD8$^-$ and TCR^{low}CD3^{low}CD4$^+$CD8$^+$, are located cortically, whereas mature TCR^{high}CD3^{high}CD4$^+$CD8$^-$ and TCR^{high}CD3^{high}CD4$^-$CD8$^+$ cells, which will leave the thymus and migrate to peripheral lymphoid organs, are found in the medulla. During their journey within the thymus,

Address for correspondence: Daniella Arêas Mendes-da-Cruz and Wilson Savino, Laboratory on Thymus Research, Oswaldo Cruz Institute, Oswaldo Cruz Foundation, Ave. Brasil 4365, Manguinhos, 21045-900, Rio de Janeiro, Brazil. Voice: 55 21 38658116; fax: 55 21 22094110. daniella@ioc.fiocruz.br or savino@fiocruz.br

[e]These authors contributed equally to this work.

Neuroimmunomodulation: Ann. N.Y. Acad. Sci. 1153: 20–28 (2009).
doi: 10.1111/j.1749-6632.2008.03980.x © 2009 New York Academy of Sciences.

developing thymocytes encounter cortical and medullary microenvironments through distinct cell–cell and cell–matrix interactions. Generally, thymocytes bearing TCR/CD3 complexes that interact with low or medium affinity with major histocompatibility complex (MHC)-presented antigens are positively selected and continue their maturation process. However, thymocytes bearing TCR/CD3 complexes that interact with high affinity with MHC-presented antigens die by apoptosis in a process called negative selection, which prevents the exit of mature T cells with autoimmune potential.[2,3] The thymic microenvironment comprises different cell types with distinct roles, including thymic epithelial cells (TEC), dendritic cells (DC), macrophages, and fibroblasts. Positive selection seems to be driven by TEC, whereas negative selection is mainly secondary to interactions involving DC with thymocytes.[2] The major function of thymic macrophages seems to be the phagocytosis of apoptotic thymocytes, and fibroblasts play a role in the TCR$^-$CD4$^-$CD8$^-$ to TCR$^+$CD4$^+$CD8$^+$ progression.[4,5] Among microenvironmental cell types, TEC correspond to the major component. They are seen in both cortex and medullary regions where they form special niches, which may be involved in specific interactions with developing thymocytes. In the outer cortex of the thymic lobules, TEC can form the so-called thymic nurse cell (TNC), a lymphoepithelial complex in which one single epithelial cell can harbor a variable number of thymocytes from two to 200.[6] Since immature as well as some mature thymocytes can be found in TNCs, it has been suggested that they can form a particular microenvironment able to support thymocyte differentiation.[6a]

Microenvironmental cells also modulate thymocyte development by the production of extracellular matrix (ECM) proteins and soluble polypeptides. TEC express thymic hormones, including thymulin, thymopoietin, and thymosin-1; cytokines, such as interleukin-1 (IL-1), IL-3, IL-6, IL-7, IL-8, and stem cell factor; and chemokines, including CXCL12, CXCL10, CCL4, CCL19, and CCL25.[1,7] Some of these soluble polypeptides are able to stimulate or inhibit thymocyte migration alone or combined with other molecules. Soluble chemokines can be presented to cells by insoluble ECM proteins, which, in turn, might modulate adhesion or de-adhesion capacities. For example, the chemokine CXCL12 is better presented to T cells when it is bound to ECM molecules as fibronectin or laminin. The combined action of these molecules in *ex vivo* migration assays has a synergic effect on thymocyte migration, resulting in a migration index greater than the sum of the migration indexes obtained by each stimulus alone.[8,9] Cell migration then derives from a balanced response to the various stimuli (positive and/or negative) provided by the microenvironment.

Intrathymic Interactions Involving Molecules Found in the Nervous System

Several molecules involved in the cross-talk between neuronal cells have been characterized. Interestingly, some of these molecules are also expressed in cells involved in the control of the immune response, suggesting their possible role as common mediators between neuroendocrine and immune systems. Several neuropeptides, such as somatostatin, neuropeptide Y (NPY), substance P, and vasointestinal polypeptide, are expressed in the brain but also in the thymus of different species from zebrafish to human and can alter thymocyte development.[10] Some of these molecules, such as NPY, which inhibits the fMLP (formyl-met-leu-phe) chemotactic effect on mouse thymocytes, can also modify thymocyte migration.[11]

Ephrins and their receptors, Ephs, are highly expressed in the nervous system during development and were described as important in growth cone collapse and cell detachment.[12] Recently, the expression of ephrins and Ephs has been reported in thymocytes and thymic

TABLE 1. Thymocyte Migration Response toward Various Stimuli

Molecule	Migratory activity	Responsive CD4/CD8-defined thymocyte subsets	References
Fibronectin	Haptotaxis	All subsets, mainly CD4*§ and CD8 SP§	20, 22
Laminin	Haptotaxis	All subsets, mainly CD4*§ and CD8 SP§	21, 22
CXCL12	Chemotaxis	All subsets, mainly DP*§	7, 18, 19
CCL4	Chemotaxis	All subsets, mainly CD4* and CD8 SP*	18, 19
CCL25	Chemotaxis	All subsets, mainly DP*§	7, 18, 19
Ephrins A1, A2, and B1	Inhibition of CXCL12-induced chemotaxis	ND§	15
Neuropeptide Y	Inhibition of fMLP-induced chemotaxis	ND*	11
Cellular prion protein	Involvement in laminin-driven migration	ND*	17

fMLP = formyl-met-leu-phe; *results observed with mouse thymocytes, which can diverge depending on the mouse strain; §results observed with human thymocytes; DP, $CD4^+CD8^+$ double-positive thymocytes; SP, single-positive thymocytes; ND, CD4/CD8-defined subsets not defined.

stromal cells. EphA4, B2, and B3 knockout mice present altered thymocyte developmentt, suggesting that these molecules could be important in the organization of the thymus and thymocyte migration.[13,14] In this respect, some Eph ligands, such as ephrins A1, A3, and B2 (but not ephrin B3), have been shown to inhibit the CXCL12-induced chemotaxis of human thymocytes by modifying CXCR4 (a CXCL12 receptor) signaling and chemokine-induced actin polymerization.[15]

Although the nervous system is the main site for the cellular prion protein [PrP(C)] expression, this molecule is also expressed in the thymus. Interestingly, mice overexpressing PrP(C) present thymic hypoplasia with accumulation of CD4-CD8 double-negative cells.[16] More recently, we showed that, in addition to a huge hypoplasia of the organ, thymocytes from PrP(C) transgenic mice do not respond to laminin in terms of cell migration.[17]

The effect of these molecules as well as chemokines and ECM molecules on thymocyte migration is summarized in Table 1.[7,11,15,17–22]

Recently, we and others described the expression of another group of molecules in the thymus originally described in the nervous system, the NPs and their respective ligands class 3 SEMAs.[23]

The Expression of Neuropilins and Class 3 Semaphorins in the Thymus

NPs are transmembrane glycoprotein receptors for secreted class 3 SEMAs and several vascular endothelial growth factor (VEGF) isoforms. They were initially described as modulators of axon guidance, angiogenesis, and organogenesis.[24,25] There are two NPs described to date (NP1 and NP2), although NP2 has several transmembrane isoforms and the two NPs have several soluble forms. NP1 binds SEMA3A, 3B, 3C, and 3D, VEGF-A_{121}, VEGF-A_{165}, and VEGF-B, C, D, and E, while NP2 binds SEMA3F, 3B, 3C, and 3D, VEGF-A_{145}, and VEGF-A_{165}, C, and D.[26–28] As NPs have a short cytoplasmic domain that lacks signaling activities, NPs also bind other transmembrane proteins called plexins, more specifically class A plexins, which act as co-receptors to transduce the effects of class 3 SEMAs.[29]

In the human thymus, NP1 is expressed at low percentages on all CD4/CD8-defined thymocyte subsets (Table 2) and at high levels on microenvironmental cells, including TEC and DC.[23]

In the mouse thymus primordium, NP1 appears later in development, at day E12.5, but

TABLE 2. Neuropilin (NP)1 Expression in Human and Mouse CD4/CD8-defined Thymocyte Subsets

	Total	DN	DP	CD4	CD8
Human	5.1 ± 1.2	10.5 ± 2.4	5.8 ± 1.3	8.4 ± 1.9	8.9 ± 2.0
Newborn mice	90.2 ± 1.1	55.5 ± 2.1	95.9 ± 0.9	54.5 ± 4.3	87.8 ± 2.8
Young adult mice	88.5 ± 0.6	25.2 ± 1.3	98.9 ± 0.7	21.9 ± 0.5	94.6 ± 2.4

Total = total thymocytes; DN, $CD4^-CD8^-$ double-negative thymocytes; DP, $CD4^+CD8^+$ double-positive thymocytes; CD4, $CD4^+CD8^-$ single-positive thymocytes; CD8, $CD4^-CD8^+$ single-positive thymocytes. Results are mean $\pm$ SE expressed as percentages from 19 human samples,[23] five newborn mice, and two young adult mice.

the expression increases with age.[30,31] When we analyzed the expression of NP1 in newborn mice (day 1) by flow cytometry, we found that thymocytes express high levels of this molecule, mainly the double-positive (DP) $CD4^+CD8^+$ and $CD4^-CD8^+$ (CD8) subpopulations (Table 2). Similar results were observed in young adults. About 88% of mouse thymocytes express NP1, mainly the DP and CD8 subpopulations (Table 2). In contrast, Corbel and colleagues[30] have shown that only a small amount of mature $CD4^+CD8^-$ (CD4) and CD8 thymocytes express this molecule. This may be due to differences in the reagents applied. In any case, in the CD4 subpopulation NP1 was described as a marker for mouse $CD4^+CD25^+Foxp3^+$ regulatory T cells (Treg), as this molecule seems to be constitutively expressed at the surface of mouse Tregs independently of their activation status.[30,32]

NP2 is also expressed in the mouse thymus primordium during development (from day E12.5 on), mainly in trabeculae and vessels.[31] In adult mice, Odaka et al. showed that the expression of NP2 was restricted to the lymphatic vessels.[33] These results are consistent with those showing that NP2-deficient mice present abnormal lymphatic vessel development.[34] The expression of the NP2 ligand SEMA3F (but not SEMA3D) in the mouse thymus is observed earlier during development, from day E10.5 in microenvironmental cells.[31]

Besides the expression of NPs and SEMAs, class A plexins can also be found in the human thymus, particularly in thymocytes (as shown in Fig. 1), suggesting that the interactions mediated by NPs/SEMAs in the thymus are functional in terms of signaling transduction.

Functional Roles of Neuropilins and Class 3 Semaphorins in the Thymus

Little is known about the function of NPs and SEMAs in the thymus. SEMA3A regulates human thymocyte adhesion onto TEC monolayers, as pre-incubation of thymocytes with this molecule resulted in 50% adhesion inhibition of all CD4/CD8-defined subsets in a dose-dependent manner. This inhibition was observed mainly in NP1-positive cells. Furthermore, SEMA3A exerts a chemorepulsive effect on human thymocytes and inhibits fibronectin and laminin-induced thymocyte migration,[23] showing the importance of SEMA3A/NP1 interactions in thymocyte guidance alone or combined with other molecules as ECM ligands.

Although the expression of NP1 in mouse thymocytes is much higher than that found in humans, thymocyte development (including Tregs) in mice deficient for NP1 in the T cell lineage was not affected.[30] These animals display normal percentages of thymocytes and peripheral CD4 and CD8 T lymphocytes, suggesting that NP1/SEMA3A in thymocyte migratory events and egress is likely replaced by other interactions, at least in this species. Interestingly, there is evidence suggesting the NP-independent direct interaction of class 3 SEMAs with plexins (in the case of SEMA3E/plexin-D1).[35] This could,

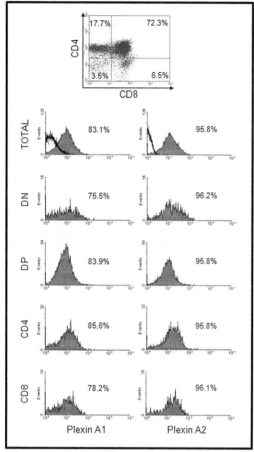

Figure 1. Expression of plexins A1 and A2 on human thymocytes by flow cytometry. Dot plots represent CD4/CD8-defined thymocyte subpopulations, and numbers indicate the classic percentage values of each subpopulation. Gray-filled histograms represent the expression of plexins, while open histograms represent fluorochrome-labeled, isotype-matched, unrelated immunoglobulins. Numbers indicate percentage values of cells expressing the respective plexins. TOTAL, total thymocyte; DN, CD4$^-$CD8$^-$ double-negative thymocytes; DP, CD4$^+$CD8$^+$ double-positive thymocytes; CD4, CD4$^+$CD8$^-$ single-positive thymocytes; CD8, CD4$^-$CD8$^+$ single-positive thymocytes.

in part, account for the normal T cell phenotype in NP1 knockout mice. Nevertheless, T cell development is normal in plexin-A1-deficient mice,[36] suggesting that the SEMA–NP–plexin combination can originate multiple cellular responses depending on the kind of interaction and the molecules involved, or other plexins could then act as compensatory

mechanisms. In any case, this issue clearly deserves further investigation.

Although the expression of SEMA3F, SEMA3D, and NP2 in the mouse thymus has been studied during development, their functional role in this organ is still largely unknown. Since the expression of NP2 in the mouse thymus primordium seems to be restricted to the vessels, it was suggested that SEMA3F and SEMA3D might be involved in guidance of T precursor cells into the thymus.[31]

Other Semaphorins Seem to Play a Role in Cell Migration in the Immune System

In addition to SEMA3A, 3D, and 3F, the expression and role of other SEMAs have been reported in the immune system. Unlike the soluble secreted class 3, class 4–7 SEMAs are transmembrane proteins that can also serve as receptors and interact with other transmembrane molecules. The first SEMA described in lymphoid tissues, especially in the thymus, was SEMA4D.[37] In this work, the authors described the expression of this SEMA in the thymus and on the surface of thymocytes, suggesting the role of this molecule in maturation-dependent thymocyte migration. SEMA4D is actually expressed by most hematopoietic cells, and the recombinant soluble molecule inhibits spontaneous migration of B cell and monocyte lineages and chemokine-driven [CCL7 or monocyte chemoattractant protein-3] monocyte migration. Interestingly, similar results were observed with SEMA3A but not with SEMA3F.[38]

SEMA7A, which is expressed by activated peripheral T cells, stimulates monocytes and macrophages to produce inflammatory cytokines through its interactions with the $\alpha 1 \beta 1$ integrin, a collagen receptor.[39] In terms of cell migration, although soluble SEMA7A is an attractant for human monocytes,[40] it seems to inhibit spontaneous human T cell migration,[41] and effector T cells can migrate normally into

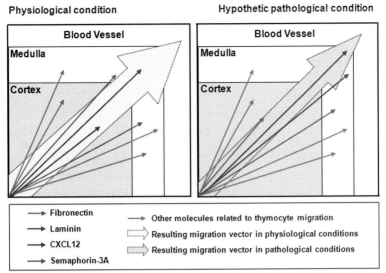

Figure 2. Concept of multivectorial thymocyte migration, including semaphorins (SEMAs) as new individual cell migration vectors. The left panel schematically defines the hypothesis stating that thymocyte migration results from a balance of several and simultaneous ligand/receptor pair interactions. Accordingly, individual vectors form a resulting vector that leads thymocytes throughout their journey within the thymic lobules from the cortex toward the medulla, with mature subsets ultimately being exported from the organ through the blood vessel walls. Right panel states that such multivectorial migration can be altered in pathological conditions if one or more individual vectors are altered. Narrow arrows represent individual migration vectors induced by specific stimuli, such as fibronectin (green), laminin (blue), CXCL12 (violet), SEMAs (red), and other molecules (gray). Large yellow and lilac-filled arrows represent the final resulting migration vector (adapted from Ref. 49). (In color in *Annals* online.)

antigen-challenged sites in SEMA7A-deficient mice.[39] Moreover, SEMA7A is expressed by mouse thymocytes at all development stages, from embryo to adult, and by human thymocytes, mainly in the DP and CD8 subpopulations.[42] Yet, its role in thymus physiology remains unknown.

Furthermore, a viral SEMA protein, known as A39R, is able to inhibit DC integrin-mediated adhesion and migration to the chemokine CCL3 (macrophage inflammatory protein-1α) in a dose-dependent manner.[43]

Given the importance of the SEMAs cited above in cell migration in the peripheral immune system (and not only in T cells), it is conceivable that they can be expressed intrathymicly and have a role in thymocyte migration and development.

Possible Role of Neuropilins and Semaphorins in Thymic Pathologies

NPs and SEMAs have been implicated in different pathologies, mainly neurodevelopmental disorders and cancer. The expression levels of NPs and SEMAs are altered in tumors of many types, and these molecules are correlated with tumor progression.[44,45] As NPs are also co-receptors for different VEGF families, several studies show the importance of this molecule in normal and tumor angiogenesis. In the human thymus, VEGF is expressed by stromal cells, mainly in the subcapsular region. This expression is altered in thymomas, depending on their type, and is correlated with the tumor microvascular density.[46] Furthermore, mouse treated with VEGF at concentrations similar to those observed in cancer patients presented thymic atrophy by a dramatic reduction in DP thymocytes without apoptosis induction, suggesting that VEGF could modulate thymocyte development.[47]

VEGF and SEMAs bind to specific sites of NPs, and a functional competition between these two molecules seems to regulate NP signaling events.[26,27] For example, SEMA3A inhibits the migration of breast cancer cell lines through NP1/plexin-A1 interactions, but this activity is antagonized by VEGF, suggesting that the ratio of endogenous VEGF and SEMA3A concentrations in carcinoma cells determines their chemotactic rate.[48]

Taking into account that VEGF and SEMA as well as their receptors are expressed in the thymus and considering the altered expression of VEGF in some types of thymomas, it is also possible that NPs and SEMAs play a role in thymic pathologic processes.

Concluding Remarks

The data discussed above reinforce the notion that thymocyte migration is a complex event, comprising multiple combined molecular interactions that lead to chemoattraction or repulsion involving various molecules, such as ECM molecules, hormones, chemokines, and the recently proposed NPs/SEMAs. As a result of all stimuli together, in a concept that we call multivectorial migration (Fig. 2), thymocytes will respond by migrating to a given direction with a given velocity. The resulting migration vector can change, depending on the concentration and combination of stimuli in each thymic region as well as the thymocyte capacity to respond via their specific receptors. In this context, SEMA3A/NP1 interactions are additional players in thymocyte migration. Accordingly, natural pathological changes in this particular molecular interaction may have consequences on the whole process of thymocyte migration. This is an exciting field that is completely open for further investigation.

Acknowledgments

This work was developed in the context of the Centre National de la Recherche Scientifique (CNRS)-Fiocruz Associated Laboratory of Immunology and Immunopathology. It was partially funded with grants by CNRS/Fiocruz French/Brazilian conjoint program, CNRS, The Foundation for Medical Research, The National League against Cancer, The National Cancer Institute (France); and Fiocruz (Brazil), Conselho Nacional de Desenvolvimento Científico e Tecnológico (CNPq; Brazil), and Coordenação de Aperfeiçoamento de Pessoal de Nível Superior (CAPES; Brazil).

Conflicts of Interest

The authors declare no conflicts of interest.

References

1. Savino, W. & M. Dardenne. 2000. Neuroendocrine control of thymus physiology. *Endocr. Rev.* **21:** 412–443.
2. Ciofani, M. & J.C. Zuniga-Pflucker. 2007. The thymus as an inductive site for T lymphopoiesis. *Annu. Rev. Cell Dev. Biol.* **23:** 463–493.
3. Petrie, H.T. & J.C. Zuniga-Pflucker. 2007. Zoned out: functional mapping of stromal signaling microenvironments in the thymus. *Annu. Rev. Immunol.* **25:** 649–679.
4. Anderson, G. *et al.* 1997. Fibroblast dependency during early thymocyte development maps to the CD25+ CD44+ stage and involves interactions with fibroblast matrix molecules. *Eur. J. Immunol.* **27:** 1200–1206.
5. Surh, C.D. & J. Sprent. 1994. T-cell apoptosis detected in situ during positive and negative selection in the thymus. *Nature* **372:** 100–103.
6a. de Waal Malefijt, R. *et al.* 1986. T- cell differentiation within thymic nurse cells. *Lab Invest.* **55:** 25–34.
6. Villa-Verde, D.M. *et al.* 1995. The thymic nurse cell complex: an in vitro model for extracellular matrix-mediated intrathymic T cell migration. *Braz. J. Med. Biol. Res.* **28:** 907–912.
7. Annunziato, F. *et al.* 2001. Chemokines and lymphopoiesis in human thymus. *Trends Immunol.* **22:** 277–281.

8. Savino, W. *et al.* 2002. Intrathymic T-cell migration: a combinatorial interplay of extracellular matrix and chemokines? *Trends Immunol.* **23:** 305–313.

9. Savino, W. *et al.* 2004. Molecular mechanisms governing thymocyte migration: combined role of chemokines and extracellular matrix. *J. Leukoc. Biol.* **75:** 951–961.

10. Silva, A.B., D. Aw & D.B. Palmer. 2006. Evolutionary conservation of neuropeptide expression in the thymus of different species. *Immunology* **118:** 131–140.

11. Medina, S. *et al.* 1998. Changes with ageing in the modulation of murine lymphocyte chemotaxis by CCK-8S, GRP and NPY. *Mech. Ageing Dev.* **102:** 249–261.

12. Pasquale, E.B. 2008. Eph-ephrin bidirectional signaling in physiology and disease. *Cell* **133:** 38–52.

13. Alfaro, D. *et al.* 2007. EphrinB1-EphB signaling regulates thymocyte-epithelium interactions involved in functional T cell development. *Eur. J. Immunol.* **37:** 2596–2605.

14. Munoz, J.J. *et al.* 2006. Thymic alterations in EphA4-deficient mice. *J. Immunol.* **177:** 804–813.

15. Sharfe, N. *et al.* 2002. Ephrin stimulation modulates T cell chemotaxis. *Eur. J. Immunol.* **32:** 3745–3755.

16. Jouvin-Marche, E. *et al.* 2006. Overexpression of cellular prion protein induces an antioxidant environment altering T cell development in the thymus. *J. Immunol.* **176:** 3490–3497.

17. Terra-Granado, E. *et al.* 2007. Is there a role for cellular prion protein in intrathymic T cell differentiation and migration? *Neuroimmunomodulation* **14:** 213–219.

18. Campbell, D.J., C.H. Kim & E.C. Butcher. 2003. Chemokines in the systemic organization of immunity. *Immunol. Rev.* **195:** 58–71.

19. Campbell, J.J., J. Pan & E.C. Butcher. 1999. Cutting edge: developmental switches in chemokine responses during T cell maturation. *J. Immunol.* **163:** 2353–2357.

20. Crisa, L. *et al.* 1996. Cell adhesion and migration are regulated at distinct stages of thymic T cell development: the roles of fibronectin, VLA4, and VLA5. *J. Exp. Med.* **184:** 215–228.

21. Vivinus-Nebot, M. *et al.* 2004. Mature human thymocytes migrate on laminin-5 with activation of metalloproteinase-14 and cleavage of CD44. *J. Immunol.* **172:** 1397–1406.

22. Yanagawa, Y., K. Iwabuchi & K. Onoe. 2001. Enhancement of stromal cell-derived factor-1alpha-induced chemotaxis for CD4/8 double-positive thymocytes by fibronectin and laminin in mice. *Immunology* **104:** 43–49.

23. Lepelletier, Y. *et al.* 2007. Control of human thymocyte migration by Neuropilin-1/Semaphorin-3A-mediated interactions. *Proc. Natl. Acad. Sci. USA* **104:** 5545–5550.

24. de Wit, J. & J. Verhaagen. 2003. Role of semaphorins in the adult nervous system. *Prog. Neurobiol.* **71:** 249–267.

25. Kruger, R.P., J. Aurandt & K.L. Guan. 2005. Semaphorins command cells to move. *Nat. Rev. Mol Cell Biol.* **6:** 789–800.

26. Geretti, E., A. Shimizu & M. Klagsbrun. 2008. Neuropilin structure governs VEGF and semaphorin binding and regulates angiogenesis. *Angiogenesis* **11:** 31–39.

27. Neufeld, G. *et al.* 2002. The neuropilins: multifunctional semaphorin and VEGF receptors that modulate axon guidance and angiogenesis. *Trends Cardiovasc. Med.* **12:** 13–19.

28. Otrock, Z.K., J.A. Makarem & A.I. Shamseddine. 2007. Vascular endothelial growth factor family of ligands and receptors: review. *Blood Cells Mol Dis.* **38:** 258–268.

29. Castellani, V. & G. Rougon. 2002. Control of semaphorin signaling. *Curr. Opin. Neurobiol.* **12:** 532–541.

30. Corbel, C. *et al.* 2007. Neuropilin 1 and CD25 co-regulation during early murine thymic differentiation. *Dev. Comp. Immunol.* **31:** 1082–1094.

31. Takahashi, K. *et al.* 2008. Expression of the semaphorins Sema 3D and Sema 3F in the developing parathyroid and thymus. *Dev. Dyn.* **237:** 1699–1708.

32. Bruder, D. *et al.* 2004. Neuropilin-1: a surface marker of regulatory T cells. *Eur. J. Immunol.* **34:** 623–630.

33. Odaka, C. *et al.* 2006. Distribution of lymphatic vessels in mouse thymus: immunofluorescence analysis. *Cell Tissue Res.* **325:** 13–22.

34. Yuan, L. *et al.* 2002. Abnormal lymphatic vessel development in neuropilin 2 mutant mice. *Development* **129:** 4797–806.

35. Gu, C. *et al.* 2005. Semaphorin 3E and plexin-D1 control vascular pattern independently of neuropilins. *Science* **307:** 265–268.

36. Takegahara, N. *et al.* 2006. Plexin-A1 and its interaction with DAP12 in immune responses and bone homeostasis. *Nat. Cell Biol.* **8:** 615–622.

37. Furuyama, T. *et al.* 1996. Identification of a novel transmembrane semaphorin expressed on lymphocytes. *J. Biol. Chem.* **271:** 33376–33381.

38. Delaire, S. *et al.* 2001. Biological activity of soluble CD100. II. Soluble CD100, similarly to H-SemaIII, inhibits immune cell migration. *J. Immunol.* **166:** 4348–4354.

39. Suzuki, K. *et al.* 2007. Semaphorin 7A initiates T-cell-mediated inflammatory responses through alpha1beta1 integrin. *Nature* **446:** 680–684.

40. Holmes, S. *et al.* 2002. Sema7A is a potent monocyte stimulator. *Scand. J. Immunol.* **56:** 270–275.

41. Vincent, P. *et al.* 2005. A role for the neuronal protein collapsin response mediator protein 2 in T lymphocyte polarization and migration. *J. Immunol.* **175:** 7650–7660.

42. Mine, T. *et al.* 2000. CDw108 expression during T-cell development. *Tissue Antigens* **55:** 429–436.

43. Walzer, T. *et al.* 2005. Plexin C1 engagement on mouse dendritic cells by viral semaphorin A39R induces actin cytoskeleton rearrangement and inhibits integrin-mediated adhesion and chemokine-induced migration. *J. Immunol.* **174:** 51–59.

44. Ellis, L.M. 2006. The role of neuropilins in cancer. *Mol. Cancer Ther.* **5:** 1099–1107.

45. Neufeld, G. & O. Kessler. 2008. The semaphorins: versatile regulators of tumour progression and tumour angiogenesis. *Nat. Rev. Cancer* **8:** 632–645.

46. Cimpean, A.M. *et al.* 2008. Immunohistochemical expression of vascular endothelial growth factor A (VEGF), and its receptors (VEGFR1, 2) in normal and pathologic conditions of the human thymus. *Ann. Anat.* **190:** 238–245.

47. Ohm, J.E. *et al.* 2003. VEGF inhibits T-cell development and may contribute to tumor-induced immune suppression. *Blood* **101:** 4878–4886.

48. Bachelder, R.E. *et al.* 2003. Competing autocrine pathways involving alternative neuropilin-1 ligands regulate chemotaxis of carcinoma cells. *Cancer Res.* **63:** 5230–5233.

49. Mendes-da-Cruz, D.A. *et al.* 2008. Multivectorial abnormal cell migration in the NOD mouse thymus. *J. Immunol.* **180:** 4639–4647.

Leptin Action in the Thymus

Lício A. Velloso,[a] Wilson Savino,[b] and Eli Mansour[a]

[a]*Department of Internal Medicine, University of Campinas, Campinas, Brazil*

[b]*Laboratory on Thymus Research, Oswaldo Cruz Institute, Oswaldo Cruz Foundation, Rio de Janeiro, Brazil*

Leptin was first characterized as a hormone that plays a central role in the control of body adiposity. A number of studies later revealed several other functions for leptin, including the capacity to modulate immune system activity. Currently, leptin occupies an important position as a unifying mechanism integrating nutritional status and immune function. Here, we will review some of the actions of leptin in the immune system, with special attention to the functions it exerts in the thymus.

Key words: **immunodeficiency; obesity; malnutrition**

Introduction

Specificity and diversity are two of the most remarkable features of the adaptive immune system.[1] Both these properties result from the adequate function of the thymus generating and selecting T lymphocytes that compose the immune repertoire.[2] Thymic function depends on the complex interactions between the anatomic and histological structures of the organ and a number of immune, endocrine, neural, and nutritional factors.[1,3]

One of the most ancient and eventually empirical concepts in medicine is that malnutrition is strongly related to defective immune function.[3,4] In fact, not only malnutrition but also another extreme nutritional dysfunction, obesity, are currently known as predisposing conditions for different forms of immune disorders ranging from severe forms of immunodeficiency to an increased risk of autoimmunity.[5] Following the discovery of the primarily adipostatic hormone leptin in 1994,[6] a number of additional important functions have been attributed to this peptide.[7] One of the most remarkable functions is the capacity of leptin to modulate immune system activity.[8] Both animal models and humans with defective leptin function present important features of immunodeficiency, which include anomalous activity of the thymus and thymic atrophy. Since leptin is produced in direct proportion to body adiposity, its concentration in the blood reflects the nutritional status at a given time.[9] The hypothalamus is one of the most important sites of action for leptin. In this organ, leptin acts in concert with insulin to modulate food intake and thermogenesis and, therefore, to control the body's stores of energy.[9–11] However, under certain environmental conditions, insufficient or excessive food consumption leads to pathological adiposity and, therefore, to anomalous leptin production. In malnutrition, leptin levels are extremely low[12] as are its functions. Conversely, in obesity, leptin levels are high, but at least some of its functions are impaired as a result of a phenomenon of molecular and functional resistance to its activity.[13,14]

As such, leptin acts simultaneously to control energy homeostasis and immune function; its activity can be impaired in malnutrition, from defective production, and in obesity, from molecular and functional resistance. Thus, a central role for leptin as a unifying mechanism to integrate the nutritional status and the

Address for correspondence: Lício A. Velloso, DCM–FCM, University of Campinas, 13084-970 Campinas – SP, Brazil. lavelloso@fcm.unicamp.br

Neuroimmunomodulation: Ann. N.Y. Acad. Sci. 1153: 29–34 (2009).
doi: 10.1111/j.1749-6632.2008.03973.x

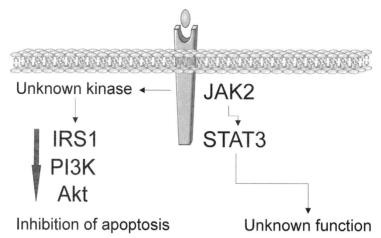

Figure 1. Leptin signal transduction in the thymus. Leptin can activate canonical signal transduction through Janus kinase (JAK)2 and signal transducer and activator of transcription (STAT)3 (right-hand side) in the thymus, but the functional outcomes of that are still unknown. A hitherto unknown tyrosine kinase links the ObR (green) to IRS1/phosphoinositide (PI)3-kinase and Akt, leading to the inhibition of apoptosis of thymic cells. (In color in *Annals* online.)

immune system has been proposed.[5] Here, we will review some of the most important advances in this field, paying special attention to the actions of leptin in the thymus.

Leptin and Leptin Receptor

Leptin, the product of the *ob* gene, is a 16-kDa protein produced predominantly by the white adipose tissue in direct proportion to whole body adiposity.[6] While initial reports regarded leptin solely as a hormone, further characterization of its structure and the identification of its receptor, the ObR, revealed that it possesses more features of a cytokine than of a hormone. In fact, the resolution of leptin's tertiary structure showed a molecule composed of four interconnected anti-parallel α-helices, which share high similarity with the cytokines interleukin (IL)-6, IL-11, IL-12, and granulocyte colony-stimulating factor.[15] Nevertheless, with regard to its multiple actions in distinct organs and tissues, leptin behaves as a hormone. Therefore, the creation of a new terminology, *adipokine*, to designate leptin and the other adipose tissue-derived substances that were identified following leptin's first appearance proved welcome.[16,17]

The *ob* gene is regulated by C/EBP-α (ccaat/enhancer binding protein-alpha), glucocorticoid responsive element, CCATT/enhancer, and specificity protein-1.[18,19] Hormones, such as glucocorticoids, testosterone, and insulin, as well as nutrients, such as fatty acids, glucosamine, and malonyl-coenzyme A are known to modulate leptin expression, which provides further support for the endocrine and metabolic roles of this peptide.[20,21] In addition, leptin expression is regulated by immunological stimuli, such as lipopolysaccharide, tumor necrosis factor-α, IL-6, and IL-1β, which illustrates its integration with the immune system.[22,23]

In the bloodstream, leptin can bind to macromolecules or circulate in a free form.[24] The ratio of free/bound leptin plays a role in its biological activity. Free leptin has direct access to receptors, but, because of proteolytic cleavage, its half-life is short. Conversely, protein bound leptin has an impaired bioavailability but a longer half-life.[25] As a peptidic signaling molecule, leptin acts through a transmembrane receptor, the ObR (Fig. 1), which belongs to the type-I cytokine receptor family because of its high similarity with the receptors for IL-2, IL-3, IL-4,

IL-6, IL-7, leukemia-inhibitory factor, granulocyte colony-stimulating factor, prolactin, growth hormone, and erythropoietin.[11,26] All receptors of this class are transmembrane proteins that transduce the incoming signal through the activation of an associated tyrosine kinase. The ObR is encoded by the *db* gene, and as a result of alternative splicing at least six isoforms of the receptor can be generated: ObRa-ObRf.[11] All forms of the receptor share the extracellular domain. The shortest isoform, ObRe, is a secreted form of the receptor, which is found in the bloodstream and plays a role in the control of leptin's biological activity.[11] The remaining forms are membrane bound and exert different roles in signal transduction. The largest isoform, ObRb, is implicated in most of leptin's actions because its intracellular portion contains various motifs required for interaction with downstream components of the leptin signaling pathway.[11]

Leptin Signal Transduction

The tyrosine kinase JAK2 (Janus kinase 2) is the most important protein involved in the transduction of the leptin signal in target cells. Upon leptin binding, ObRb undergoes dimerization, which accompanies JAK2 autophosphorylation and the tyrosine phosphorylation of two residues (Tyr985 and Tyr1138) in the receptor.[27,28] These events lead to the activation of at least three distinct intracellular signaling pathways.[28] Tyrosine phosphorylation of Tyr985 recruits the tyrosine phosphatase SHP2 (Src homology 2 domain-containing protein tyrosine phosphatase), which mediates the activation of the p21ras/extracellular signal-regulated kinase signaling pathway.[28] Tyrosine phosphorylation of Tyr1138 recruits signal transducer and activator of transcription (STAT)3 to the ObRb, leading to STAT3 tyrosine phosphorylation and translocation to the nucleus, providing a rapid path for leptin-induced control of gene expression.[28] Finally, the autophosphorylation of JAK2 leads to the recruitment and tyrosine phosphorylation of insulin receptor substrate (IRS)1/2 adaptor proteins, which promote the activation of phosphoinositide (PI)3-kinase and its downstream signaling.[28] It is possible that several other signaling pathways are also activated through the ObRb. These may include other substrates for JAK2, as a large number of Tyr residues may be phosphorylated following kinase activation,[27] and the engagement of as yet unknown tyrosine kinases because signal transduction through IRS1/PI3-kinase/Akt can occur even in the absence of JAK2 activation.[29]

The Thymus in Animal Models of Defective Leptin Activity

There are three animal models frequently employed to evaluate the outcomes of defective leptin activity. The ob/ob mouse is a monogenic model with a defect in the *ob* gene that leads to no production of leptin. The db/db mouse and the Zucker rat have truncated and nonfunctional forms of the ObR from monogenic defects of the *db* gene. All three models were developed long before 1994, the year when leptin was first described, and from the very beginning of their characterization, evidence for thymic dysfunction was noticed.

Reduction of thymic size is a common feature of all three models. In the Zucker rat, the thymus is about 30% smaller than in the lean control,[30] while in ob/ob and db/db mice the difference may reach up to 50%.[31–33] As ascertained in db/db mice, this precocious atrophy of the organ is accompanied by an incipient depletion of T cells in the cortex and an increased number of Hassall's corpuscles.[32] The epithelial cells present an increased number of vacuoles and granules of different aspects at the ultrastructural level.[32,34] Functionally, there is a precocious age-dependent decrease in the intrathymic contents and serum levels of the thymic epithelial cell-derived hormone thymulin.[32]

Besides anatomical and structural differences, the thymi of obese mice present a considerably different distribution of thymocyte subpopulations compared to lean mice. The absolute number of thymocytes are reduced by about 10-fold, which is accompanied by a relative increase in CD4$^-$ CD8$^-$ and CD4$^+$ CD8$^-$ cells and by a relative decrease in CD4$^+$ CD8$^+$, resulting in a decreased ratio of CD4$^+$ CD8$^+$/ CD4$^-$ CD8$^-$.[35] Moreover, thymocytes from obese mice proliferate significantly less than cells from lean-mice counterparts when exposed to unspecific stimulus.[33]

Immunological Features of Humans with Defective Leptin Function

There are only a few reported cases of defective leptin function in humans.[36–38] These patients present extreme obesity from early in life and some features of immunodeficiency. Some of these individuals report frequent upper respiratory tract infections.[36] The relative and absolute numbers of CD4$^+$ cells in peripheral blood are reduced, while CD8$^+$ and CD19$^+$ are increased. The ratio CD4$^+$/CD8$^+$ is about 0.5 (normal 1.0–2.6). In addition, the *in vitro* proliferative response of peripheral lymphocytes from leptin-deficient patients is severely compromised.[36]

Effects of Leptin in the Thymus

Leptin plays an important role in thymic mass maintenance. In acutely starved mice (48-h fasting) the relative mass of the thymus decreases up to 60%, an effect that is completely suppressed by leptin treatment.[35] In addition, in ob/ob mice an increase in thymic cellularity, as high as 18-fold compared to untreated animals, is achieved with chronic leptin infusion.[35] Apparently, both direct and indirect mechanisms take place in this regulation. The modulation of glucocorticoid levels by leptin and by changes in body adiposity seems to be one of the most important indirect mechanisms involved in this regulation.[33] However, leptin acts directly, both acutely and chronically, to inhibit apoptosis in the thymus,[29] and this may be one of the most remarkable features of leptin as a factor that controls immune function.

In order to exert its apoptosis-controlling effects in the thymus, leptin depends on the presence of the long form of the leptin receptor.[29] Upon ligand binding, the ObRb undergoes tyrosine phosphorylation, which is dependent on at least one associated tyrosine kinase, JAK2. Following JAK2 activation, the leptin signal generated intracellularly is rapidly driven to the control of gene expression by the engagement and activation of STAT3.[29] In addition, leptin signaling in the thymus leads to IRS1 phosphorylation and the activation of PI3-kinase activity, which induces the activation of the serine kinase Akt.[29] Therefore, at least some of the canonical steps of leptin signal transduction, originally described in the hypothalamus, are present and active in the thymus. However, in contrast to its actions in the central nervous system, at least one event controlled by leptin in the thymus is not dependent on JAK2 activation. The chemical inhibition of JAK2 activity does not modify the capacity of leptin to inhibit thymic apoptosis. Interestingly, inhibiting IRS1 expression or PI3-kinase activity completely suppresses the anti-apoptotic effects of leptin in this organ.[29] Therefore, it is expected that another, hitherto unknown, kinase links the ObRb to the IRS1/PI3-kinase/Akt signaling system and controls apoptosis through this path (Fig. 1).

Last, it remains to be defined whether leptin acts upon the thymus only through an endocrine circuit or if there is an intrathymic production of this molecule. As previously reviewed,[3] several peptidic hormones, classically known to be produced in endocrine glands, are also produced in the thymus. Moreover, preliminary data derived from microarray analyses indicate a constitutive expression of leptin by the human thymic epithelium (L. Lacerda and W. Savino, unpublished data). Thus, one can conceive of a paracrine effect of leptin upon the thymus, and this hypothesis represents an interesting point that deserves further investigation.

Concluding Remarks

Unraveling leptin action in the immune system is helping to progress the characterization of the mechanisms involved in the common association between nutritional dysfunctions and anomalous immune activity. Moreover, even in primary immunodeficiency[39] or in HIV-infected hosts, which also exhibit a severe thymic atrophy,[40] leptin serum levels are low, suggesting that not only leptin modulates immune function but also the immune system can exert some control in leptin production. Advances in this field may reveal novel targets for therapeutics of distinct forms of immune diseases.

Acknowledgments

The authors works are supported by grants from Fundação de Amparo à Pesquisa do Estado de São Paulo, Fundação Oswaldo Cruz, Conselho Nacional de Desenvolvimento Científico e Tecnológico, and Fundação de Amparo à Pesquisa do Estado do Rio de Janeiro. We thank Dr. N. Conran for editing the English grammar.

Conflicts of Interest

The authors declare no conflicts of interest.

References

1. Gill, J. *et al.* 2003. Thymic generation and regeneration. *Immunol. Rev.* **195:** 28–50.
2. Ladi, E. *et al.* 2006. Thymic microenvironments for T cell differentiation and selection. *Nat. Immunol.* **7:** 338–343.
3. Savino, W. & M. Dardenne. 2000. Neuroendocrine control of thymus physiology. *Endocr. Rev.* **21:** 412–443.
4. Savino, W. 2002. The thymus gland is a target in malnutrition. *Eur. J. Clin. Nutr.* **56**(Suppl 3): S46–S49.
5. Matarese, G., S. Moschos & C.S. Mantzoros. 2005. Leptin in immunology. *J. Immunol.* **174:** 3137–3142.
6. Zhang, Y. *et al.* 1994. Positional cloning of the mouse obese gene and its human homologue. *Nature* **372:** 425–432.
7. Otero, M. *et al.* 2005. Leptin, from fat to inflammation: old questions and new insights. *FEBS Lett.* **579:** 295–301.
8. Lord, G.M. *et al.* 1998. Leptin modulates the T-cell immune response and reverses starvation-induced immunosuppression. *Nature* **394:** 897–901.
9. Friedman, J.M. & J.L. Halaas. 1998. Leptin and the regulation of body weight in mammals. *Nature* **395:** 763–770.
10. Carvalheira, J.B. *et al.* 2001. Insulin modulates leptin-induced STAT3 activation in rat hypothalamus. *FEBS Lett.* **500:** 119–124.
11. Myers, M.G. Jr. 2004. Leptin receptor signaling and the regulation of mammalian physiology. *Recent Prog. Horm. Res.* **59:** 287–304.
12. Cederholm, T., P. Arner & J. Palmblad. 1997. Low circulating leptin levels in protein-energy malnourished chronically ill elderly patients. *J. Intern. Med.* **242:** 377–382.
13. De Souza, C.T. *et al.* 2005. Consumption of a fat-rich diet activates a proinflammatory response and induces insulin resistance in the hypothalamus. *Endocrinology* **146:** 4192–4199.
14. Carvalheira, J.B. *et al.* 2003. Selective impairment of insulin signalling in the hypothalamus of obese Zucker rats. *Diabetologia* **46:** 1629–1640.
15. Baumann, H. *et al.* 1996. The full-length leptin receptor has signaling capabilities of interleukin 6-type cytokine receptors. *Proc. Natl. Acad. Sci. USA* **93:** 8374–8378.
16. Plata-Salaman, C.R. 1998. Cytokine-induced anorexia. Behavioral, cellular, and molecular mechanisms. *Ann. N. Y. Acad. Sci.* **856:** 160–170.
17. Mora, S. & J.E. Pessin. 2002. An adipocentric view of signaling and intracellular trafficking. *Diabetes Metab. Res. Rev.* **18:** 345–356.
18. Miller, S.G. *et al.* 1996. The adipocyte specific transcription factor C/EBPalpha modulates human ob gene expression. *Proc. Natl. Acad. Sci. USA* **93:** 5507–5511.
19. Hwang, C.S. *et al.* 1996. Transcriptional activation of the mouse obese (ob) gene by CCAAT/enhancer binding protein alpha. *Proc. Natl. Acad. Sci. USA* **93:** 873–877.
20. Fried, S.K. *et al.* 2000. Regulation of leptin production in humans. *J. Nutr.* **130:** 3127S–3131S.
21. Lee, M.J. *et al.* 2007. Acute and chronic regulation of leptin synthesis, storage, and secretion by insulin

and dexamethasone in human adipose tissue. *Am. J. Physiol. Endocrinol. Metab.* **292:** E858–E864.

22. Sarraf, P. *et al.* 1997. Multiple cytokines and acute inflammation raise mouse leptin levels: potential role in inflammatory anorexia. *J. Exp. Med.* **185:** 171–175.

23. Finck, B.N. *et al.* 1998. In vivo and in vitro evidence for the involvement of tumor necrosis factor-alpha in the induction of leptin by lipopolysaccharide. *Endocrinology* **139:** 2278–2283.

24. Houseknecht, K.L. *et al.* 1996. Evidence for leptin binding to proteins in serum of rodents and humans: modulation with obesity. *Diabetes* **45:** 1638–1643.

25. Sinha, M.K. *et al.* 1996. Evidence of free and bound leptin in human circulation. Studies in lean and obese subjects and during short-term fasting. *J. Clin. Invest.* **98:** 1277–1282.

26. Bazan, J.F. 1989. A novel family of growth factor receptors: a common binding domain in the growth hormone, prolactin, erythropoietin and IL-6 receptors, and the p75 IL-2 receptor beta-chain. *Biochem. Biophys. Res. Commun.* **164:** 788–795.

27. Myers, M.G., M.A. Cowley & H. Munzberg. 2008. Mechanisms of leptin action and leptin resistance. *Annu. Rev. Physiol.* **70:** 537–556.

28. Munzberg, H. & M.G. Myers Jr. 2005. Molecular and anatomical determinants of central leptin resistance. *Nat. Neurosci.* **8:** 566–570.

29. Mansour, E. *et al.* 2006. Leptin inhibits apoptosis in thymus through a janus kinase-2-independent, insulin receptor substrate-1/phosphatidylinositol-3 kinase-dependent pathway. *Endocrinology* **147:** 5470–5479.

30. Walker, C.D. *et al.* 1992. Obese Zucker (fa/fa) rats exhibit normal target sensitivity to corticosterone and increased drive to adrenocorticotropin during the diurnal trough. *Endocrinology* **131:** 2629–2637.

31. Hick, R.W. *et al.* 2006. Leptin selectively augments thymopoiesis in leptin deficiency and lipopolysaccharide-induced thymic atrophy. *J. Immunol.* **177:** 169–176.

32. Dardenne, M. *et al.* 1983. Thymic dysfunction in the mutant diabetic (db/db) mouse. *J. Immunol.* **130:** 1195–1199.

33. Palmer, G. *et al.* 2006. Indirect effects of leptin receptor deficiency on lymphocyte populations and immune response in db/db mice. *J. Immunol.* **177:** 2899–2907.

34. Nabarra, B. & I. Andrianarison. 1986. Thymic reticulum of autoimmune mice. I. Ultrastructural studies of the diabetic (db/db) mouse thymus. *Exp. Pathol.* **29:** 45–53.

35. Howard, J.K. *et al.* 1999. Leptin protects mice from starvation-induced lymphoid atrophy and increases thymic cellularity in ob/ob mice. *J. Clin. Invest.* **104:** 1051–1059.

36. Farooqi, I.S. *et al.* 2002. Beneficial effects of leptin on obesity, T cell hyporesponsiveness, and neuroendocrine/metabolic dysfunction of human congenital leptin deficiency. *J. Clin. Invest.* **110:** 1093–1103.

37. Strobel, A. *et al.* 1998. A leptin missense mutation associated with hypogonadism and morbid obesity. *Nat. Genet.* **18:** 213–215.

38. Clement, K. *et al.* 1998. A mutation in the human leptin receptor gene causes obesity and pituitary dysfunction. *Nature* **392:** 398–401.

39. Ferraroni, N.R. *et al.* 2005. Severe hypoleptinaemia associated with insulin resistance in patients with common variable immunodeficiency. *Clin. Endocrinol. (Oxf).* **63:** 63–65.

40. Savino, W. *et al.* 1986. Thymic epithelium in AIDS. An immunohistologic study. *Am. J. Pathol.* **122:** 302–307.

Nitric Oxide at the Crossroad of Immunoneuroendocrine Interactions

Valeria Rettori,[a] Javier Fernandez-Solari,[a] Claudia Mohn,[a] María A. Zorrilla Zubilete,[b] Carolina de la Cal,[a] Juan Pablo Prestifilippo,[a] and Andrea De Laurentiis[a]

[a]*Center of Pharmacological and Botanical Studies, School of Medicine, University of Buenos Aires, Buenos Aires, Argentina*

[b]*Department of Neuropharmacology, School of Medicine, University of Buenos Aires, Buenos Aires, Argentina*

Nitric oxide (NO) was initially described as a mediator of endothelial relaxation, and now its participation is recognized in numerous physiological and pathological processes. It was demonstrated that lipopolysaccharide-stimulated corticotropin-releasing factor release involves NO production. Furthermore, it has been shown that interleukin (IL)-1, tumor necrosis factor (TNF)-α, IL-6, and IL-2 can stimulate adrenocorticotropic hormone release from anterior pituitary via NO. Also, we found that NO released from hypothalamic NOergic neurons in response to norepinephrine diffuses to luteinizing hormone-releasing hormone (LHRH) neurons that activate cyclooxygenase and guanylate cyclase. This activation results in an increase in prostaglandin E2 and cyclic guanosine monophosphate, respectively, which leads to the exocytosis of LHRH granules. During pathological conditions, such as manganese intoxication, NO production is increased, leading to an increase in LHRH secretion that can advance puberty. In another study we demonstrated that NO reduces oxytocin as well as vasopressin secretion from the posterior pituitary, suggesting it has a modulatory role during dehydration. An increase in NO synthase (NOS) activity and protein in the hippocampus and cerebellum was found in offspring of rats that were subjected to prenatal stress, and this was correlated with behavioral changes in adults. Also NO participates in signal transduction pathways in peripheral tissue in physiological processes, such as in corticosterone release from the adrenal gland. Pathological conditions, such as tumors of the head and neck, that are treated with radiation are followed by xerostomy. In a rat model, radiation diminished NOS activity in the submandibulary gland, and this was followed by inhibition in salivary secretion. In summary, this review describes the wide participation of NO in the cross-talk between neuroendocrine and neuroimmune systems in physiological and pathological processes.

Key words: luteinizing hormone-releasing hormone; oxytocin; corticosterone; hypothalamus; posterior pituitary; adrenal gland; radiation; submandibulary gland; prenatal stress

Introduction

At the end of the 1980s, it was clearly demonstrated that cells can produce nitric oxide (NO) and that this gaseous molecule is a highly reactive free radical with multiple and complex roles within many biological systems. In the present review our particular aim is to describe the role of NO in the field known as neuroimmunomodulation in which central nervous system (CNS) activity modulates the immune system and, in turn, the immune system modulates the activity of the nervous system. In fact, during the past

Address for correspondence: Dr. Andrea De Laurentiis, Centro de Estudios Farmacológicos y Botánicos, Facultad de Medicina, Paraguay 2155 piso 16, Ciudad Autónoma de Buenos Aires, AR 1121ABG, Buenos Aires, Argentina. Voice: +54-11-4508-3680 int 112; fax: +54-11-4508-3680 int 106. andredelaurentiis@yahoo.com

Neuroimmunomodulation: Ann. N.Y. Acad. Sci. 1153: 35–47 (2009).
doi: 10.1111/j.1749-6632.2008.03968.x © 2009 New York Academy of Sciences.

years NO has been recognized as a key player in the cross-talk between both systems.

The first example of neuroimmunomodulation was from the pioneer work of Selye in 1936 in which a noxious stimulus, called *stress*, induced the release of adrenocorticotrophic hormone (ACTH) from the pituitary, which in turn released adrenal cortical steroids.[1] The introduction of bacteria into the body causes the release of toxic soluble products from the bacteria's cell wall, such as lipopolysaccharide (LPS), that induce fever and a concomitant increase in plasma cortisol as well as the synthesis and release of various cytokines, such as interleukin-1 (IL-1), tumor necrosis factor-alpha (TNF-α), IL-6, IL-2, interferon-gamma, and others. These cytokines can release corticotrophin-releasing hormone (CRH) that activates ACTH, followed by cortisol release.[2] The cytokines can be produced not only by immune cells, particularly monocytes and macrophages, but also within the brain by glial elements and neurons.[3] We have shown an IL-1 immunoreactive neuronal system with cells bodies in the dorsal preoptic area and anterior hypothalamus and relatively short axons that could not be traced to the median eminence (ME).[4] In addition, these substances are synthesized within the pituitary.[5]

The research of the last decade indicates that cytokines induce NO production and that NO has a powerful influence on the secretion of hypothalamic peptides and classic synaptic transmitters, such as catecholamines and γ-aminobutyric acid (GABA); NO can also suppress or stimulate the release of pituitary hormones directly.[6]

One of the main physiological effects of NO is a result of its binding to a heme moiety of guanylate cyclase (GC) by altering its conformation and increasing its activity, causing the conversion of guanosine triphosphate (GTP) to cyclic guanosine monophosphate (cGMP). NO also reacts with several other metalloproteins, such as cytochrome P450 side-chain cleavage, which is essential for steroidogenic reactions.[7] Another target for NO action is the heme

group of the enzyme cyclooxygenase (COX). COX metabolizes free arachidonic acid (AA) to prostaglandins (PGs) and thromboxanes. There are two known COX forms; COX-1 is constitutively expressed whereas COX-2 is strongly induced during inflammation, but COX-2 also has been shown to be expressed constitutively in the brain.[7]

NO is synthesized by NO synthase (NOS), an enzyme that converts arginine in the presence of oxygen and several cofactors into equimolar quantities of citrulline and NO. There are three variants of the enzyme; two of these are constitutively expressed while the other must be induced. The inducible NOS (iNOS) is formed mainly in immune cells, such as macrophages. LPS combines with its receptors on the surface of macrophages and other cells, inducing the synthesis of iNOS mRNA. LPS also induces mRNA expression of various cytokines, such as IL-1, IL-6, and TNF-α.[8]

One of the constitutive forms of NOS was originally characterized in endothelial cells and was therefore known as endothelial NOS (eNOS), while the other constitutive form, originally characterized in neurons, was known as neuronal NOS (nNOS). These two isoforms have been found to be distributed more widely than originally thought. The eNOS is found in the caveoli of endothelial cells and is activated following cholinergic stimulation and the consequent increase of intracellular calcium. This produces NO, which diffuses to overlying smooth muscle and activates GC, converting GTP to cGMP, which produces vasodilatation.[9] nNOS is found in the cerebellum and various regions of the cerebral cortex and also in various ganglion cells of the autonomic nervous system. Large numbers of nNOS-containing neurons were also found in the hypothalamus, particularly in the paraventricular nucleus (PVN) and supraoptic nuclei (SON), with axons projecting to the ME and neural lobe, which also contains large amounts of nNOS.[10] Because of this distribution in the hypothalamus in regions that contain peptidergic neurons that control pituitary hormone secretion, we studied the role of NO in the hypothalamic–pituitary axis.

Role of NO in the Hypothalamic–Pituitary Axis during Infection

As was previously described, the hypothalamic–pituitary response to infection can be mimicked by the intravenous or intraperitoneal (i.p.) injection of bacterial LPS. There is a rapid increase in plasma ACTH and prolactin (PRL) within a few minutes, accompanied by a rapid inhibition of luteinizing hormone (LH) and thyroid-stimulating hormone.[11] Growth hormone secretion is stimulated in humans but not in rats.[4] Also, LPS causes the induction of cytokine synthesis and release from cells of the immune system. The first cytokine to be released in the rat and in large quantities is TNF-α, which apparently causes the induction of IL-1 synthesis and release, which in turn induces secretion of IL-6.[12] Because the response of the pituitary hormones occurs within a few minutes, it is obvious that the secretion of cytokines from immune cells in the periphery cannot be responsible for the immediate alterations in pituitary hormone secretion triggered by LPS. Our research demonstrated that i.p. injection of LPS induced IL-1β and iNOS mRNA in the brain, anterior pituitary, and pineal glands. The induction of both mRNAs occurred in the meninges, the choroids plexus, the circumventricular organs (such as the subfornical organ and the ME), and in the parvocellular neurons of the PVN and arcuate nucleus, areas of particular interest since they contain the hypothalamic-releasing and inhibiting hormone producing neurons and also other neurotransmitters controlled by NO. The greatest induction of iNOS occurred in the anterior lobe of the pituitary.[8] This massive increase in NO production should further increase the effects of NO to maintain the pattern of hypothalamic hormone secretion already induced by LPS.[13,14]

The initial response to LPS is mediated in the brain by nNOS. There is no participation of iNOS in this initial response. Indeed, the initial response must be a result of LPS receptors in areas where the blood–brain barrier is not present, such as the choroid plexus, ME, organum vasculosum laminae terminalis, and other circumventricular organs. LPS-induced input to the hypothalamus occurs, at least in part, by activation of the locus coeruleus, which sends noradrenergic axons to the hypothalamus; these axons synapse on cholinergic interneurons in the PVN, activating CRH release.[15,16] LPS-stimulated CRH release involves NO production because it can be blocked by inhibitors of all forms of NOS. Also it has been shown that NO activates COX I, leading to the generation of prostaglandin E2 (PGE2), which activates adenylyl cyclase (AC) and therefore increases cAMP. This cyclic nucleotide activates protein kinase A (PKA), which induces exocytosis of CRH secretory granules into hypophyseal portal vessels, activating ACTH release from the corticotrophs of the anterior pituitary gland.[15] NO activates not only COX but also lipoxygenase (LOX)[17,18] and GC, which produces cGMP; cGMP, in turn, increases intracellular calcium that converts membrane phospholipids into AA, the substrate for COX and LOX, generating PGs and leukotrienes, respectively. Activation of CRH by cytokines can be blocked by cyclosporine, probably by the blockade of dephosphorylation of NOS by calcineurin, rendering NOS inactive.[19] Furthermore, it has been shown that IL-1, TNF-α, IL-6, and IL-2 can directly stimulate ACTH release from the anterior pituitary via NO.[8,20]

Role of NO in the Control of Luteinizing Hormone-releasing Hormone Release

The control of gonadotropin secretion is extremely complex (Fig. 1), as revealed by research since the discovery of luteinizing hormone-releasing hormone (LHRH),[21] now commonly called gonadotropin-releasing

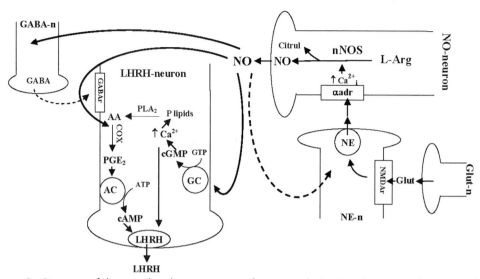

Figure 1. Diagram of the postulated participation of nitric oxide (NO) in luteinizing hormone-releasing hormone (LHRH) release. Glutamic acid (Glut) released from its neurons binds to N-methyl-D-aspartate (NMDA) receptors located on catecholaminergic neurons inducing norepinephrine (NE) release, which acts on α-adrenergic receptors activating neuronal NO synthase (nNOS) and therefore the production of NO. NO exerts its stimulatory actions on LHRH release by the interaction with the heme group of at least two enzymes. One is the activation of cyclooxygenase (COX), present in LHRH neurons, producing the conversion of arachidonic acid (AA) into prostaglandin E2 (PGE2), which stimulates adenylyl cyclase (AC) activity with the consequent increase in cAMP production, which induces LHRH secretion via cAMP-dependent protein kinase (PK) A. The other is activation of guanylate cyclase (GC), increasing cyclic guanosine monophosphate (cGMP) production, which stimulates LHRH secretion via cGMP-dependent PKG. Also, releasing AA from membrane phospholipids enhances PGE2 production. On the other hand, NO can produce inhibitory actions on LHRH release. NO depolarizes γ-aminobutyric acid (GABA)ergic neurons and therefore increases GABA release that acts on GABA receptors located on LHRH neurons producing the inhibition of LHRH release. Also, NO blocks the depolarization of the catecholaminergic terminals, inhibiting NE release and therefore the NE-stimulatory pathway. Both inhibitory actions of NO probably are necessary to terminate LHRH pulses. Solid arrows indicate stimulation; dashed arrows indicate inhibition.

hormone. LHRH controls the release of LH and follicle-stimulating hormone (FSH) from the pituitary and also induces mating behavior and penile erection in rats.[22,23] We demonstrated that intracerebroventricular microinjections of NOS inhibitors inhibited pulsatile LH release and mating behavior, which indicates that NO controls the pulsatile release of LHRH and mating behavior.[23,24] In *in vitro* experiments we showed that NO, released from sodium nitroprusside (NP), promoted LHRH release from medial basal hypothalamus (MBH) and that this action was blocked by hemoglobin, a scavenger of NO. NP also increases the release of PGE2 and LOX products that have been shown to play a role in LHRH release.[25] More-

over, inhibitors of COX blocked the release of LHRH induced by norepinephrine (NE), providing further evidence for the role of NO in the control of LHRH release via the activation of COX, as we mentioned above.[26,27] We postulate that the NO released from the NOergic neurons, near the LHRH neuronal terminals, increases the intracellular free calcium required to activate phospholipase A that converts membrane phospholipids to AA, which then can be converted to PGE2 via COX. The released PGE2 activates AC, increasing cAMP, which activates PKA, leading to exocytosis of LHRH secretory granules into the hypophyseal portal vessels for transport to the anterior pituitary gland.[28]

NE plays a controlling role in LHRH release by acting on hypothalamic NOergic neurons.[26–28] We determined that the release of NO from the NOergic neurons has a tonic inhibitory action to decrease the release of NE from hypothalamic explants. Presumably, the NO produced by NOergic neurons diffuses to the terminals of the catecholaminergic neurons where it acts on GC within the terminals to activate the enzyme and cause the production of cGMP. This cGMP may cause a decrease in intracellular free calcium in the cell, which may block the depolarization of the catecholaminergic terminals, inhibiting NE release from storage vesicles.[29] We have shown that NO is increased by NE by α_1 receptor stimulation as it can be blocked by prazosine, an α_1 receptor blocker.[28] The NO diffuses to the noradrenergic terminals and inhibits them, generating a negative feedback to terminate the release of NE and consequently contributing to finalize LHRH surge.[29]

The principal excitatory transmitter in the CNS is glutamic acid (Glut). We demonstrated that the mechanism by which Glut stimulates LHRH release involves NE release from noradrenergic neurons because the α receptor blocker, phentolamine, blocked the Glut-induced LHRH release.[30–32] Therefore, Glut neurons synapse with the noradrenergic terminal, which, in turn, synapses with the NOergic neuron, which then generates NO that diffuses to the LHRH terminal to stimulate LHRH release.

GABA plays a dual role in the control of LHRH release in rats.[33,34] In female rats it inhibits LHRH secretion by acting on LHRH neurons in the medial preoptic area and it has a stimulatory effect on LHRH secretion from the arcuate nucleus-ME region.[33] NO stimulates GABA release from the hypothalamus of adult male rats, and GABA inhibits LHRH release. We have shown that this inhibition is mediated by NO because the inhibitory effect was prevented by hemoglobin or by NG-monomethyl-L-arginine, a competitive inhibitor of NOS. Therefore, NO is involved not only in the stimulation of LHRH release induced by NE but also in its inhibition by inducing GABA release.[35]

Dopamine (DA) is another catecholamine that, as well as NE, stimulates LHRH release; however, the role of DA in pulsatile LHRH release is less clear. There are tuberoinfundibular dopaminergic neurons in the hypothalamus that have been shown to stimulate LHRH release from male rat hypothalami *in vitro*[36]; however, other studies indicate that at certain concentrations and in different hormonal states, such as in the castrate rat, both DA and NE can inhibit LHRH release.[37] The release of NO from the NOergic neurons in the hypothalamus has a tonic inhibitory action to decrease the release of DA from the tissue. Whether DA is released prior to each LH pulse to stimulate NO and LHRH release has yet to be determined, but this catecholamine may contribute to the release of NO and augment pulsatile LHRH release since DA receptor blockers can block LH release.[38]

The presence of an ultra-short negative feedback that controls the episodic secretion of LHRH was suggested for the first time by Hyppa *et al.* studying FSH secretion.[39] Morphological and molecular evidence show that LHRH receptors are expressed in LHRH hypothalamic neurons.[40] However, there is not much evidence for the signal transduction pathways triggered by the activation of these receptors *in vivo*. Krsmanovic *et al.* reported a signal transduction mechanism in GT1–7 neurons, driven by inositol trisphosphate-induced Ca^{2+} mobilization, responding to LHRH receptor activation.[41] We demonstrated that LHRH produces differential effects on the mediators of its own release, in MBH incubated *in vitro*, depending on its concentration in the intersynaptic space. LHRH 10^{-11} mol/L produced an increase in GABA release but inhibited Glut release at 10^{-7} mol/L, in both cases leading to the inhibition of LHRH release. Based on our results, we propose the existence of different populations of LHRH receptors that respond with a distinct threshold, activating different signal transduction pathways. Also, it is possible that LHRH affects its own release by activating an additional neurotransmitter-independent mechanism. Moreover, it was shown that the inhibitory effect of buserelin on LHRH release started before changes on neurotransmitter releases were observed.[42] These findings led us to study the effect of LHRH on cellular messengers involved in LHRH release, such as NO and PGE2. LHRH at 10^{-7} and 10^{-11} mol/L decreased PGE content after the incubation of MBH explants for 30 min. However, LHRH 10^{-7} mol/L stimulated NOS activity but at 10^{-11} mol/L had no effect. Although NO is a known promoter of LHRH release, the stimulatory effect of the higher concentration of LHRH on NOS activity is not contradictory to the ultra-short negative-feedback theory, since, as was described above, it was proposed that NO has a dual function inducing LHRH exocytosis during the normal surge but also increasing GABA release and decreasing NE and DA release to promote the termination of LHRH pulse.[35] Additionally, LHRH 10^{-7} mol/L but not 10^{-11} mol/L increased phosphatidylinositol breakdowns, suggesting that LHRH receptors coupled to PLC are involved in this NO-dependent mechanism. Although the mechanism of episodic release of LHRH is not clear to date, the NO-dependent pathway described could be one of the different existing mechanisms that provide redundancy for this important cycle that controls the physiology of reproduction.

These data together with those described above indicate that the NO released from NO-ergic neurons stimulates LHRH release and initiates the pulse but also acts back on the NE and dopaminergic neurons to terminate the pulse. This is coupled with the negative feedforward of GABA released by NO to bring about the termination of the pulse.

Participation of NO on the effect of Manganese on LHRH Release

Manganese (Mn^{2+}) is an essential metal that acts as a cofactor for many enzymes and therefore plays an important role in biological functions.[43] Nevertheless, high doses of Mn^{2+} can cause reproductive dysfunction.[44] It was reported that chronic administration of low doses of Mn^{2+} to female rats resulted in increased serum levels of puberty-related hormones, such as LH, FSH, and estradiol, and advanced the time of vaginal opening, indicating an advance in puberty.[45] We demonstrate that manganese chloride ($MnCl_2$) is capable of stimulating LHRH secretion from MBH and this effect is accompanied by an increase in plasma LH levels. Also, $MnCl_2$ is capable of stimulating DA secretion and NOS activity in the MBH. Because it was shown that DA can induce NOS/NO[46] and based on the important role of NO in the control of LHRH,[25] this suggests that DA/NO activation may mediate the $MnCl_2$-stimulated secretion of LHRH. We have also found an action of this metal stimulating the inhibitory transmitter GABA. Furthermore, when GABA-A receptors were blocked by bicuculline, the release of LHRH elicited by $MnCl_2$ was doubled. We suggest that the action of $MnCl_2$ to induce GABA secretion may represent a neurotoxic effect to ultimately inhibit LHRH secretion. Also, it was shown that $MnCl_2$ stimulates LHRH release from prepubertal female[45] and male[47] rats via the activation of guanylyl cyclase and subsequent stimulation of the cGMP/PKG pathway.[48] In concordance with that, our recent experiments demonstrate that $MnCl_2$ is capable of stimulating LHRH secretion through the activation of the hypothalamic NO/cGMP/PKG pathway.[49]

The Role of NO in Control of Posterior Pituitary Function

In the rat, the neural lobe of the pituitary is one of the regions richest in NOS, with a predominance of the nNOS isoform, suggesting that NO may play a role in controlling the release of neuropeptides and neurotransmitters from the posterior pituitary.[10,50] NADPH-diaphorase, used as a marker of NOS, was co-localized with vasopressin (VP) and oxytocin (OT) in the hypothalamic nuclei that synthesized these hormones.[51,52] The synthesis of NO by oxytocinergic or vasopressinergic neurons suggests that NO may participate in autoregulation and/or cross-regulation of OT and VP secretion. Our studies indicate that NO donors reduce OT secretion from the neural pituitary lobe, and we postulated that released NO may suppress OT secretion through an ultra-short negative-feedback mechanism.[53] It has been reported that intracerebroventricular administration of L-NAME enhanced plasma levels of both OT and VP.[54] Because NOS activity increases following salt loading and dehydration, it has been suggested that this increase may provide a negative feedback to prevent over stimulation of OT and VP release.[55] In conclusion, NO may intervene in the control of OT response to osmotic stimuli. Also, chronic saline ingestion increases hypothalamic tachykinin concentration in SON.[56] Tachykinins belong to a family of peptides that include substance P and neurokinin A (NKA). They are contained in hypothalamic neurons and nerve fibers and secretory cells of the posterior and anterior pituitary lobes, suggesting that these peptides may have a physiological role in the control of pituitary function.[57] Some actions of tachykinins are known to be exerted through NO release.[58] We observed an inhibitory effect of NKA on OT release by activation of NO-ergic neurons, thus suggesting that NKA may have a dual effect on OT release, decreasing it through NO and increasing OT release by an NO-independent mechanism.[59] Nevertheless, the net effect of NKA on OT release from posterior pituitary seems to be inhibitory. As we mentioned above, NO has been linked to the release of several neurotransmitters, including glutamate, DA, and GABA. Results on the effect of NO on GABA release are contradictory. Our study showed that endogenous NO has an inhibitory effect on GABAergic activity in posterior pituitary,[59] contrary to the effect that we have reported at the hypothalamic level.[35] GABAergic terminals in the neural and inter-

mediate lobes participate in the control of OT and VP release,[60,61] raising the possibility that NO modulation of GABAergic activity in the posterior pituitary may be involved in the regulation of the secretory function of this pituitary lobe. However, since NO decreased both OT and GABA release from the posterior pituitary and GABA was reported to inhibit OT release from nerve terminals of the neural lobe, it is possible that NO might influence the release of OT at the level of the cell bodies and on nerve terminals of the neural lobe by different mechanisms. NO is involved, at least partially, in the reduction of the GABAergic activity induced by NKA. The reduction in GABA release may contribute to the stimulatory effect of NKA on lactotroph function.[62] This effect will increase the release of PRL, considered a pro-inflammatory factor, which could participate in the regulation of the immune response during the acute phase of endotoxemia.

Role of NO on Corticosterone Release from the Adrenal Gland

ACTH is the major regulator of steroid secretion and synthesis from the adrenal cortex, inducing an acute secretory response within a few minutes and an increase in steroid synthesis, including the transcription of steroidogenic genes.[63] Many clinical and experimental observations indicate that there could be dissociation between plasma ACTH concentrations and cortisol/corticosterone secretion.[64] Since the sympathetic nervous system responds earlier than the hypothalamic–pituitary–adrenal (HPA) axis to stressors, corticosterone release prior to ACTH action may be a result of earlier stimulation of the adrenal cortex via the splachnic nerves, possibly via NO release. The effect of ACTH on adrenal function may involve NO[65] since NOS was found expressed in the adrenal gland.[66] Endothelial and neuronal cells have a close anatomical proximity to steroidogenic cells in the adrenal gland, and these cells release NO. In fact, one study suggested that the production of NO by eNOS or nNOS could be effective in regulating the blood flow and steroid release.[67] Moreover, NO can also be generated within steroid-producing cells and may be involved in steroidogenesis.[68]

On the other hand there are controversial reports on the effects of NO and PGs on the steroidogenic pathway.[68] All of these studies used dispersed cells, thereby eliminating the normal architecture of the gland. NO has been postulated as an autocrine/paracrine regulator of steroidogenesis in several tissues, with effects on adrenal steroid secretion.[64,68] We investigated the role of NO and the participation of PGE2 in corticosterone release stimulated from rat adrenal glands by ACTH *in vitro*.[69] Our results indicate that NO stimulates corticosterone release from adrenals. We hypothesize that NO leads to a rapid release of stored corticosterone from the adrenals because the amount released at 15 min was nearly as great as at 30 min and corticosterone adrenal content was lower than the control, indicating that any *de novo* synthesis of corticosterone occurred during this period. The effect of NO and ACTH on acute release of corticosterone could be mediated by PGE2 because PGE2 can release corticosterone and this effect is blocked by indomethacin, a COX inhibitor.[69]

We hypothesize that ACTH activates NOS, which increases NO, which activates COX, which generates PGE2, which in turn releases corticosterone. The mechanism by which PGE2 causes exocytosis remains to be determined.

Effect of Radiation on NO Production in the Submandibular Gland

The exposure to ionizing radiation during therapy for head and neck tumors results in alterations of salivary glands, such as sialoadenitis and xerostomia followed by dysphagia, mucositis, rampant dental caries, increased tooth decay, oral infections, oesophagitis, and gustatory dysfunction.[70,71] There has been a continuous effort to understand this salivary gland dysfunction; however, the specific mechanisms that underline such damage remain poorly understood. Salivary glands are composed of highly differentiated almost non-cycling cells, and differences in radiosensitivity of the various cell types have been observed.[72] In the submandibular gland (SMG), it has been shown that serous cells are far more radiosensitive, and this is in concordance with the observed decrease in salivary flow after irradiation.[71]

NOS is widely distributed in different regions of SMG.[73] In previous publications of our group we have shown that nNOS is clearly present in nerve terminals and together with iNOS in the apical membrane of the excretory and striated ducts of SMG. Interestingly, NOS was absent in the acinar cells.[74] Previously reported results from our group indicate that NO has a stimulatory effect on salivary secretion,[75] therefore we hypothesize that radiation could affect salivary secretion by modulating the NOS activity in the SMG. The inducible NOS expressed in immune cells produces the greatest quantities of NO, and many macrophages were seen within the gland.[75] We observed that iNOS activity was significantly reduced after radiation, indicating that the decrease in the levels of NO in SMG could mediate the decreased salivary secretion.[76] Also we found an increase in the PGE content in the SMG that could contribute to the decrease in salivary secretion, as we have shown previously.[77] Furthermore, we found an increase in lipid peroxidation, oxidative stress, and an increase in mitochondrial NOS expression in SMG that could lead to tissue damage observed 180 days after radiation. At 365 days post radiation, there were structural changes that could account for irreversible damage, such as fibrosis with loss of salivary secretion.

Effect of Prenatal Stress on NO Production in the CNS of the Offspring

The developing CNS is especially vulnerable to stress-induced damages. The effect of stress during the first stages of development induces both immediate and later alterations, which reflect changes in the neuroendocrine, cognitive, and behavioral systems. Stress during pregnancy triggers physiological and behavioral abnormalities in the offspring.[78]

The hippocampus is one of the classic structures associated with cognitive processes. However, recently the cerebellum has been redefined as a structure with a much wider functionality. Certain investigations in humans and animal models involve the cerebellum in cognitive functions. We evaluated the effect of stress during pregnancy in the offspring at 30, 60, and 90 postnatal days on nNOS and iNOS activities and protein content in the hippocampus and cerebellum and on learning and memory capabilities.

When protein levels from cerebellum and hippocampus were studied in the offspring of stressed animals, an increase in nNOS was found in both tissues at different ages. At the same time, iNOS expression did not vary in a significant manner in the analyzed tissues. Also, we found an increase in the activity in calcium-dependent NOS in cerebellum homogenates in prenatal-stressed animals with respect to controls.

When a spatial memory test was performed, it showed that offspring from stressed mothers needed more time to complete the task than offspring from control animals. The differences were highly significant at postnatal day 30 and were maintained at day 60s and 90. Also, prenatal stress induced a deficit in the inhibitory avoidance task. As predicted, the latency for the control group increased in a significant manner, which reflects that both information acquisition and consolidation provided by the context were successful. In the prenatal-stressed group, no significant differences were observed when the training latency was compared with the test latency. Also, significant differences were found between control and stressed animals for the test latency values from postnatal day 45. It has, therefore, been demonstrated that, from a behavioral point of view, prenatal stress induced a decrease in the ability to resolve spatial

navigation tasks and a learning deficit in the inhibitory avoidance test.[79]

The results indicate that the prenatal-stress model used is able to induce a decrease in offspring learning and memory capabilities. These alterations correlate with an increase in the expression and activity of the enzyme NOS in different parts of the brain of stressed rats.

Therefore, we conclude that the changes in NOS profiles and activities might constitute primary events during the development of the nervous system that may manifest as significant changes in animal behavior in adulthood.

Conclusions

NO regulates numerous and diverse physiological processes, including reproduction and neurotransmission. The data presented above indicate that there are many areas in the brain where there is regular, periodic, physiological release of NO throughout the life span. This occurs in the hippocampus, cerebellum, and, in particular, in the hypothalamus where NO controls most of the hypothalamic peptidergic neurons (such as CRH, LHRH, GHRH, somatostatin, OT, and VP) and also activates the release of GABA and inhibits that of NE and DA.

Because of the ubiquitous nature of NO, the inappropriate release of this mediator has been linked to pathogenesis of a number of disease states, including stress, neurodegenerative disorders, inflammation, and septic shock. It is already well known that stress and infections with release of viral or bacterial products, such as LPS, cause the induction of cytokines, which are released and travel through the bloodstream. LPS and the released cytokines combine with their receptors to induce iNOS expression in neurons, glia, and many other immune cells, producing high amounts of NO than would be released in basal conditions. NO itself or combined to other free radicals and other substances produces toxic effects in cells, which cause cell injury and death. On the other hand, there appears to be a temporal and functional relation between the HPA axis response and NO formation at every level of the axis, suggesting a fundamental role of NO as a key modulator of the HPA to maintain homeostasis in these pathological states.

Acknowledgments

Most of this work was inspired by Professor Dr. Samuel M. McCann who spent the last years of his life with us—our deepest gratitude to our Maestro. Also we thank Ana Ines Casella for her administrative assistance. This work was supported by Agencia Nacional de Promoción Científica y Tecnológica, Argentina, grant PICT 14264 and Consejo Nacional de Investigaciones Científicas y Técnicas (CONICET) Grant PIP 6149.

Conflicts of Interest

The authors declare no conflicts of interest.

References

1. Selye, H. 1937. The significance of the adrenals for adaptation. *Science* **85:** 247–248.
2. Chowers, I., H.T. Hammel, J. Eiseman, *et al*. 1996. A comparision of the effects of environmental and pre-optic heating and pyrogen on plasma cortisol levels. *Am. J. Physiol.* **210:** 606–610.
3. Breder, C.D., C.A. Dinarello & C.B. Saper. 1988. Interleukin-1 immunoreactive innervation of the human hypothalamus. *Science* **240:** 321.
4. Rettori V., W.L. Dees, J.K. Hiney, *et al*. 1994. An interleukin-1-alpha-like neuronal system in the preoptic-hypothalamic region and its induction by bacterial lipopolysaccharide in concentrations which alter pituitary hormone release. *Neuroimmunomodulation* **1:** 251–258.
5. Spangelo, B.L., P.C. Isakson & R.M. MacLeod. 1990. Production of interleukin-6 by anterior pituitary cells is stimulated by increased intracellular adenosine 3', 5'-monophosphate and vasoactive intestinal peptide. *Endocrinology* **127:** 403–409.
6. McCann, S.M., M. Kimura, S. Karanth, *et al*. 1998. Role of nitric oxide in the neuroendocrine responses to cytokines. *Ann. N. Y. Acad. Sci.* **840:** 174–184.

7. Hobbs, A.J., A. Higgs & S. Moncada. 1999. Inhibition of nitric oxide synthase as a potential therapeutic target. *Annu. Rev. Pharmaco.l Toxicol.* **39:** 191–220.
8. McCann, S.M., K. Lyson, S. Karanth, *et al*. 1995. Mechanism of action of cytokines to induce the pattern of pituitary hormone secretion in infection. *Ann. N. Y. Acad. Sci.* **771:** 386–395.
9. Förstermann, U., I. Gath, P. Schwarz, *et al*. 1995. Isoforms of nitric oxide synthase. Properties, cellular distribution and expressional control. *Biochem. Pharmacol.* **50:** 1321–1332.
10. Bredt, D.S., P.M. Hwang & S.H. Snyder. 1990. Localization of nitric oxide synthase indicating a neural role for nitric oxide. *Nature* **347:** 768–70.
11. McCann, S.M., J. Antunes-Rodrigues, C.R. Franci, *et al*. 2000. Role of the hypothalamic pituitary adrenal axis in the control of the response to stress and infection. *Braz. J. Med. Biol. Res.* **33:** 1121–1131.
12. McCann, S.M., M. Kimura, W.H. Yu, *et al*. 2001. Cytokines and pituitary hormone secretion. *Vitam. Horm.* **63:** 29–62.
13. Wong, M.L., P.B. Bongiorno, V. Rettori, *et al*. 1997. Interleukin (IL) 1 beta, IL-1 receptor antagonist, IL-10, and IL-13 gene expression in the central nervous system and anterior pituitary during systemic inflammation: pathophysiological implications. *Proc. Natl. Acad. Sci. USA* **94:** 227–232.
14. Wong, M.L., V. Rettori, A. al-Shekhlee, *et al*. 1994. Inducible nitric oxide synthase gene expression in the brain during systemic inflammation. *Nat. Med.* **2:** 581–584.
15. Karanth, S., K. Lyson & S.M. McCann. 1993. Role of nitric oxide in interleukin 2-induced corticotropin-releasing factor release from incubated hypothalami. *Proc. Natl. Acad. Sci. USA* **90:** 3383–3387.
16. McCann, S.M., J. Antunes-Rodrigues, C.R. Franci, *et al*. 2000. Role of the hypothalamic pituitary adrenal axis in the control of the response to stress and infection. *Braz. J. Med. Biol. Res.* **33:** 1121–1131.
17. Karanth, S., K. Lyson, M.C. Aguila, *et al*. 1995. Effects of luteinizing-hormone-releasing hormone, alpha-melanocyte-stimulating hormone, naloxone, dexamethasone and indomethacin on interleukin-2-induced corticotropin-releasing factor release. *Neuroimmunomodulation* **2:** 166–173.
18. Lyson, K. & S.M. McCann. 1992. Involvement of arachidonic acid cascade pathways in interleukin-6-stimulated corticotropin-releasing factor release *in vitro. Neuroendocrinology* **55:** 708–713.
19. Karanth, S., K. Lyson & S.M. McCann. 1994. Cyclosporin A inhibits interleukin-2-induced release of corticotropin-releasing hormone. *Neuroimmunomodulation* **1:** 82–85.

20. McCann, S.M., S. Karanth, A. Kamat, *et al.* 1994. Induction by cytokines of the pattern of pituitary hormone secretion in infection. *Neuroimmunomodulation* **1:** 2–13.

21. McCann, S.M., S. Taleisnik & H.M. Fridman. 1960. LH-releasing activity in hypothalamic explants. *Proc. Soc. Exp. Biol. Med.* **104:** 432–434.

22. McCann, S.M. & S.R. Ojeda. 1996. The anterior pituitary and hypothalamus. In *Textbook of Endocrine Physiology.* J.E. Griffin & S.R. Ojeda, Eds.: 101–133. Oxford University Press. Oxford, England.

23. Mani, S.K., J.M. Allen, V. Rettori, *et al.* 1994. Nitric oxide mediates sexual behavior in female rats by stimulating LHRH release. *Proc. Natl. Acad. Sci. USA* **91:** 6468–6472.

24. McCann, S.M., M. Kimura, S. Karanth, *et al.* 2002. Role of nitric oxide in the neuroendocrine response to cytokines. *Front. Horm. Res.* **29:** 117–129.

25. Rettori, V., N. Belova, W.L. Dees, *et al.* 1993. Role of nitric oxide in the control of luteinizing hormone-releasing hormone release in vivo and in vitro. *Proc. Natl. Acad. Sci. USA* **90:** 10130–10134.

26. Canteros, G., V. Rettori, A. Franchi, *et al.* 1995. Ethanol inhibits luteinizing hormone-releasing hormone (LHRH) secretion by blocking the response of LHRH neuronal terminals to nitric oxide. *Proc. Natl. Acad. Sci. USA* **92:** 3416–3420.

27. Rettori, V., M. Gimeno, K. Lyson, *et al.* 1992. Nitric oxide mediates norepinephrine-induced prostaglandin E2 release from the hypothalamus. *Proc. Natl. Acad. Sci. USA* **89:** 11543–11546.

28. Canteros, G., V. Rettori, A. Genaro, *et al.* 1996. Nitric oxide synthase content of hypothalamic explants: increase by norepinephrine and inactivated by NO and cGMP. *Proc. Natl. Acad. Sci. USA* **93:** 4246–4250.

29. Seilicovich, A., M. Lasaga, M. Befumo, *et al.* 1995. Nitric oxide inhibits the release of norepinephrine and dopamine from the medial basal hypothalamus of the rat. *Proc. Natl. Acad. Sci. USA* **92:** 11299–11302.

30. McCann, S.M. & L. Krulich. 1989. Role of transmitters in control of anterior pituitary hormone release. In *Endocrinology*, 2nd en. L. DeGroot, Ed.: 117–130. W. B. Saunders. Philadelphia.

31. Rettori, V., A. Kamat & S.M. McCann. 1994. Nitric oxide mediates the stimulation of luteinizing-hormone releasing hormone release induced by glutamic acid in vitro. *Brain Res. Bull.* **33:** 501–503.

32. Kamat, A., W.H. Yu, V. Rettori & S.M. McCann. 1995. Glutamic acid induces luteinizing hormone releasing hormone release via alpha receptors. *Brain Res. Bull.* **37:** 233–235.

33. McCann, S.M. & V. Rettori. 1986. Gamma amino butyric acid (GABA) controls anterior pituitary hormone secretion. *Adv. Biochem. Psychopharmacol.* **42:** 173–179.

34. Masotto, C., G. Wisnieski & A. Negro-Vilar. 1989. Different gamma-aminobutyric acid receptor subtypes are involved in the regulation of opiate-dependent and independent luteinizing hormone-releasing hormone secretion. *Endocrinology* **125:** 548–553.

35. Seilicovich, A., B.H. Duvilanski, D. Pisera, *et al.* Nitric oxide inhibits hypothalamic luteinizing hormone-releasing hormone release by releasing gamma-aminobutyric acid. *Proc. Natl. Acad. Sci. USA* **92:** 3421–3424.

36. Ojeda, S.R., A. Negro-Vilar & S.M. McCann. 1979. Catecholaminergic modulation of luteinizing hormone-releasing hormone release by median eminence terminals in vitro. *Endocrinology* **104:** 617–624.

37. Vijayan, E. & S.M. McCann. 1978. Re-evaluation of the role of catecholamines in control of gonadotropin and prolactin release. *Neuroendocrinology* **25:** 221–235.

38. Ojeda, S.R., P.G. Harms, S.M. McCann. 1974. Effect of blockade of dopaminergic receptors on prolactin and LH release: median eminence and pituitary sites of action. *Endocrinology* **94:** 1650–1657.

39. Hyppa, M., M. Motta & L. Martini. 1971. 'Ultrashort' feedback control of follicle-stimulating hormone-releasing factor secretion. *Neuroendocrinology* **7:** 227–235.

40. Krsmanovic, L.Z., S.S. Stojilkovic, L.M. Mertz, *et al.* 1993. Expression of gonadotropin-releasing hormone receptors and autocrine regulation of neuropeptide release in immortalized hypothalamic neurons. *Proc. Natl. Acad. Sci. USA* **90:** 3908–3912.

41. Krsmanovic, L.Z., N. Mores, C.E. Navarro, *et al.* 2001. Regulation of Ca2+-sensitive adenylyl cyclase in gonadotropin-releasing hormone neurons. *Mol. Endocrinol.* **15:** 429–440.

42. Feleder, C., H. Jarry, S. Leonhardt, *et al.* 1996. Evidence to suggest that gonadotropin-releasing hormone inhibits its own secretion by affecting hypothalamic amino acid neurotransmitter release. *Neuroendocrinology* **64:** 298–304.

43. Keen, C.L., B. Lönnerdal & L.S. Hurley. 1984. Manganese. In *Biochemistry of the Essential Ultratrace Elements*. E. Frieden, Ed.: 89–132. Plenum Publishing Co. New York.

44. Grey, L.E. & J.W. Laskey. 1980. Multivariate analysis of the effects of manganese on the reproductive physiology and behavior of the male house mouse. *J. Toxicol. Environ. Health* **6:** 861–867.

45. Pine, M., B. Lee, R. Dearth, *et al.* 2005. Manganese acts centrally to stimulate luteinizing hormone secretion: a potential influence on female pubertal development. *Toxicol. Sci.* **85:** 880–885.

46. Melis, M.R., S. Succu & A. Argiolas. 1996. Dopamine agonists increase nitric oxide production in the paraventricular nucleus of the hypothalamus: correlation with penile erection and yawning. *Eur. J. Neurosci.* **8:** 2056–2063.

47. Lee, B., M. Pine, L. Johnson, *et al*. 2006. Manganese acts centrally to activate reproductive hormone secretion and pubertal development in male rats. *Reprod. Toxicol.* **22:** 580–85.

48. Lee, B., J.K. Hiney, M.D. Pine, *et al*. 2007. Manganese stimulates luteinizing hormone releasing hormone secretion in prepubertal female rats: hypothalamic site and mechanism of action. *J. Physiol.* **578:** 765–772.

49. Prestifilippo, J.P., J. Fernández-Solari, C. Mohn, *et al*. 2007. Effect of manganese on luteinizing hormone-releasing hormone secretion in adult male rats. *Toxicol. Sci.* **97:** 75–80.

50. Sagar, S.M. & D.M. Ferreiro. 1987. NADPH diaphorase activity in the posterior pituitary: relation to neuronal function. *Brain Res.* **400:** 348–352.

51. Calka, J. & C.H. Block. 1993. Relationship of vasopressin with NADPH-diaphorase in the hypothalamo-neurohypophyseal system. *Brain Res. Bull.* **32:** 207–210.

52. Miyagagua, A., H. Okamura & Y. Ibata. 1994. Coexistence of oxytocin and NADPHdiaphorase in magnocellular neurons of the paraventricular and supraoptic nuclei of the rat hypothalamus. *Neurosci. Lett.* **171:** 13–16.

53. Rettori, V., G. Canteros, R. Reynoso, *et al*. 1997. Oxytocin stimulates the release of luteinizing hormone–releasing hormone from medial basal hypothalamic explants by releasing nitric oxide. *Proc. Natl. Acad. Sci. USA* **94:** 2741–2744.

54. Kadekaro, M., M.L. Terrell, H. Liu, *et al*. 1998. Effects of L-NAME on cerebral, vasopressin, oxytocin, and blood pressure responses in hemorrhaged rats. *Am. J. Physiol.* **274:** 1070–1077.

55. Liu, Q.S., Y. Jia & G. Ju. 1997. Nitric oxide inhibits neuronal activity in the supraoptic nucleus of the rat hypothalamic slices. *Brain Res. Bull.* **43:** 121–125.

56. Larsen, P.J., D.S. Jessop, S.L. Lightman, *et al*. 1993. Preprotachykinin A gene expression in distinct hypothalamic and brain stem regions of the rat is affected by chronic osmotic stimulus: a combined immunohistochemical and in situ hybridization histochemistry study. *Brain Res. Bull.* **30:** 535–545.

57. Nussdorfer, G.G. & L.K. Malendowicz. 1998. Role of tachykinins in the regulation of the hypothalamo-pituitary-adrenal axis. *Peptides* **19:** 949–968.

58. Eutamene, H., V. Theodorou, J. Fioramonti, *et al*. 1995. Implication of NK1 and NK2 receptors in rat colonic hypersecretion induced by interleukin 1 beta: role of nitric oxide. *Gastroenterology* **109:** 483–489.

59. De Laurentiis, A., D. Pisera, B. Duvilanski, *et al*. 2000. Neurokinin A inhibits oxytocin and GABA release from the posterior pituitary by stimulating nitric oxide synthase. *Brain Res. Bull.* **53:** 325–330.

60. Crowley, W. & W. Armstrong. 1992. Neurochemical regulation of oxytocin secretion in lactation. *Endocr. Rev.* **13:** 33–65.

61. Sladek, C. & W. Armstrong. 1987. Gamma-aminobutyric acid antagonists stimulate vasopressin release from organ cultured hypothalamo-neurohypophyseal explants. *Endocrinology* **120:** 1576–1580.

62. Pisera, D., A. De Laurentiis, B. Duvilanski, *et al*. 1996. Neurokinin A affects the tubero-hypophyseal GABAergic system. *Neuroreport* **7:** 2236–2240.

63. Sewer, M.B. & M.R. Waterman. 2003. ACTH modulation of transcription factors responsible for steroid hydroxylase gene expression in the adrenal cortex. *Microsc. Res. Tech.* **61:** 300–307.

64. Bornstein, S.R. & G.P. Chrousos. 1999. Clinical review 104: Adrenocorticotropin (ACTH)- and non-ACTH-mediated regulation of the adrenal cortex: neural and immune inputs. *J. Clin. Endocrinol. Metab.* **84:** 1729–1736.

65. Nakayama, T., Y. Izumi, M. Soma, *et al*. 1996. A nitric oxide synthesis inhibitor prevents the ACTH-stimulated production of aldosterone in rat adrenal gland. *Endocrin. J.* **43:** 157–162.

66. Cymeryng, C.B., S.P. Lotito, C. Colonna, *et al*. 2002. Expression of nitric oxide synthases in rat adrenal zona fasciculata cells. *Endocrinology* **143:** 1235–1242.

67. Riquelme, R.A., G. Sánchez, L. Liberona, *et al*. 2002. Nitric oxide plays a role in the regulation of adrenal blood flow and adrenocorticomedullary functions in the llama fetus. *J. Physiol.* **544:** 267–276.

68. Cymeryng, C.B., L.A. Dada, C. Colonia, *et al*. 1999. Effects of L-arginine in rat adrenal cells: involvement of nitric oxide synthase. *Endocrinology* **140:** 2962–2967.

69. Mohn, C.E., J. Fernandez-Solari, A. De Laurentiis, *et al*. 2005. The rapid release of corticosterone from the adrenal induced by ACTH is mediated by nitric oxide acting by prostaglandin E2. *Proc. Natl. Acad. Sci. USA* **102:** 6213–6218.

70. Valdez, I.H., J.C. Atkinson, J.A. Ship, *et al*. 1993. Major salivary gland function in patients with radiation-induced xerostomia: flow rates and sialochemistry. *Int. J. Radiat. Oncol. Biol. Phys.* **25:** 41–47.

71. Nagler, R.M., B.J. Baum, G. Miller, *et al*. 1998. Long term salivary effects of single-dose head and neck irradiation in the rat. *Archs. Oral Biol.* **43:** 297–303.

72. O'Connell, A., R. Redman, L. Evans, *et al*. 1999. Radiation-induced progressive decrease in fluid secretion in rat submandibular gland is related to decrease acinar volume and not impaired calcium signaling. *Rad. Res.* **151:** 150–158.

73. Lohinai, Z., A.D. Szekely, L. Soos, *et al.* 1995. Distribution of nitric oxide synthase containing elements in the feline submandibular gland. *Neurosci. Lett.* **192:** 9–12.

74. Lomniczi, A., A.M. Suburo, J.C. Elverdin, *et al.* 1998. Role of nitric oxide in salivary secretion. *Neuroimmunomodulation* **5:** 226–233.

75. Rettori, V., A. Lomniczi, J.C. Elverdin, *et al.* 2000. Control of salivary secretion by nitric oxide and its role in neuroimmunomodulation. *Ann. N. Y. Acad. Sci.* **917:** 258–267.

76. de la Cal, C., A. Lomniczi, C.E. Mohn, *et al.* 2006. Decrease in salivary secretion by radiation mediated by nitric oxide and prostaglandins. *Neuroimmunomodulation* **13:** 19–27.

77. Lomniczi, A., C. Mohn, A. Faletti, *et al.* 2001. Inhibition of salivary secretion by lipopolisaccharide: possible role of prostaglandins. *Am. J. Physiol. Endocrinol. Metab.* **281:** E405–E411.

78. Ruiz, R. & C. Avant. 2005. Effects of maternal prenatal stress on infant outcomes. *Adv. Nurs. Sci.* **28:** 345–355.

79. Martin, L., D. Goldowitz & G. Mittleman. 2003. The cerebellum and spatial ability: dissection of motor and cognitive components with a mouse model system. *Eur. J. Neurosci.* **18:** 2002–2010.

Cytokine Control of Adult Neural Stem Cells

Chronic versus Acute Exposure

Sylvian Bauer

Département de Physiologie Neurovégétative, Centre de Recherche en Neurobiologie et Neurophysiologie de Marseille (CRN2M), Unité Mixte de Recherche (UMR) 6231, Centre National de la Recherche Scientifique (CNRS)-Universités Aix-Marseille I and II, Marseille, France

The neuropoietic cytokine family includes interleukin-6 (IL-6), leukemia inhibitory factor (LIF), and ciliary neurotrophic factor (CNTF), among others. These cytokines have been shown to alter neural stem cell (NSC) self-renewal and progenitor cell division and differentiation, which could be mediated by the Janus kinase-signal transducer and activator of transcription (JAK/STAT) pathway. Using neurospheres from the adult mouse subventricular zone (SVZ), we found that acute or chronic exposure to LIF or CNTF differentially affects sphere development and sphere growth. Both cytokines also favor the amplification of NSCs. Contrasting results were obtained with IL-6 or leptin, although both cytokines also activate the JAK/STAT pathway. Stimulating NSC self-renewal *in vivo* could be of therapeutic interest for treating neurodegeneration. When applied to the adult mouse brain, chronic LIF stimulates NSC self-renewal but prevents the emergence of more differentiated progeny. On the other hand, acute LIF treatment stimulates SVZ regeneration, most likely through an increase in NSCs. These results reveal that cytokine effects could vary as a function of exposure duration and suggest that, in the search for strategies to promote brain repair, *in vivo* acute LIF treatment could promote cell replacement.

Key words: gp130; neurogenesis; gliogenesis; cell fate

Introduction

Neurogenesis persists in at least two regions of the normal adult brain: the hippocampal dentate gyrus and the olfactory bulb (OB) (reviewed in Ref. 1). In the OB, new neurons are generated from distant neural stem cells (NSCs) located in the subventricular zone (SVZ). The cell lineage from adult NSCs to new neurons in the OB has been well described *in vivo*[2–5] and could also be studied *in vitro* using the neurosphere assay.[6,7]

Despite persisting NSCs, the adult brain shows a very limited capacity for cell replace-ment after lesion or injury.[8–10] Understanding NSC biology *in vivo* could thus lead to new therapeutic strategies for promoting brain repair from endogenous progenitors.

In this context, one cytokine of particular interest is leukemia inhibitory factor (LIF), which is well known for maintaining mouse embryonic stem (ES) cell phenotype.[11] LIF is a member of the interleukin-6 (IL-6) cytokine family, which also includes ciliary neurotrophic factor (CNTF) and IL-6, among others.[12,13]

In the nervous system, endogenous LIF expression is very low under normal physiological conditions but it is systematically induced following various types of injuries, including trauma, seizures, and ischemia[14–21] (see Table 1). Relevance of this rise of LIF has been emphasized in the regenerating adult olfactory epithelium where it is necessary for the lesion-induced proliferation of neuronal

Address for correspondence: Sylvian Bauer, CRN2M-UMR 6231, CNRS-Université Aix-Marseille, Département de Physiologie Neurovégétative, Fac. St-Jérôme – BP 351-352, Av. Escadrille Normandie-Niemen, Marseille 13397 cedex 20, France. Voice: 33-4-91-28-87-31; fax: 33-4-91-28-88-85. sylvian.bauer@univ-cezanne.fr

Neuroimmunomodulation: Ann. N.Y. Acad. Sci. 1153: 48–56 (2009).
doi: 10.1111/j.1749-6632.2009.03986.x © 2009 New York Academy of Sciences.

TABLE 1. Leukemia Inhibitory Factor (LIF) Is Induced after Various Types of Brain Injuries[a]

Type of injury	Mode of detection	Timing of LIF induction	References
Adult rat – sciatic nerve section	Quantitative RNAse protection assay	Strong induction seen at 24 h, maintained for up to 5 days, followed by gradual decreased expression	14
Adult rat – cortical lesion	Quantitative RNAse protection assay	Induction starts at 6 h, expression peaks at 24 h and returns to near baseline at 48 h	15
Adult mouse – olfactory bulb ablation	Semiquantitative RT-PCR + Western blot	Induction starts at 4 h, expression peaks at 8 h and returns to near baseline at 48 h	16
Postnatal rat – hypoxia/ischemia	Quantitative real-time PCR	Strong induction at 24 and 48 h, decreased expression at 72 h	17
Adult rat – pilocarpine-induced seizures	Quantitative RNAse protection assay	Induction starts at 2 h, expression peaks at 12 h and returns to near baseline by 72 h	18
Young rat – kainic acid-induced seizures	Northern blot	Induction starts at 2–4 h, expression peaks at 8–24 h and returns to baseline by 48 h	19
Adult mouse – MPTP intoxication	Quantitative real-time PCR	Induction starts at 4 h, expression peaks at 12 h and starts declining at 24 h	20
Adult rats – middle cerebral artery occlusion (MCAO)	Immunohistochemistry	Induction starts at 12 h, expression peaks at 24 h and starts declining by 48 h	21

[a]Lesion-induced LIF expression occurs very rapidly after the lesion and is always transient in the central nervous system.

Abbreviations: MPTP, 1-methyl-4-phenyl-1,2,3,6-tetrahydropyridine.

progenitors.[16] In the normal adult brain, we recently showed that exogenous LIF promotes NSC self-renewal *in vivo*,[22] suggesting that the very rapid and transient overexpression of endogenous LIF observed after lesion could constitute a signal that recruits and amplifies NSCs, making their regenerative potential available for brain repair.

Here, we present both *in vitro* and *in vivo* data aimed at exploring the effects of LIF under various conditions in order to better understand how LIF could be used to promote brain repair. Parts of these results are unpublished, whereas other parts were recently published in other forms[22] (see this reference for technical details).

Chronic LIF Exposure *in Vitro* Prevents Neurosphere Formation and Growth

As NSCs cannot be identified with specific markers, a functional assay *in vitro* is used to study the main characteristics of NSCs, which are proliferation, multipotentiality (the ability to generate neurons, astrocytes, and oligodendrocytes), and self-renewal. To generate neurospheres, dissociated cells from the adult mouse SVZ are cultured in medium supplemented with growth factors [epidermal growth factor (EGF) and/or basic fibroblast growth factor (bFGF)]. Some cells, presumably the NSCs, will proliferate and generate free-floating spheres that contain progenitors of the three neural cell types, demonstrating proliferation and multipotentiality. These neurospheres can be passaged multiple times; after dissociation, some cells will generate secondary neurospheres, demonstrating self-renewal.

The effects of continuous LIF exposure were studied by adding mouse recombinant LIF protein on single cells obtained from dissociated fully grown neurospheres derived from the adult mouse SVZ. LIF was added to the culture medium every 2 days, and neurospheres were quantified after 8 days *in vitro* (DIV).

Compared to control neurospheres, addition of LIF to the culture medium at 20 ng/mL

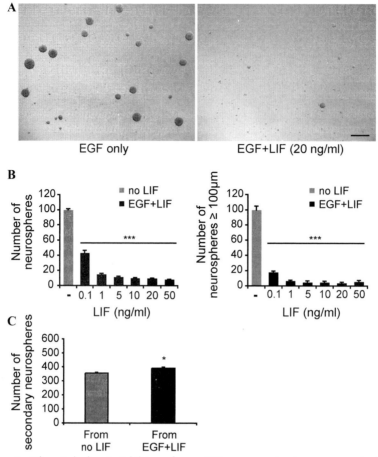

Figure 1. Chronic leukemia inhibitory factor (LIF) exposure *in vitro* prevents the formation and growth of adult mouse subventricular zone (SVZ)-derived neurospheres, even at a very low dose, but does not alter secondary sphere-forming potential. (**A**) Photomicrographs showing neurosphere cultures after 8 days *in vitro* (DIV) in control conditions [epidermal growth factor (EGF) only] or in EGF supplemented with recombinant mouse LIF protein (20 ng/mL). Scale bar = 300 μm. (**B**) Dose – response study of the effects of chronic LIF on sphere number (left graph) and on sphere size (right graph) after 8 DIV. Total number of neurospheres and neurospheres with a diameter ≥ 100 μm were quantified; data are shown as percent of control. (**C**) Number of secondary spheres derived from single cells dissociated from spheres grown for 8 DIV in EGF only or in EGF supplemented with LIF (20 ng/mL). Secondary spheres were grown in regular culture medium (EGF only) for 8 DIV. *P < 0.05 and ***P < 0.001, Student's *t*-test.

profoundly impaired the formation and growth of neurospheres; fewer and smaller spheres developed (Fig. 1A). In a dose – response study, similar effects were found with concentrations of LIF as low as 0.1 ng/mL (Fig. 1B).

To test the potential of cells contained in neurospheres exposed to LIF (20 ng/mL) for 1 week, these spheres were dissociated and plated as single cells in regular culture medium without LIF. After 8 DIV, the number of secondary spheres grown from cells exposed to LIF was slightly higher than the control condition (Fig. 1C), and similar numbers of multipotent spheres were found in both conditions (data not shown). This indicates that chronic exposure to LIF does not alter NSC potential in this model.

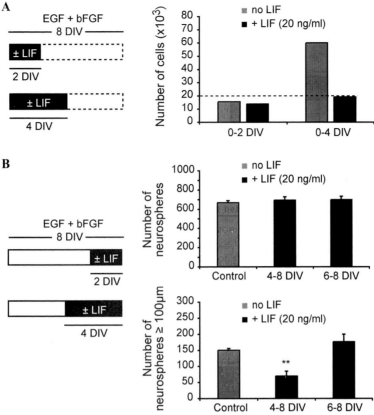

Figure 2. Acute exposure to LIF during the first or the last 2 DIV does not change cell number or sphere number and size, respectively. Time-course analysis of the effects of LIF on sphere development and growth: (**A**) Recombinant mouse LIF (20 ng/mL) was added on single cells immediately at the beginning of the neurosphere culture, and cell numbers were quantified after 2 and 4 DIV. Experiments started with 20,000 cells/well. (**B**) Recombinant mouse LIF (20 ng/mL) was added on neurospheres that were grown without LIF for 4 or 6 DIV. Total number of spheres and spheres with a diameter $\geq$ 100 μm were quantified at 8 DIV. **$P < 0.01$, Student's t-test. Control conditions consisted in culture medium containing EGF and basic fibroblast growth factor (bFGF).

Thus, although chronic LIF exposure produces very small neurospheres, these spheres do contain similar numbers of sphere-forming cells compared to those grown in control conditions, suggesting that LIF could promote NSC self-renewal *in vitro*.

Acute LIF Exposure Stimulates NSC Self-renewal *in Vitro*

To test if LIF stimulates NSC self-renewal *in vitro*, conditions in which sphere formation and growth are not altered are necessary.

Indeed, because chronic LIF exposure alters sphere number and size, the increased number of secondary spheres obtained from cells exposed to LIF could simply reflect NSC enrichment from the lack of other cell types that normally grow in neurospheres. We thus performed a time-course analysis by varying the duration and initiation of incubation in LIF. In some experiments, LIF was applied on single cells at the beginning of the neurosphere culture, and cell numbers were quantified after 2 and 4 DIV. In other experiments, LIF was added at 4 or 6 DIV, and neurosphere number and size were quantified at 8 DIV (see Fig. 2).

The first stage of neurosphere formation *in vitro* is the survival and proliferation of single cells (NSCs) that will generate other NSCs as well as more differentiated progeny. Comparing single cells exposed to LIF with controls, no difference was found after the first 2 DIV (Fig. 2A). However, the number of cells dramatically increased during the first 4 DIV in controls, whereas almost no change was detected in the presence of LIF (Fig. 2A). These data suggest that LIF does not induce cell death in the early phase of sphere formation but rather prevents the emergence of more differentiated progenies.

When LIF was applied during the last 4 DIV, no change in sphere number was detected but spheres were smaller (Fig. 2B), again suggesting that LIF prevents the formation of cells in the neurosphere. However, no change was detected when LIF was applied during the last 2 DIV (Fig. 2B).

These data indicate that acute exposure to LIF during the first or the last 2 DIV does not change cell number or sphere number and size, respectively. These conditions were used to address the effects of LIF on NSC self-renewal by analyzing secondary sphere formation. After dissociating and replating single cells without LIF, significantly more secondary spheres were generated from cultures exposed to LIF during the first (+18%) or the last (+66%) 2 DIV (Fig. 3), indicating that acute LIF exposure promotes NSC self-renewal *in vitro*.

Thus, chronic LIF could favor NSC self-renewing divisions *in vitro*, which would prevent the formation of more differentiated progenies and alter the growth of neurospheres.

CNTF but Not IL-6 or Leptin Has Similar Effects As LIF *in Vitro*

LIF is known to activate intracellular pathways linked to the membrane co-receptor gp130, such as signal transducer and activator of transcription 3 (STAT3). Intracellular phosphorylation of STAT3 is essential for the

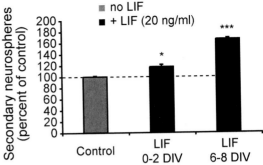

Figure 3. Acute exposure to LIF during the first or the last 2 DIV promotes NSC self-renewal. Recombinant mouse LIF (20 ng/mL) was incubated for 2 DIV on single cells (0–2 DIV) or 6-day-old neurospheres (6–8 DIV), after which spheres were dissociated and grown in regular culture medium (EGF+bFGF) without LIF. Secondary spheres were quantified after 8 DIV. Data are shown as percent of control; significantly more secondary spheres are generated from cultures exposed to LIF during the first (+18%) or the last (+66%) 2 DIV. $*P < 0.05$ and $***P < 0.001$, Student's *t*-test.

effects of LIF in maintaining ES cell phenotype[23] as well as for the astrocyte-promoting effects of LIF.[24] Furthermore, STAT3 is essential for the maintenance of NSCs.[25,26] We thus tested the effects of other cytokines known to activate STAT3, such as cytokines in the IL-6 family (including IL-6 itself and CNTF), as well as leptin, which activates STAT3 after binding to the leptin receptor.[27]

Chronic exposure to CNTF impaired sphere number and size, similar to the effects of LIF, whereas IL-6 did not change sphere number, although it produced smaller spheres (Fig. 4). Testing for NSC self-renewal, acute exposure to CNTF for the last 2 DIV produced an increased secondary sphere formation, as observed with LIF (Fig. 4). In contrast, leptin slightly decreased secondary sphere formation (Fig. 4). These data indicate that LIF and CNTF, which have comparable effects on neurosphere growth, both stimulate NSC self-renewal *in vitro*. This is not true, however, for all cytokines that activate intracellular STAT3, such as leptin.

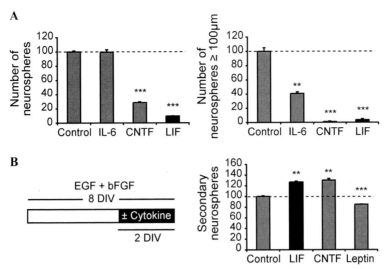

Figure 4. Ciliary neurotrophic factor (CNTF) has similar effects as LIF, unlike other cytokines that also signal through activation of signal transducer and activator of transcription 3 (STAT3). (**A**) Chronic incubation in recombinant rat CNTF (20 ng/mL) reduces the total number of spheres and the number of spheres with a diameter ≥ 100 μm after 8 DIV, similar to the effects of LIF (20 ng/mL). In contrast, recombinant rat interleukin-6 (IL-6) (20 ng/mL) reduces sphere size but does not alter sphere number. (**B**) Acute incubation in CNTF (20 ng/mL) for the last 2 DIV promotes secondary sphere formation, as observed with LIF (20 ng/mL). In contrast, acute incubation in recombinant mouse leptin (100 ng/mL) in similar conditions reduces secondary sphere formation. All data are shown as percent of control. **P < 0.01 and ***P < 0.001, Student's t-test.

Chronic Exposure to LIF *in Vivo* Alters the Formation of NSC Progenies and Promotes NSC Self-renewal

In the context of brain repair, understanding the effects of exogenous LIF *in vivo* could lead to the development of new therapeutic strategies. We thus analyzed the effects of chronic (4 weeks) exposure to LIF in adult mice injected with a recombinant adenovirus in the lateral ventricle. Compared to control animals, chronic exposure to LIF reduced cell proliferation in the SVZ as well as neurogenesis in the OB by about 50%.[22] Chronic LIF *in vivo* also depleted NSC progenies, identified in the SVZ by immunohistochemistry,[22] suggesting that chronic LIF could prevent the formation of these cells *in vivo* as it does *in vitro*.

To test if chronic LIF prevents the emergence of more differentiated progenies from adult NSCs *in vivo*, we used the model of SVZ regeneration after infusion of the antimitotic drug AraC, developed by Doetsch and collaborators.[4] When LIF was infused after AraC, cell proliferation during SVZ regeneration was altered at all time points analyzed (Fig. 5). Furthermore, there was a delay in the reappearance of specific populations of progenitors during the regeneration process,[22] suggesting that chronic LIF could indeed slow the emergence of NSC progenies *in vivo*.

An explanation for this effect is that LIF could promote NSC self-renewal *in vivo*, as seen on neurosphere cultures. By using a dual thymidine analogue-labeling strategy, we found that long-term label-retaining cells that re-entered the cell cycle, likely corresponding to NSCs *in vivo*, were more numerous in the SVZ of animals treated with LIF-adenovirus compared to controls.[22] These data indicate that LIF does indeed stimulate NSC self-renewal *in vivo*, as observed *in vitro*.

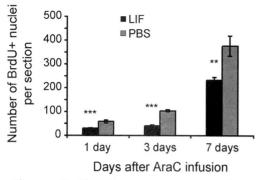

Figure 5. Chronic exposure to recombinant mouse LIF *in vivo* prevents SVZ regeneration. Adult mice were infused with the antimitotic drug AraC in the lateral ventricle for 6 days, after which the mini-pump was replaced with a new one containing either LIF or PBS as control. Animals were sacrificed after 1, 3, or 7 days after AraC removal, 1–2 h after an i.p. injection of bromodeoxyuridine (BrdU; 100 mg/kg). The dose of LIF delivered was 120 ng/day for the 1- and 3-day time points and 60 ng/day for the 7-day condition. Infusion of LIF during SVZ regeneration significantly reduces cell proliferation at all time points analyzed. ** $P < 0.01$ and *** $P < 0.001$, Student's *t*-test.

Thus, chronic exposure to LIF *in vivo* promotes NSC self-renewal, preventing at the same time the emergence of more differentiated progenies.

Comparison between *in Vitro* and *in Vivo* Data: Acute LIF Exposure *in Vivo* Promotes SVZ Regeneration

The most intriguing results from these studies come from comparing *in vitro* and *in vivo* data. Indeed, changes in cell numbers *in vitro* during neurosphere formation or changes in proliferating cells *in vivo* during SVZ regeneration show a very conserved increase during the first 3–4 experimental days in control conditions, whereas application of exogenous LIF abrogates these changes (see Fig. 6). These observations suggest that SVZ regeneration *in vivo* and neurosphere formation *in vitro* could involve similar mechanisms. In fact, in both conditions isolated NSCs proliferate and undergo clonal expansion, reforming the characteristic SVZ "niche"

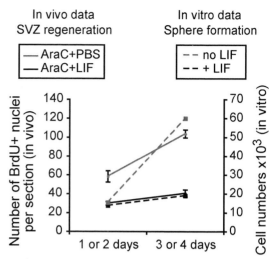

Figure 6. Comparison between *in vivo* and *in vitro* effects of LIF suggests that similar mechanisms are involved in SVZ regeneration *in vivo* and neurosphere formation *in vitro*. Data are redrawn from Figure 2 (*in vitro*; dashed lines) and Figure 5 (*in vivo*; continuous lines). Note that in control conditions (gray lines), number of cells *in vitro* or number of BrdU+ nuclei *in vivo* increases dramatically between 2 and 4 days (*in vitro*) and 1 and 3 days (*in vivo*). In contrast, almost no increase is found after exposure to exogenous LIF (black lines) in both types of experiment.

in vivo or generating neurospheres *in vitro*. During this process, NSCs self-renew and generate immediate progenies. Both *in vivo* and *in vitro*, exogenous LIF promotes NSC self-renewal at the expense of more differentiated progenies, thereby slowing the clonal expansion.

Because acute exposure to exogenous LIF *in vitro* before dissociating neurospheres stimulates subsequent neurosphere formation, we tested whether acute LIF exposure *in vivo*, before inducing SVZ degeneration/regeneration, could stimulate subsequent SVZ regeneration. Exogenous LIF was infused for 3 days into the lateral ventricle before a 6-day AraC infusion. Mini-pumps containing AraC were then removed to allow SVZ regeneration, which was analyzed at 3 days. In this experiment, animals receiving acute exogenous LIF treatment before AraC showed an increased SVZ cell proliferation (Fig. 7), suggesting that LIF does

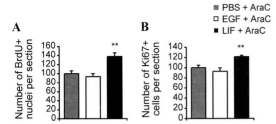

Figure 7. Infusion of recombinant mouse LIF before AraC promotes subsequent SVZ regeneration, whereas EGF has no effect. Adult mice were infused with LIF, EGF, or PBS as control for 3 days before a 6-day infusion of AraC in the lateral ventricle. Minipumps containing AraC were then removed, and animals were sacrificed 3 days later, 1–2 h after an i.p. injection of BrdU (100 mg/kg). The dose of LIF delivered was 120 ng/day. Infusion of LIF before AraC increases the number of BrdU+ nuclei (**A**) and the number of Ki67+ cells (**B**) in the SVZ, but EGF produces no effect compared to control. Data are shown as percent of control. ****$P < 0.01$, Student's *t*-test. PBS, phosphate-buffered saline.

indeed promote SVZ regeneration in these conditions. In contrast, infusing EGF before AraC had no effect on subsequent SVZ regeneration (Fig. 7).

These data suggest that acute exogenous LIF treatment could be used to stimulate NSC self-renewal and promote brain repair.

Conclusions

These data highlight the potential use of exogenous LIF to promote adult brain repair. However, they also indicate the need to have a full understanding of the effects of a cytokine to develop efficient therapeutic strategies. In fact, although exogenous LIF stimulates NSC self-renewal *in vivo*, chronic application of LIF does not promote adult neurogenesis or SVZ regeneration, most likely because LIF maintains NSCs in a mode of self-renewing division. Hence, the pool of adult NSCs could be augmented, but in the continued presence of LIF, no progeny is available for brain repair. Thus, acute but not chronic administration of exogenous LIF could perhaps be used to trig-

ger increased NSC self-renewal as a first step to promote cell replacement in the injured brain. Physiologically, the early induction of endogenous LIF expression after brain injury and its later downregulation could be viewed as an attempt for self-repair.

Acknowledgments

Financial support is provided by the Centre National de la Recherche Scientifique, Universités Aix-Marseille II and III, Institut National de la Recherche Agronomique, and Fondation Fyssen.

Conflicts of Interest

The author declares no conflicts of interest.

References

1. Gould, E. 2007. How widespread is adult neurogenesis in mammals? *Nat. Rev. Neurosci.* **8:** 481–488.
2. Doetsch, F., J.M. Garcia-Verdugo & A. Alvarez-Buylla. 1997. Cellular composition and three-dimensional organization of the subventricular germinal zone in the adult mammalian brain. *J. Neurosci.* **17:** 5046–5061.
3. Doetsch, F. *et al.* 1999. Subventricular zone astrocytes are neural stem cells in the adult mammalian brain. *Cell* **97:** 703–716.
4. Doetsch, F., J. M. Garcia-Verdugo & A. Alvarez-Buylla. 1999. Regeneration of a germinal layer in the adult mammalian brain. *Proc. Natl. Acad. Sci. USA* **96:** 11619–11624.
5. Doetsch, F. *et al.* 2002. EGF converts transit-amplifying neurogenic precursors in the adult brain into multipotent stem cells. *Neuron* **36:** 1021–1034.
6. Reynolds, B.A. & S. Weiss. 1992. Generation of neurons and astrocytes from isolated cells of the adult mammalian central nervous system. *Science* **255:** 1707–1710.
7. Reynolds, B.A. & R.L. Rietze. 2005. Neural stem cells and neurospheres—re-evaluating the relationship. *Nat. Methods.* **2:** 333–336.
8. Arvidsson, A. *et al.* 2002. Neuronal replacement from endogenous precursors in the adult brain after stroke. *Nat. Med.* **8:** 963–970.
9. Magavi, S.S., B.R. Leavitt & J.D. Macklis. 2000. Induction of neurogenesis in the neocortex of adult mice. *Nature* **405:** 951–955.

10. Nakatomi, H. *et al.* 2002. Regeneration of hippocampal pyramidal neurons after ischemic brain injury by recruitment of endogenous neural progenitors. *Cell* **110:** 429–441.

11. Williams, R.L. *et al.* 1988. Myeloid leukaemia inhibitory factor maintains the developmental potential of embryonic stem cells. *Nature* **336:** 684–687.

12. Heinrich, P.C. *et al.* 2003. Principles of interleukin (IL)-6-type cytokine signalling and its regulation. *Biochem. J.* **374:** 1–20.

13. Bauer, S., B.J. Kerr & P.H. Patterson. 2007. The neuropoietic cytokine family in development, plasticity, disease and injury. *Nat. Rev. Neurosci.* **8:** 221–232.

14. Banner, L.R. & P.H. Patterson. 1994. Major changes in the expression of the mRNAs for cholinergic differentiation factor/leukemia inhibitory factor and its receptor after injury to adult peripheral nerves and ganglia. *Proc. Natl. Acad. Sci. USA* **91:** 7109–7113.

15. Banner, L.R., N.N. Moayeri & P.H. Patterson. 1997. Leukemia inhibitory factor is expressed in astrocytes following cortical brain injury. *Exp. Neurol.* **147:** 1–9.

16. Bauer, S. *et al.* 2003. Leukemia inhibitory factor is a key signal for injury-induced neurogenesis in the adult mouse olfactory epithelium. *J. Neurosci.* **23:** 1792–1803.

17. Covey, M.V. & S.W. Levison. 2007. Leukemia inhibitory factor participates in the expansion of neural stem/progenitors after perinatal hypoxia/ischemia. *Neuroscience* **148:** 501–509.

18. Jankowsky, J.L. & P.H. Patterson. 1999. Differential regulation of cytokine expression following pilocarpine-induced seizure. *Exp. Neurol.* **159:** 333–346.

19. Minami, M. *et al.* 2002. Kainic acid induces leukemia inhibitory factor mRNA expression in the rat brain: differences in the time course of mRNA expression between the dentate gyrus and hippocampal CA1/CA3 subfields. *Brain Res. Mol. Brain Res.* **107:** 39–46.

20. Sriram, K. *et al.* 2004. Induction of gp130-related cytokines and activation of JAK2/STAT3 pathway in astrocytes precedes up-regulation of glial fibrillary acidic protein in the 1-methyl-4-phenyl-1,2,3,6-tetrahydropyridine model of neurodegeneration: key signaling pathway for astrogliosis in vivo? *J. Biol. Chem.* **279:** 19936–19947.

21. Suzuki, S. *et al.* 2000. Immunohistochemical detection of leukemia inhibitory factor after focal cerebral ischemia in rats. *J. Cereb. Blood Flow Metab.* **20:** 661–668.

22. Bauer, S. & P.H. Patterson. 2006. Leukemia inhibitory factor promotes neural stem cell self-renewal in the adult brain. *J. Neurosci.* **26:** 12089–12099.

23. Burdon, T., A. Smith & P. Savatier. 2002. Signalling, cell cycle and pluripotency in embryonic stem cells. *Trends Cell Biol.* **12:** 432–438.

24. He, F. *et al.* 2005. A positive autoregulatory loop of Jak-STAT signaling controls the onset of astrogliogenesis. *Nat. Neurosci.* **8:** 616–625.

25. Androutsellis-Theotokis, A. *et al.* 2006. Notch signalling regulates stem cell numbers *in vitro* and in vivo. *Nature* **442:** 823–826.

26. Yoshimatsu, T. *et al.* 2006. Non-cell-autonomous action of STAT3 in maintenance of neural precursor cells in the mouse neocortex. *Development* **133:** 2553–2563.

27. Bjorbaek, C. & B.B. Kahn. 2004. Leptin signaling in the central nervous system and the periphery. *Recent Prog. Horm. Res.* **59:** 305–331.

Neuronal Cell Survival

The Role of Interleukins

Elizabeth Giestal de Araujo,[a] Gustavo Mataruna da Silva,[a] and Aline Araujo dos Santos[a,b]

[a] *Departamento de Neurobiologia, Programa de Neuroimunologia, Instituto de Biologia, Universidade Federal Fluminense, Niterói, Rio de Janeiro, Brazil*

[b] *Departamento de Fisiologia e Farmacologia, Instituto Biomédico, Universidade Federal Fluminense, Niterói, Rio de Janeiro, Brazil*

One of the central issues in neuroscience today is the study of the mechanisms of neuronal survival. Since the discovery of nerve growth factor (almost 60 years ago), many groups have clearly demonstrated the central role of neurotrophins on the regulation of neuronal cell survival during developmental stages as well as during adult life. However, neurotrophins are not alone in regulating neuronal survival, and many groups have demonstrated the effect of different cytokines on this phenomenon. In this brief review we will address the effect of interleukins (IL), particularly IL-2, IL-6, and IL-4, on the survival of neuronal cells.

Key words: neuronal survival; IL-2; IL-4; IL-6; trophic factors; development

Introduction

Studies of the development of the nervous system show that a great number of neurons are generated at an early phase of this process. After a selective period, the same neuronal population is constantly maintained during life. Accordingly, mammalian neurons are the most long-lived cell types in the body. This particular characteristic stimulated many research groups to investigate the mechanisms regulating neuronal survival or, in other words, how neuronal death is inhibited.

The investigation involving cell death can be divided into at least two groups (natural cell death and neurodegeneration). Researchers want to know how natural cell death occurs during development. This regressive phenomenon plays a key role in regulating the number of neurons in the nervous system from the earliest stages of its development. For this reason, the importance of unveiling the mechanisms underlying this regressive event is widely recognized. During adult life, neuronal death is mainly related to pathological conditions, such as trauma, ischemia, and neurodegenerative diseases. Inhibition of neuronal death related to pathological conditions is the main goal of investigations focused on the adult stage. It is well accepted that if we have the knowledge of the molecular mechanisms involved in natural neuronal death we will be able to establish new therapeutic strategies to inhibit—or at least to delay—neuronal degeneration.

Since the pioneering study of Hamburger and Levi-Montalcini (1949), natural cell death within the nervous system has been extensively studied. It has been well established that this regressive phenomenon is ubiquitously distributed within the nervous system. During development approximately half the neurons initially generated die. It has been assumed that a surplus number of neuronal cells are generated to promote the

Address for correspondence: Elizabeth Giestal de Araujo, Departamento de Neurobiologia, Programa de Neuroimunologia, Instituto de Biologia, Universidade Federal Fluminense, Caixa Postal 100180, Niterói – RJ, Brazil. CEP: 24001-970. Voice: 55 21 26292276; fax: 26292268. egiestal@vm.uff.br

Neuroimmunomodulation: Ann. N.Y. Acad. Sci. 1153: 57–64 (2009).
doi: 10.1111/j.1749-6632.2008.03974.x

appropriate neuronal connections to adjust their projections to the size and function of target cells. Neuronal cell death is concomitant with synaptogenesis and neurotrophins released by target cells during this period play a fundamental role controlling this cell death.[1] Neurotrophins are a family of small polypeptides that include nerve growth factor (NGF),[2] brain-derived neurotrophic factor (BDNF),[3] neurotrophin-3 (NT-3),[4–6] NT-4/5,[7,8] NT-6[9] and NT-7.[10,11] All neurotrophins bind to the low-affinity receptor p75.[12] They also bind to high-affinity receptors represented by the Trk (tropomyosin-related kinase) family that includes TrkA, TrkB, and TrkC receptors. NGF binds to TrkA; BDNF and NT4/5 bind to TrkB; NT-3 binds to TrkC; and NT 6/7 binds to TrkA.[13] High-affinity receptors signal through a rapid dimerization and autophosphorylation following neurotrophin binding.[13,14] The interaction of neurotrophin with their high-affinity receptors plays a fundamental role during development as knockout of Trk receptors induces neuronal degeneration and animal death in a few weeks after birth.[15]

Afferent cells also play an important role in controlling natural cell death. It has been extensively demonstrated that the blockade of electrical activity of afferent cells induces degeneration either during early stages of development or in the adult phase.[16–19] The importance of both the electrical activity and the release of trophic factors by afferent and glial cells on the control of neuronal cell death is quite evident.[20,21]

Naturally occurring cell death is an active process of self destruction with distinctive and biochemical features. It has been demonstrated by different groups that neuronal cell death is executed, at least in part, through apoptosis.[22] Apoptosis is characterized by cytoplasmic condensation, nuclear pyknosis, chromatin condensation, DNA fragmentation, cell rounding, membrane bledding, cytoskeletal collapse, and the formation of membrane-bound apoptotic bodies that are rapidly phagocytosed and digested by macrophages or neighboring cells, avoiding a significant inflammatory response.[23]

Past investigations have clearly shown that the balance between cell survival and cell death is regulated by different signals, including other trophic molecules. Today it is well known that several cytokines can indeed rescue neurons from death. Cytokines are a large group of polypeptides comprising interleukins (ILs), chemokines, tumor necrosis factors (TNFs), transforming growth factors, interferons (IFNs), growth promoting factors, hematopoietic factors, and neurotrophins.[24]

Concerning the nervous system, the role of cytokines during inflammatory responses is well characterized. However, data from the literature demonstrate that cytokines are synthesized and their receptors are also present in the normal brain. This suggests a role for these molecules during developmental stages as well as during adult life. Many authors have suggested that pro-inflammatory cytokines are involved in injury and cell death and also that anti-inflammatory cytokines are involved in protection and cell survival. It is important to emphasize that this classification is academic and several results indicate that both anti- and pro-inflammatory cytokines can mediate regressive and progressive phenomena. What is very important to stress is that the regulation of cytokine balance plays a crucial role in homeostasis.[25]

Several groups have demonstrated that ILs can indeed regulate events during developmental stages as well as during adult life, in spite of their role during the inflammatory process. Proliferation, survival, and differentiation can be modulated by several ILs. In this brief review we will address the role of IL-2, IL-6, and IL-4 in the survival of neuronal cells.

Interleukin-2

IL-2 was initially described in 1976 as a growth factor for bone marrow-derived T lymphocytes.[26] Nowadays the role of IL-2 is well established as a mediator of activation-induced cell death[27] and in the generation and function of CD4$^+$CD25$^+$ regulatory T cells.[28] Biological effects of IL-2 are mediated through binding to specific IL-2 receptor (IL-2R) complexes.[29] IL-2 binds to IL-2Rα with low affinity and does not induce any known signaling response. IL-2Rβ and IL-2Rγ bind together to IL-2 as a dimer with intermediate affinity. The trimeric αβγ combination represents the functional high-affinity IL-2R complex.[29]

In the nervous system IL-2 plays a pivotal role during development of the normal brain as well as in neurodegenerative processes and neuronal injury responses.[30–32] The effect of IL-2 on the control of growth and differentiation of oligodendrocytes was one of the earliest reports concerning the role of this cytokine in cultured neural cells. IL-2 has been shown to inhibit the proliferation of progenitor cells. When a concomitant treatment with IL-2 and IL-1 was performed, the cell number was changed.[33] IL-2 increases the survival of hippocampal, cortical, septal, and cerebellar neurons.[34–36] Treatment with IL-2 also increases the survival of axotomized retinal ganglion cells in culture.[37] Moreover, several biological effects in the normal brain have been extensively described *in vitro*, such as modulation of acetylcholine release from hippocampal cells, stimulation of choline acetyltransferase activity of septal neurons,[38,39] regulation of catecholamine release from hypothalamus,[31,40] and modulation of dopamine release either from cultured mesencephalic cells[41] or from striatal slices.[42] IL-2 is also able to regulate the release of both pituitary[43] and hypothalamic hormones[32,44] and to inhibit long-term potentiation in the hippocampus.[45] IL-2 can also modulate the function of N-methyl-D-aspartate (NMDA) receptors through an inhibitory mechanism in mesolimbic and hippocampal neurons.[46,47]

The synthesis of IL-2 in the rodent brain is widely distributed. Both IL-2 and IL-4 mRNA were detected in various neuronal populations, especially concentrated in the septum, hippocampus, and various hypothalamic nuclei.[48–50] In parallel, the presence of IL-2R was also observed in the same regions.[49,50]

Interleukin-6

IL-6 was originally described as a T cell factor responsible for the maturation of Ig-releasing B cells, and in 1986 the molecule was cloned.[51] Since then, this molecule was referred to as IL-6.[52] IL-6 is a multifunctional cytokine regulating cell growth, differentiation, and cellular functions in many lineages and may play a role in the pathogenesis of a variety of diseases.[53] IL-6 belongs to the neuropoietic cytokine family, which also includes ciliary neurotrophic factor (CNTF), leukemia inhibitory factor (LIF), oncostatin M (OSM), IL-11, cardiotrophin 1 (CT-1),[54] neurotrophin-1 (NNT-1),[55] IL-27,[56] neuropoietin,[57] and B-cell-stimulating factor 3.[58] These cytokines have been grouped in a family because all their receptor complexes contain the signal transducing receptor subunit gp130 that activates the Janus kinase-signal transducer activator of transcription (JAK-STAT) and mitogen-activated protein kinase signal transduction pathways.[59] IL-6, IL-11, and CNTF bind to specific nonsignaling α-receptor subunits and subsequently associate with two gp130 subunits (IL-6 and IL-11) or a gp130/LIFβR heterodimer (CNTF). CT-1 signals via a gp130/LIFβR heterodimer probably involving a specific glycosylphosphatidylinositol-linked receptor component. LIF binds directly to LIFβR and heterodimerizes with gp130. OSM binds to gp130 and forms a heterodimer with LIFβR or with OSMR.[54] NNT-1 stimulates tyrosine phosphorylation of gp130 and LIFβR.[55]

IL-6 produces its biological effects through a specific binding protein, the α-receptor subunit, which induces the homodimerization of gp130 subunits followed by the activation of JAK (a family of tyrosine kinases).[60] Then, the activated JAKs lead to the activation of the transcription factors STAT3 and STAT1.[60]

STAT dimers translocate into the nucleus and induce transcription of immediate early genes, such as *jun*B, and the rapid activation of a nuclear factor, termed acute-phase response factor.[60,61] Besides the membrane-bound IL-6R, there is a naturally occurring soluble IL-6R (sIL-6R) that retains its ligand-binding capacity.[62,63] sIL-6R can be generated by limited proteolysis of the membrane protein or by differential splicing of the IL-6R mRNA.[62,63] The soluble α-receptor can be released from the surface in a biologically active form, imparting sensitivity to the ligands on cells that do not express IL-6R by themselves.[54] This process has been named *trans*-signaling.[62]

IL-6 is a pro-inflammatory cytokine produced by a variety of cells, including monocytes, fibroblasts, and endothelial cells. In the central nervous system (CNS) it is synthesized mainly by microglial cells and astrocytes but also by neurons.[64,65] IL-6 synthesis can be induced by a variety of stimuli, but its major inducers are lipopolysaccharides, IL-1, and TNF.[66] Much attention has been focused on the functional role of neuropoietic cytokines, such as IL-6, in the CNS. IL-6 has been implicated as an important regulator of cellular function in the CNS, either as a mediator of chemical signals between cells of the immune system and cells of the CNS or as a mediator of chemical signals between cells of the CNS.[53] IL-6 promotes the differentiation of oligodendrocytes and cortical precursor cells into astrocytes, activates astrocytes, and also functions as a neurotrophic and differentiation factor for neurons of the peripheral and CNS.[65,67,68] IL-6 can induce the differentiation of pheochromocytoma cells (PC)12 cells into sympathetic-like neurons inducing elaboration of neuritis and electrical excitability.[69] IL-6 can also support the survival of PC12 cells under adverse conditions in culture, such as deprivation of NGF or serum withdrawal[70,71] or addition of a calcium ionophore.[72] In 2002, Nakajima and co-workers demonstrated that IL-6 protects PC12 cells from 4-hydroxynonenal-induced cytotoxicity, an effect mediated by the increase in intracellular glutathione levels.[73] More recently it was demonstrated that in PC12 cells, IL-6 is co-localized with dense-core vesicle marker secretogranin-II and can be released by a secretory pathway.[74]

Chronic treatment (48 h) with IL-6 has been shown to increase the survival of axotomized retinal ganglion cells *in vitro*. This effect was independent of the addition of IL-6 soluble receptors, suggesting that retinal cells express α-IL-6R and can promptly respond to this interleukin.[75] Inomata and co-workers in 2003 showed that concomitant treatment with IL-6 and sIL-6R induces a neuroprotective effect on NMDA-induced rat retinal damage. The authors observed a significant decrease in the apoptosis induced by NMDA in the ganglion cell layer and outer nuclear layer.[76] More recently it was shown that IL-6 protects retinal ganglion cells from death induced by high pressure, suggesting a neuroprotective effect for this cytokine.[77] It was recently demonstrated that treatment with methylmercury induces the release of IL-6 by glial cells, suggesting a potential neuroprotector effect of this cytokine.[78]

Interleukin-4

IL-4 is a typical anti-inflammatory cytokine primarily related to the regulation of proliferation of anti-IgM co-activated B lymphocytes,[79] and its cDNA was cloned in 1986.[80] It has been demonstrated that glial cells are the major target of this cytokine in the nervous system, although IL-4 is also able to enhance the survival of hippocampal neurons *in vitro*.[81,82] IL-4 inhibits the release of neurotoxic molecules (e.g., TNF-α and nitric oxide) by IFN-γ-activated microglia[83] and prevents antigen presentation reducing the expression of induced class II major histocompatibility complex by IFN-γ-activated astrocytic cells.[84] In addition, this cytokine controls the synthesis and release of NGF *in vitro* as well as glial cell proliferation.[81] In 2000 the expression of IL-4 in the brain of neonatal mice, but not in adult mice, was demonstrated.[85]

During brain injury, infection, and neurodegenerative diseases, high levels of IL-4 are expressed. It is produced either by the glial environment or by invading T cells.[86] Constitutive expression of IL-4 receptor γC subunit (IL-4RγC) mRNA was demonstrated *in vitro* in unstimulated astrocytes.[87] The IL-4Rα mRNA expression in the nervous system is controversial, but its presence has been reported in isolated glial cells as well as in a neuronal cell line.[88]

IL-4 is able to enhance the survival of axotomized retinal ganglion cells either in culture[37] or *in vivo*.[89] IL-4 is also able to protect motoneurons from toxicity induced by activated microglia.[90] It was demonstrated that IL-4 is involved in the immune-mediated neuroprotection of axotomized mouse facial motoneurons,[91] and more recently it was shown that IL-4, by downregulation of glial cell activation, attenuates the neuroinflammation induced by amyloid-beta both *in vivo* or *in vitro*.[92] Interesting data showed that treatment of rats with atorvastatin (an anti-inflammatory drug) increases IL-4 concentration, which antagonizes the increase in microglial activation and leads to a neuroprotective effect.[93]

Conclusion

Having summarized the data present in the literature concerning the effects of IL-2, IL-4, and IL-6 in the nervous system, we can observe that these molecules not only play a role during pathological conditions but also play an important role during normal development. Future studies will show how these small proteins can contribute to the survival of neuronal cells, further broadening this new and important field of investigation.

Acknowledgments

We would like to thank Arnaldo Paes de Andrade for his helpful discussions. We also thank all researchers for giving us much to write about in this review and apologize to those whose work has not been included because of constraints on space or ignorance on our part. Gustavo Mataruna da Silva is the recipient of a Coordenação de Aperfeiçoamento de Pessoal de Nível Superior (CAPES) fellowship. The results from our group presented in this review were supported by grants from CAPES, Conselho Nacional de Desenvolvimento Científico e Tecnológico, Programa de Apoio a Núcleos de Excelência—Ministério de Ciência e Tecnologia, and Fundação de Amparo à Pesquisa do estado do Rio de Janeiro.

Conflicts of Interest

The authors declare no conflicts of interest.

References

1. Oppenheim, R.W. 1991. Cell death during development of the nervous system. *Annu. Rev. Neurosci.* **14:** 453–501.
2. Levi-Montalcini, R. 1987. The nerve growth factor 35 years later. *Science* **237:** 1154–1162.
3. Barde, Y.A., D. Edgar & H. Thoenen. 1982. Purification of a new neurotrophic factor from mammalian brain. *EMBO J.* **1:** 549–553.
4. Hohn, A., J. Leibrock, K. Bailey, *et al.* 1990. Identification and characterization of a novel member of the nerve growth factor/brain-derived neurotrophic factor family. *Nature* **344:** 339–341.
5. Maisonpierre, P.C., L. Belluscio, S. Squinto, *et al.* 1990. Neurotrophin-3: a neurotrophic factor related to NGF and BDNF. *Science* **247:** 1446–1451.
6. Rosenthal, A., D.V. Goeddel, T. Nguyen, *et al.* 1990. Primary structure and biological activity of a novel human neurotrophic factor. *Neuron* **4:** 767–773.
7. Berkemeier, L.R., J.W. Winslow, D.R. Kaplan, *et al.* 1991. Neurotrophin-5: a novel neurotrophic factor that activates trk and trkB. *Neuron* **7:** 857–866.
8. Hallbook, F., C.F. Ibanez & H. Persson. 1991. Evolutionary studies of the nerve growth factor family reveal a novel member abundantly expressed in Xenopus ovary. *Neuron* **6:** 845–858.
9. Gotz, R., R. Koster, C. Winkler, *et al.* 1994. Neurotrophin-6 is a new member of the nerve growth factor family. *Nature* **372:** 266–269.
10. Lai, K.O., W.Y. Fu, F.C. Ip, *et al.* 1998. Cloning and expression of a novel neurotrophin, NT-7, from carp. *Mol. Cell Neurosci.* **11:** 64–76.

11. Nilsson, A.S., M. Fainzilber, P. Falck, *et al*. 1998. Neurotrophin-7: a novel member of the neurotrophin family from the zebrafish. *FEBS Lett.* **424:** 285–290.

12. Carter, B.D. & G.R. Lewin. 1997. Neurotrophins live or let die: does p75NTR decide? *Neuron* **18:** 187–190.

13. Barbacid, M. 1994. The Trk family of neurotrophin receptors. *J. Neurobiol.* **25:** 1386–1403.

14. Miller, F.D. & D.R. Kaplan. 2001. On Trk for retrograde signaling. *Neuron* **32:** 767–770.

15. Snider, W.D. 1994. Functions of the neurotrophins during nervous system development: what the knockouts are teaching us. *Cell* **77:** 627–638.

16. Baker, R.E., J.M. Ruijter & D. Bingmann. 1991. Elevated potassium prevents neuronal death but inhibits network formation in neocortical cultures. *Int. J. Dev. Neurosci.* **9:** 339–345.

17. Lipton, S.A. 1986. Blockade of electrical activity promotes the death of mammalian retinal ganglion cells in culture. *Proc. Natl. Acad. Sci. USA* **83:** 9774–9778.

18. Maderdrut, J.L., R.W. Oppenheim & D. Prevette. 1988. Enhancement of naturally occurring cell death in the sympathetic and parasympathetic ganglia of the chicken embryo following blockade of ganglionic transmission. *Brain Res.* **444:** 189–194.

19. Okado, N. & R.W. Oppenheim. 1984. Cell death of motoneurons in the chick embryo spinal cord. IX. The loss of motoneurons following removal of afferent inputs. *J. Neurosci.* **4:** 1639–1652.

20. Araujo, E.G. & R. Linden. 1993. Trophic factors produced by retinal cells increase the survival of retinal ganglion cells in vitro. *Eur. J. Neurosci.* **5:** 1181–1188.

21. Linden, R. 1994. The survival of developing neurons: a review of afferent control. *Neuroscience* **58:** 671–682.

22. Yuan, J., M. Lipinski & A. Degterev. 2003. Diversity in the mechanisms of neuronal cell death. *Neuron* **40:** 401–413.

23. Kerr, J.F., A.H. Wyllie & A.R. Currie. 1972. Apoptosis: a basic biological phenomenon with wide-ranging implications in tissue kinetics. *Br. J. Cancer* **26:** 239–257.

24. Rothwell, N.J. 1999. Annual review prize lecture cytokines—killers in the brain? *J. Physiol.* **514**(Pt 1): 3–17.

25. Szelényi, J. 2001. Cytokines and the central nervous system. *Brain Res. Bull.* **54:** 329–338.

26. Morgan, D.A., F.W. Ruscetti & R. Gallo. 1976. Selective in vitro growth of T lymphocytes from normal human bone marrows. *Science* **193:** 1007–1008.

27. Green, D.R., N. Droin & M. Pinkoski. 2003. Activation-induced cell death in T cells. *Immunol. Rev.* **193:** 70–81.

28. Malek, T.R. & A.L. Bayer. 2004. Tolerance, not immunity, crucially depends on IL-2. *Nat. Rev. Immunol.* **4:** 665–674.

29. Minami, Y., T. Kono, T. Miyazaki, *et al*. 1993. The IL-2 receptor complex: its structure, function, and target genes. *Annu. Rev. Immunol.* **11:** 245–268.

30. Otero, G.C. & J.E. Merrill. 1997. Response of human oligodendrocytes to interleukin-2. *Brain Behav. Immun.* **11:** 24–38.

31. Hanisch, U.K. & R. Quirion. 1995. Interleukin-2 as a neuroregulatory cytokine. *Brain Res. Brain Res. Rev.* **21:** 246–284.

32. Raber, J. & F.E. Bloom. 1994. IL-2 induces vasopressin release from the hypothalamus and the amygdala: role of nitric oxide-mediated signaling. *J. Neurosci.* **14:** 6187–6195.

33. Saneto, R.P., A. Altman, R.L. Knobler, *et al*. 1986. Interleukin 2 mediates the inhibition of oligodendrocyte progenitor cell proliferation in vitro. *Proc. Natl. Acad. Sci. USA* **83:** 9221–9225.

34. Sarder, M., H. Saito & K. Abe. 1993. Interleukin-2 promotes survival and neurite extension of cultured neurons from fetal rat brain. *Brain Res.* **625:** 347–350.

35. Sarder, M., K. Abe, H. Saito, *et al*. 1996. Comparative effect of IL-2 and IL-6 on morphology of cultured hippocampal neurons from fetal rat brain. *Brain Res.* **715:** 9–16.

36. Awatsuji, H., Y. Furukawa, M. Nakajima, *et al*. 1993. Interleukin-2 as a neurotrophic factor for supporting the survival of neurons cultured from various regions of fetal rat brain. *J. Neurosci. Res.* **35:** 305–311.

37. Sholl-Franco, A., K.G. Figueiredo & E.G. De Araujo. 2001. Interleukin-2 and interleukin-4 increase the survival of retinal ganglion cells in culture. *Neuroreport* **12:** 109–112.

38. Seto, D., S. Kar & R. Quirion. 1997. Evidence for direct and indirect mechanisms in the potent modulatory action of interleukin-2 on the release of acetylcholine in rat hippocampal slices. *Br. J. Pharmacol.* **120:** 1151–1157.

39. Mennicken, F. & R. Quirion. 1997. Interleukin-2 increases choline acetyltransferase activity in septal-cell cultures. *Synapse* **26:** 175–183.

40. Lapchak, P.A. & D.M. Araujo. 1993. Interleukin-2 regulates monoamine and opioid peptide release from the hypothalamus. *Neuroreport* **4:** 303–306.

41. Alonso, R., I. Chaudieu, J. Diorio, *et al*. 1993. Interleukin-2 modulates evoked release of [3H]dopamine in rat cultured mesencephalic cells. *J. Neurochem.* **61:** 1284–1290.

42. Lapchak, P.A. 1992. A role for interleukin-2 in the regulation of striatal dopaminergic function. *Neuroreport* **3:** 165–168.

43. Karanth, S. & S.M. McCann. 1991. Anterior pituitary hormone control by interleukin 2. *Proc. Natl. Acad. Sci. USA* **88:** 2961–2965.

44. Raber, J., G.F. Koob & F.E. Bloom. 1995. Interleukin-2 (IL-2) induces corticotropin-releasing factor (CRF)

release from the amygdala and involves a nitric oxide-mediated signaling; comparison with the hypothalamic response. *J. Pharmacol. Exp. Ther.* **272:** 815–824.

45. Tancredi, V., C. Zona, F. Velotti, *et al*. 1990. Interleukin-2 suppresses established long-term potentiation and inhibits its induction in the rat hippocampus. *Brain Res.* **525:** 149–151.

46. Ye, J.H., L. Tao & S.S. Zalcman. 2001. Interleukin-2 modulates N-methyl-D-aspartate receptors of native mesolimbic neurons. *Brain Res.* **894:** 241–248.

47. Shen, Y., L.J. Zhu, S.S. Liu, *et al*. 2006. Interleukin-2 inhibits NMDA receptor-mediated currents directly and may differentially affect subtypes. *Biochem. Biophys. Res. Commun.* **351:** 449–454.

48. Sawada, M., A. Suzumura & T. Marunouchi. 1995. Cytokine network in the central nervous system and its roles in growth and differentiation of glial and neuronal cells. *Int. J. Dev. Neurosci.* **13:** 253–264.

49. Petitto, J.M. & Z. Huang. 1994. Molecular cloning of a partial cDNA of the interleukin-2 receptor-beta in normal mouse brain: in situ localization in the hippocampus and expression by neuroblastoma cells. *Brain Res.* **650:** 140–145.

50. Araujo, D.M., P.A. Lapchak, B. Collier, *et al*. 1989. Localization of interleukin-2 immunoreactivity and interleukin-2 receptors in the rat brain: interaction with the cholinergic system. *Brain Res.* **498:** 257–266.

51. Hirano, T., K. Yasukawa, H. Harada, *et al*. 1986. Complementary DNA for a novel human interleukin (BSF-2) that induces B lymphocytes to produce immunoglobulin. *Nature* **324:** 73–76.

52. Kishimoto, T. 2006. Interleukin-6: discovery of a pleiotropic cytokine. *Arthritis Res. Ther.* **8**(Suppl 2): S2.

53. Gruol, D.L. & T.E. Nelson. 1997. Physiological and pathological roles of interleukin-6 in the central nervous system. *Mol. Neurobiol.* **15:** 307–339.

54. Taga, T. & T. Kishimoto. 1997. Gp130 and the interleukin-6 family of cytokines. *Annu. Rev. Immunol.* **15:** 797–819.

55. Senaldi, G., B.C. Varnum, U. Sarmiento, *et al*. 1999. Novel neurotrophin-1/B cell-stimulating factor-3: a cytokine of the IL-6 family. *Proc. Natl. Acad. Sci. USA* **96:** 11458–11463.

56. Pflanz, S., L. Hibbert, J. Mattson, *et al*. 2004. WSX-1 and glycoprotein 130 constitute a signal-transducing receptor for IL-27. *J. Immunol.* **172:** 2225–2231.

57. Derouet, D., F. Rousseau, F. Alfonsir, *et al*. 2004. Neuropoietin, a new IL-6-related cytokine signaling through the ciliary neurotrophic factor receptor. *Proc. Natl. Acad. Sci. USA* **101:** 4827–4832.

58. Murakami, M., D. Kamimura & T. Hirano. 2004. New IL-6 (gp130) family cytokine members, CLC/NNT1/BSF3 and IL-27. *Growth Factors* **22:** 75–77.

59. Bauer, S., B.J. Kerr & P.H. Patterson. 2007. The neuropoietic cytokine family in development, plasticity, disease and injury. *Nat. Rev. Neurosci.* **8:** 221–232.

60. Carpenter, L.R., G.D. Yancopoulos & N. Stahl. 1998. General mechanisms of cytokine receptor signaling. *Adv. Protein Chem.* **52:** 109–140.

61. Hibi, M., K. Nakajima & T. Hirano. 1996. IL-6 cytokine family and signal transduction: a model of the cytokine system. *J. Mol. Med.* **74:** 1–12.

62. Rose-John, S. & P.C. Heinrich. 1994. Soluble receptors for cytokines and growth factors: generation and biological function. *Biochem. J.* **300**(Pt 2): 281–290.

63. Marz, P., U. Otten & S. Rose-John. 1999. Neural activities of IL-6-type cytokines often depend on soluble cytokine receptors. *Eur. J. Neurosci.* **11:** 2995–3004.

64. Schöbitz, B., D.A. Voorhuis & E.R. de Kloet. 1992. Localization of interleukin 6 mRNA and interleukin 6 receptor mRNA in rat brain. *Neurosci. Lett.* **136:** 189–192.

65. Gadient, R.A. & U.H. Otten. 1997. Interleukin-6 (IL-6)—a molecule with both beneficial and destructive potentials. *Prog. Neurobiol.* **52:** 379–390.

66. Lotz, M. 1993. Interleukin-6. *Cancer Invest.* **11:** 732–742.

67. Marz, P., J.G. Cheng, R.A. Gadient, *et al*. 1998. Sympathetic neurons can produce and respond to interleukin 6. *Proc. Natl. Acad. Sci. USA* **95:** 3251–3256.

68. Thier, M., P. Marz, U. Otten, *et al*. 1999. Interleukin-6 (IL-6) and its soluble receptor support survival of sensory neurons. *J. Neurosci. Res.* **55:** 411–422.

69. Wagner, J.A. 1996. Is IL-6 both a cytokine and a neurotrophic factor? *J. Exp. Med.* **183:** 2417–2419.

70. Satoh, T., S. Nakamura, T. Taga, *et al*. 1988. Induction of neuronal differentiation in PC12 cells by B-cell stimulatory factor 2/interleukin 6. *Mol. Cell Biol.* **8:** 3546–3549.

71. Kunioku, H., K. Inoue & M. Tomida. 2001. Interleukin-6 protects rat PC12 cells from serum deprivation or chemotherapeutic agents through the phosphatidylinositol 3-kinase and STAT3 pathways. *Neurosci. Lett.* **309:** 13–16.

72. Umegaki, H., K. Yamada, M. Naito, *et al*. 1996. Protective effect of interleukin-6 against the death of PC12 cells caused by serum deprivation or by the addition of a calcium ionophore. *Biochem. Pharmacol.* **52:** 911–916.

73. Nakajima, A., K. YamadA, L.B. Zou, *et al*. 2002. Interleukin-6 protects PC12 cells from 4-hydroxynonenal-induced cytotoxicity by increasing intracellular glutathione levels. *Free Radic. Biol. Med.* **32:** 1324–1332.

74. Moller, J.C., A. Kruttgen, R. Burmester, *et al*. 2006. Release of interleukin-6 via the regulated secretory pathway in PC12 cells. *Neurosci. Lett.* **400:** 75–79.

75. Mendonça Torres, P.M. & E.G. de Araujo. 2001. Interleukin-6 increases the survival of retinal ganglion cells in vitro. *J. Neuroimmunol.* **117:** 43–50.

76. Inomata, Y., A. Hirata, N. Yonemura, *et al.* 2003. Neuroprotective effects of interleukin-6 on NMDA-induced rat retinal damage. *Biochem. Biophys. Res. Commun.* **302:** 226–232.

77. Sappington, R.M., M. Chan & D.J. Calkins. 2006. Interleukin-6 protects retinal ganglion cells from pressure-induced death. *Invest Ophthalmol. Vis. Sci.* **47:** 2932–2942.

78. Chang, J.Y. 2007. Methylmercury causes glial IL-6 release. *Neurosci. Lett.* **416:** 217–220.

79. Farrar, J.J., M. Howard, J. Fuller-Farrar, *et al.* 1983. Biochemical and physicochemical characterization of mouse B cell growth factor: a lymphokine distinct from interleukin 2. *J. Immunol.* **131:** 1838–1842.

80. Noma, Y., P. Sideras, T. Naito, *et al.* 1986. Cloning of cDNA encoding the murine IgG1 induction factor by a novel strategy using SP6 promoter. *Nature* **319:** 640–646.

81. Brodie, C., A. Oshiba, H. Renz, *et al.* 1996. Nerve growth-factor and anti-CD40 provide opposite signals for the production of IgE in interleukin-4-treated lymphocytes. *Eur. J. Immunol.* **26:** 171–178.

82. Araujo, D.M. & C.W. Cotman. 1993. Trophic effects of interleukin-4, -7 and -8 on hippocampal neuronal cultures: potential involvement of glial-derived factors 81. *Brain Res.* **600:** 49–55.

83. Chao, C.C., T.W. Molitor & S. Hu. 1993. Neuroprotective role of IL-4 against activated microglia. *J. Immunol.* **151:** 1473–1481.

84. Morga, E. & P. Heuschling. 1996. Interleukin-4 down-regulates MHC class II antigens on cultured rat astrocytes. *Glia* **17:** 175–179.

85. Lovett-Racke, A.E., M.E. Smith, L.R. Arredondo, *et al.* 2000. Developmentally regulated gene expression of Th2 cytokines in the brain 83. *Brain Res.* **870:** 27–35.

86. Mizuno, T., M. Sawada, A. Suzumura, *et al.* 1994. Expression of cytokines during glial differentiation. *Brain Res.* **656:** 141–146.

87. Pousset, F., S. Cremona, R. Dantzer, *et al.* 1999. Interleukin-4 and interleukin-10 regulate IL1-beta induced mouse primary astrocyte activation: a comparative study. *Glia* **26:** 12–21.

88. Sawada, M., Y. Itoh, A. Suzumura, *et al.* 1993. Expression of cytokine receptors in cultured neuronal and glial cells. *Neurosci. Lett.* **160:** 131–134.

89. Koeberle, P.D., J. Gauldie & A.K. Ball. 2004. Effects of adenoviral-mediated gene transfer of interleukin-10, interleukin-4, and transforming growth factor-beta on the survival of axotomized retinal ganglion cells. *Neuroscience* **125:** 903–920.

90. Zhao, W., W. Xie, Q. Xiao, *et al.* 2006. Protective effects of an anti-inflammatory cytokine, interleukin-4, on motoneuron toxicity induced by activated microglia. *J. Neurochem.* **99:** 1176–1187.

91. Deboy, C.A., J. Xin, S.C. Byram, *et al.* 2006. Immune-mediated neuroprotection of axotomized mouse facial motoneurons is dependent on the IL-4/STAT6 signaling pathway in CD4(+) T cells. *Exp. Neurol.* **201:** 212–224.

92. Lyons, A., R.J. Griffin, C.E. Costelloe, *et al.* 2007. IL-4 attenuates the neuroinflammation induced by amyloid-beta in vivo and n vitro. *J. Neurochem.* **101:** 771–781.

93. Clarke, R.M., A. Lyons, F. O'Connell, *et al.* 2008. A pivotal role for interleukin-4 in atorvastatin-associated neuroprotection in rat brain. *J. Biol. Chem.* **283:** 1808–1817.

Interleukin-4 as a Neuromodulatory Cytokine

Roles and Signaling in the Nervous System

**Alfred Sholl-Franco, Ana Gabriela Ledo Santos da Silva,
and Juliana Adão-Novaes**

*Instituto de Biofísica Carlos Chagas Filho, Centro de Ciências da Saúde, Universidade
Federal do Rio de Janeiro, Rio de Janeiro, Brazil*

Although interleukin (IL)-4 is described as a prototypical anti-inflammatory cytokine,
in recent years its role as a neuromodulatory cytokine has been extensively discussed.
This review highlights the pivotal contributions of IL-4 during the development and
normal physiology of neural cells as well as IL-4 connections with the pathophysiology of
degenerative or inflammatory processes observed in the central and peripheral nervous
system.

Key words: interleukin-4; nervous system; development; cell signaling; neuroimmunomodulation; neuroinflammation

Introduction

Cytokines are multifunctional pleiotropic proteins that play crucial roles in cell-to-cell communication and cellular activation. Functionally, cytokines have been classified as being either pro-inflammatory (Th1-type, stimulatory) or anti-inflammatory (Th2-type, inhibitory), depending on the final balance of their effects on the immune system.[1] However, cytokines are involved not only in the immune system response but also in a variety of physiological and pathological processes, including events in the central nervous system (CNS) and peripheral nervous system (PNS), as immunoregulator and neuromodulator factors.[2] This review attempts to explore the cytokine interleukin-4 (IL-4) as a key player in neuromodulation and will particularly focus on its effects on neural cells. By understanding the physiological effects of IL-4 on neuronal and glial cells as well as the consequences of ele-

vated IL-4 levels in cerebrospinal fluid (CSF) or within the nervous tissue, its therapeutic application becomes more relevant. When compared with other neuroregulatory cytokines, the suggested CNS and PNS functions of IL-4 are relatively recent findings. Herein, we show an integrative overview of IL-4, pointing out the main effects of IL-4 and intracellular pathways activated through the IL-4 receptor (IL-4R). The function of IL-4 in the physiology of neural cells and, more specifically, on neuromodulatory actions of several pathological conditions in the CNS and PNS are also discussed.

The IL-4/IL-4 Receptor System

IL-4 is a typical anti-inflammatory cytokine primarily related to Th2 cells, basophil, mast cells, and natural killer1 T cells, with pleiotropic actions on different cell types, which act in various stages of cell differentiation.[3] This cytokine is a glycoprotein with a molecular weight of 20 kDa and composed of 129 amino acids. IL-4 has a unique molecular structure formed by 4-α propellers targeted way "up-down-up-down" and two long-handle terminals.[4,5] It plays

Address for correspondence: Dr. Alfred Sholl-Franco, Laboratório de
Neurogênese, Programa de Neurobiologia, IBCCF, Bl. G, Sl. G2-019/032,
CCS, UFRJ, Cidade Universitária, Rio de Janeiro, RJ 21949-900, Brazil.
Voice: +55-21-25626562; fax: +55-21-22808193. asholl@biof.ufrj.br

Neuroimmunomodulation: Ann. N.Y. Acad. Sci. 1153: 65–75 (2009).
doi: 10.1111/j.1749-6632.2008.03962.x © 2009 New York Academy of Sciences.

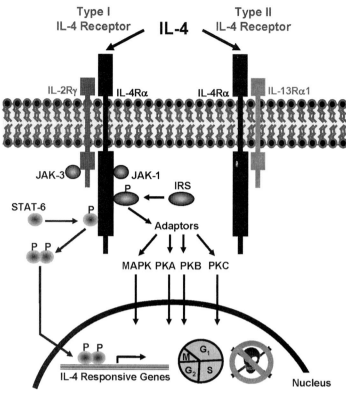

Figure 1. Schematic representation of classes I and II interleukin (IL)-4 receptors and signaling pathways activated. The binding of IL-4 to the IL-4Rα induces heterodimerization with the IL-2Rγ (class I IL-4 receptor) or the IL-13Rα1 (class II IL-4 receptor). This dimerization activates members of the janus kinase (JAK) family that initiate the phosphorylation cascade. Phosphorylated residues in the cytoplasmic tail of the IL-4Rα act as docking sites for adaptors and signaling molecules. After phosphorylation, signal transducer and activator of transcription (STAT) dimerizes, migrates to the nucleus, and binds to different gene promoters. The recruitment of insulin receptor substrate (IRS) and other adaptors can orchestrate the activation of several signaling pathways. Indeed, protein kinase A (PKA), protein kinase B (PKB), protein kinase C (PKC), or mitogen-activated protein kinase (MAPK) activities have been shown to participate in several cellular events controlled by IL-4, such as proliferation, differentiation, survival, and protection from apoptosis. G1, G1 phase; G2, G2 phase; S, synthesis phase; M, mitotic phase; P, phosphate.

an important role in the function of various immunocompetent cells as well as in the pathophysiology of various disorders in the CNS.

IL-4 exerts its biological activities through interaction with cell surface receptors,[6] which consists of two transmembrane proteins.[7,8] The cellular response to this cytokine depends on the presence of the α subunit (IL-4Rα), also called CD124,[9] which has a molecular weight of 140 kDa[10] and is responsible for the process of dimerization of the two types of receptors for IL-4, as illustrated in Figure 1.

IL-4R type I, which is present in hematopoietic cell lines, is formed by the interaction of IL-4Rα with the other forming subunit, the IL-2γc chain (CD132),[7,9,11] which is also shared by receptors for others cytokines (such as IL-2, IL-7, IL-9, IL-15, and IL-21).[5,12] IL-4R type II is present in nonhematopoietic cell lines and is formed by the interaction of IL-4Rα with IL-13Rα1, instead of IL-2Rγc.[5,12] Thus, IL-13 is also able to bind to the complex formed by heterodimerization of IL-4Rα with IL-3Rα1.[12]

After dimerization of IL-4R, tyrosine residues present in cytoplasmic tails of receptors become phosphorylated and act as docking sites for different signaling molecules.[5,7,12] Signal transduction through IL-4 receptors involves three major pathways: JAK (janus kinase)-STAT (signal transducer and activator of transcription)-6, Raf-MAPKK-MAPK (mitogen-activated protein kinase), and phosphatidylinositol-3′-kinase-Akt (PKB).[6,12] Furthermore, an increase of intracellular calcium and cAMP[13] and of protein kinase C (PKC) activity can also mediate the effects of IL-4.[14] These various signal transduction pathways account for the pleiotropic and differential effects exerted by IL-4 on distinct cell types.

IL-4 and the Physiology of the Nervous System

During the last decade, several groups investigated developmentally related actions of IL-4 on processes, such as neurogenesis and neuronal and glial differentiation and activity, as well as on events, such as phenotypic plasticity, growth, and programmed cell death.[15–17] In developing rat retina, IL-4 was shown to regulate retinal progenitor proliferation and rod photoreceptor differentiation[15] as well as cholinergic and GABAergic amacrine differentiation *in vitro*.[16,17] These results clearly show an important role for this cytokine on the normal development of retinal circuitry.

Poor recovery from acute insults or chronic degenerative disorders in the CNS has been attributed to lack of neurogenesis, limited regeneration of injured neurons, and extreme vulnerability to degenerative conditions.[18] However, Eriksson *et al.*[19] showed that the brain is capable of neurogenesis throughout life, albeit to a limited extent. Recent studies have shown that although an uncontrolled local immune response impairs neuronal survival and blocks the repair process, a properly controlled local immune response can support survival and promote recovery.[18,20]

IL-4 has been shown to induce expression of nerve growth factor (NGF) in astrocytes.[21] NGF is expressed in the developing nervous system and plays a critical role in the survival, growth, and differentiation of peripheral sympathetic neurons.[22] NGF is only expressed in adult brains following injury.[23] Since astrocytes have been shown to express functional IL-4R, IL-4 may be a regulatory factor in NGF expression in the developing CNS.[21] Indeed, direct neurotrophic effects of IL-4 have also been demonstrated on hippocampal neurons *in vitro*.[24] It is interesting to notice that during the course of brain trauma and inflammation there is activation of astrocytes and microglia cells in the vicinity of the insult.[25] These cells, as well as various lymphoid cells that gain access to the CNS, secrete a large number of cytokines that act on glial and neuronal cells.[26] IL-4 is produced during such lesions either by infiltrating Th2 lymphocytes or by mast cells in the brain but not by astrocytes or microglia cells.[27] In such circumstances IL-4 can inhibit the production of either tumor necrosis factor (TNF)-α or nitric oxide (NO) by astrocytes and microglia,[28,29] suggesting that IL-4 exerts immunosuppressive effects in the CNS.

The direct effects of IL-4 in neuronal survival of different cell populations, such as hippocampal neurons from rat embryos or rat retinal ganglion cells,[24,30] were evaluated *in vitro*. A neuroprotective effect of IL-4 on retinal ganglion cells after axotomy *in vivo* was confirmed by studies using adenovirus-associated vector-transgene expression of this cytokine in the superior colliculus or intravitreally.[31] Degenerative retinopathies, such as retinitis pigmentosa, have been shown to promote photoreceptor apoptosis in humans.[32] In this case, photoreceptor cell death control is poorly understood. Recently, Adão-Novaes[33] investigated the action of IL-4 on the blockage of thapsigargin-induced rod photoreceptor death *in vitro* and showed that the IL-4 neuroprotective effect was mediated by cAMP/protein kinase A (PKA) activation.

Functional IL-4Rs are expressed on granule cells of the dentate gyrus of hippocampus where a significant decrease in the expression of IL-4 is associated with aging.[34] These data are corroborated by Maher *et al.*[35] who proposed that an imbalance between pro- and anti-inflammatory cytokines in the aged brain significantly contributes to age-related deficits in synaptic function. Among nervous system cells the constitutive expression of the IL-2Rγc subunit mRNA had previously been demonstrated only in unstimulated astrocytes *in vitro*,[36] and no consistent data about the presence of IL-4Rα had been found in brain.[21,34,37] Both neural and non-neural retinal cells express IL-4Rα during early postnatal development,[15] and expression becomes restricted to outer and inner photoreceptor segments in adult mice, indicating a possible role of IL-4 in the maintenance of these structures. However, neither expression of IL-4 molecule[15] nor of IL-4 mRNA were detected during the developing or adult rodent retina.[38] Conversely, Silva *et al.*[15] showed that IL-4 is abundantly present in mice non-neural cells of eyeball (pigmented epithelia, choroids, and sclera) during postnatal development, and this was previous demonstrated by Zheng and Atherton for pigmented epithelia of adult rats submitted to retinitis.[39] In view of these findings, the expression pattern of IL-4/IL-4Rα in neural and non-neural retinal tissue suggests that IL-4 may be secreted by retinal pigmented epithelia (RPE) and contribute as a modulator of retina neural development as well as an RPE-derived maintenance factor for photoreceptor outer segments in the mature retina. It is interesting that IL-4 mRNA expression in neural retina of adult rats was only detected during autoimmune uveoretinitis experimental models, and the detection declined in parallel with lymphocyte number as a result of the end of the inflammatory process.[38]

IL-4 Effects during Inflammatory Processes in the Nervous System

Microglia and astrocytes play central roles during CNS inflammatory responses because they produce a variety of cytokines, some of which seem to be unique while others are complementary and redundant.[2,40,41] Microglia cells are considered as intrinsic, immune, effector cells of CNS that are activated in response to brain injury[42,43] and initiate the CNS cytokine reactions. Astrocytes are involved in intermediate/late responses and, thus, may expand the CNS cytokine reactions. These two cells types control cellular activities including growth, viability, cytokine production, morphological transformation, and differentiation in paracrine and/or autocrine fashions.[44] Cytokines produced by these cells may also contribute to the growth and differentiation of other CNS cells, including neurons and oligodendrocytes.[40,41] Sawada *et al.*[37] summarized and reviewed the results concerning the expression of mRNA for IL-4 receptors in mouse neuronal cells line, microglia-, astrocyte-, and oligodendrocyte-enriched cultures. Its results showed that IL-4Rα mRNA is expressed in microglia and oligodendrocytes, but not in astrocytes.

Activated microglia can produce and release inflammatory mediators leading to brain damage,[43] suggesting that brain inflammation is involved in the pathogenesis of various neurodegenerative diseases, including Alzheimer's and Parkinson's diseases.[40,41,45] The ability of activated microglia-induced inflammation to exacerbate brain damage underscores the pathophysiological importance of understanding how the extent and duration of brain inflammation is controlled *in vivo*. Little is known about the underlying mechanisms responsible for the death of activated microglia and the functional consequences of the death of these cells, especially *in vivo*. Park *et al.*[46] performed an elegant study *in vivo* that suggested that IL-4 regulates brain inflammation, inducing the death of activated microglia and therefore increasing neuronal survival. Surprisingly, they also found that IL-4 immunoreactivity was detected in microglia but not in astrocytes or neurons.[46] Some lines of evidence indicate that downregulation of inflammatory mediators and removal of activated microglia may be the underlying mechanism by which brain inflammation is controlled in the CNS.[47] Accumulating evidence has indicated that IL-4 reduces the production of inflammatory mediators by activated microglia *in vivo* and *in vitro*, including NO, TNF-α, cyclooxygenase-2, IL-1β, macrophage chemo-attractant protein (MCP)-1, and indoleamine 2,3-dioxygenase.[48,49] The IL-4-activated microglia can also induce oligodendrogenesis, which is, at least in part, mediated by insulin growth factor I (IGF-1) or directly by IL-4.[50] It thus appears that microglial phenotype critically affects its ability to support or impair cell renewal in the nervous system from adult stem cells.[18,51]

IL-4, Alzheimer's Disease, and Other Related Diseases

Alzheimer's disease (AD) is a common form of dementia characterized by a progressive loss of select neuronal population, the appearance of structurally abnormal neurons containing paired helical filaments of tau protein, and the formation of extracellular amyloide β (Aβ) peptide plaque deposits and cytokine production.[41,52] A hallmark of the immunopathology associated with AD is the presence of activated microglia surrounding plaque deposits of Aβ peptides. In response to Aβ, microglia secrete complement proteins,[53] the inflammatory cytokines IL-1,[54] and TNF-α.[55] Microglial cells responded to Aβ or lipopolysaccharide by producing the prototypical pro-inflammatory cytokines IL-1α, IL-1β, TNF-α, IL-6, and chemokine MCP-1. The induction of these pro-inflammatory proteins was inhibited by IL-4, and this effect was attributed to downregulation of TNF-α and upregulation of IGF-1.[20,56] These results indicate that the capacity of Aβ to activate microglial cells may be modulated by endogenous anti-inflammatory cytokines, such as IL-4. Consistent with these data, cytokines are able to modulate Aβ-induced neurodegeneration in an *in vitro* model with human fetal brain cells. This process was

TABLE 1. Levels of Interleukin (IL)-4 in Cerebrospinal Fluid (CSF) during Different Central Nervous System Inflammatory Conditions

Disease	CSF IL-4 Level
Parkinson's Disease[61,62]	↑
Complex Region Pain Syndrome[63]	↓
Creutzfeldt-Jakob Disease[64]	↑
Multiple Sclerosis[65–68]	↑
Neuroborreliosis[69]	↑

↑, increased; ↓, decreased.

accompanied by microglia cell proliferation and enhanced release of IL-1, IL-6, and TNF-α. Once again, IL-4 also proved to be neuroprotective.[57] It is remarkable that TNF-α upregulated the expression of formyl peptide receptor 2 (mFPR2), a receptor for Aβ fragment 1–42, in mouse microglial cells. Iribarren et al.[58] showed that IL-4 markedly inhibited TNF-α-induced expression of mFPR2 in microglial cells by attenuating activation of extracellular signal-regulated kinase and p38 MAPK as well as nuclear factor-κB. The effect of IL-4 was not dependent on STAT-6 but rather required the protein phosphatase 2A (PP2A). Since both IL-4 and TNF-α are produced in the CNS under pathophysiological conditions, these results suggest that IL-4 may play an important role in the maintenance of CNS homeostasis by limiting microglia activation caused by proinflammatory stimulants.

Parkinson's disease (PD) is the most common and debilitating degenerative disease and is characterized by severe motor symptoms of tremor, bradykinesia, rigidity, and postural instability, which result from a massive loss of dopamine (DA) neurons in the *substantia nigra*.[59,60] One hypothesis to explain the degeneration of the DA neurons is that PD is caused by programmed cell death (apoptosis) from increased levels of cytokines and/or a decrease in neurotrophins. A marked increased level of IL-4 was found in the *nigrostriatal* dopaminergic regions and in the CSF of PD patients (Table 1). This is in agreement with higher levels of IL-4 and other cytokines found in the *striatum* of postmortem human brain.[62] Furthermore, the levels of apoptosis-related proteins, such as bcl-2 and soluble Fas (sFas), were also elevated in PD. These results suggest that the changes in the levels of cytokines and apoptosis-related proteins may be involved in degeneration of the dopaminergic neurons and the changes in cytokine and neurotrophin levels may be initiated by activated microglia.[62,70] Similar to that observed for PD, some other diseases present modified IL-4 levels in CSF as demonstrated in Table 1.

IL-4, Multiple Sclerosis, and Experimental Autoimmune Encephalomyelitis

Multiple sclerosis (MS) is a disabling, inflammatory, demyelinating disease of the CNS involving numerous soluble mediators secreted by different cell populations[65,71] that could be reproduced on the animal model of experimental autoimmune encephalomyelitis (EAE).[72] It has been shown that IL-4 is increased in CSF (Table 1), derived from infiltrating peripheral blood cells or produced by CNS resident cells.[65,73–75] The pattern of IL-4 secretion by peripheral blood cells in both relapsing–remitting MS and chronic progressive MS is similar. Thus, it has been proposed that IL-4 acts inhibiting IFNγ-actions upon microglia cells and thus attenuates the IFNγ-associated tissue destructive response in MS.[29]

Hulshof *et al.*[75] examined the expression of IL-4 and IL-4Rα and other cytokines in postmortem human brain tissue obtained from MS patients and showed that the IL-4/IL-4Rα system has a specific pattern of localization, which is restricted to the MS lesion sites. In accordance with this, it was demonstrated that during MS microglial cells express Th2-cytokines and oligodendrocytes present IL-4Rα.[50] IL-4-activated microglia cells injected into CSF in EAE animals produce a significant increase in oligodendrogenesis in the spinal cord and improved clinical symptoms.[51]

Thus, IL-4 could certainly contribute to regulation of MS disease. Indeed, in EAE, subcutaneous administration of IL-4 has an ameliorating effect,[76,77] and, using delivered therapeutic *IL-4* gene in the CNS of EAE animals, Furlan *et al.*[78,79] showed protection from EAE progression in IL-4-treated mice. It was also showed that the system of *Herpes simplex* type 1 (HSV)-derived vector engineered to carried the *IL-4* gene (i) diminished microglia activation and migration in spinal cord areas, (ii) decreased the expression of MCP-1 and Rantes (regulated on activation normal T cell expressed and secreted), and (iii) decreased the demyelinated areas and axon loss. The same type of improvement in EAE animals was observed with gene therapy applied prior to immunization.[80,81]

IL-4, Pain, and Peripheral Nerve Regeneration

Peripheral inflammatory conditions are products of environmentally triggered reactions to antigens that activate the immune response. Neuropathic pain is a classical pathological condition where neural–immune interactions mediated by IL-4 could be observed and analyzed. In models of inflammatory pain, intraplantar administration of the IL-4 molecule reduces pain caused by subsequent intraplantar injection of carageeninin, bradykinin, or TNF-α,[82] and intraperitoneal administration of IL-4 produces a transient reduction in pain-related behavior measured by the writhing response in mice and by zymosan-induced knee joint incapacitation in rats.[83] It has also been demonstrated, in the neuropathic pain model induced by peripheral nerve injury (PNI), that expression of IL-4 stimulated by HSV vector transgene in dorsal root ganglia (DRG) significantly reduces pain-related behaviors (mechanical allodynia and thermal hyperalgesia) and inhibits expression of IL-1β and Prostaglandin E2 (PGE2) in spinal cord[84]; this could be a product of macrophage activity reduction through global suppression of pro-inflammatory cytokine production.[85,86] On the other hand, IL-4 was shown to positively regulate the transcription of opioid receptors, through the activation of STAT-6, in blood cells and primary sensory rat neurons,[87,88] implicating IL-4 as a neuroimmunomodulatory cytokine in pain relief.

The presence of IL-4 after PNI is also important for increasing DRG response to endogenous neurotrophin-4 during axon regrowth,[89] and this could reflect modulating activity of IL-4 on migration and activation of macrophages and class II major histocompatibility complex-positive cells.[90] In addition, Deboy et al.[91] demonstrated that IL-4 supports facial motoneuron survival after nerve axotomy, which further supports a Th2-mediated mechanism of neuroprotection in PNI. The modulation of immune response in the lesion site is a controversial question, but using a model of experimental allergic neuritis (EAN) it was possible to analyze the role of IL-4 in the complex cytokine network produced during inflammation in the PNS.[92,93]

IL-4 and Autonomic Nervous System

The autonomic imbalance observed during allergic bronchial asthma and others airway pathologies are related to the local inflammatory state[94]; this could be compared, at least in part, with the chronic inflammation detected in several bowel diseases.[95] The mechanisms controlling the recruitment and activity of immune cells to the lung involves production of eotaxin by parasympathetic neurons in response to IL-4 stimulation.[96] Afferent and efferent neural fibers change the activity to produce bronchoobstruction and hyper-reactivity in response to neurotrophins and others cytokines produced by infiltrating and resident lung cells, such as Th-2-derived cytokines.[94,97] In this way, IL-4, eotaxin, and neurotrophins are strong candidates to mediate the cross-talk communication between immune cells, neurons, epithelial cells, and muscle cells present in the airways.

The enteric nervous system (ENS), a specific subdivision of the autonomic nervous system, is formed by a complex network of neurons (motor, sensory, and interneurons) and enteric glial cells (satellite cells) responsible for the normal motor and secretory functions of the digestive system. Pathological changes in enteric homeostasis (e.g., during Crohn's disease, necrotizing enterocolitis, parasite infection, and inflammation) could be controlled by cytokines present in this microenvironment. In reality, the presence of inflammation induces severe changes in enteric neural circuitry, contributing to intestinal dysmobility and diarrhea.[98] Shea-Donohue et al.[99] showed that IL-4 acts on nerves of ENS during gastrointestinal nematode (Heligmosomoides polygyrus) infection, regulating enteric mobility directly on nonlymphoid cells (intestinal epithelial cells) and indirectly on nerve cells. However, no IL-4 effect in enteric glial fibrillary acidic protein expression or NGF secretion in vitro was observed.[100] IL-4 secreted by peripheral blood cells during inflammation was able to increase neurotrophin-3 mRNA expression,[101] and this could be effective in regulating neuronal synaptic activity in the ENS.

Conclusions

Much has been learned during the last 15 years about the presence of IL-4/IL-4R pathways in the nervous system. This review was an attempt to capture some of the highlights of what is known about the integration of events triggered by IL-4 in neural and non-neural cells that may contribute to the control of normal development, and maintenance of homeostasis of the nervous system. It was also a challenge to look for direct and indirect immune responses mediated by IL-4 within the nervous system. The role of endogenous and/or exogenous IL-4 in neurodegenerative (AD, PD), autoimmune and inflammatory (MS, EAE, PNI, EAN), and other pathological conditions must be investigated as it could be useful in the development of new therapeutic strategies.

Acknowledgments

We would like to thank Dr. Paula Campello-Costa, Dr. Lucianne Fragel-Madeira, and Dr. Marcelo Einicker Lamas for their helpful discussions and critical review. J. Adão-Novaes is the recipient of a Conselho Nacional de Desenvolvimento Científico e Tecnológico (CNPq) fellowship. Research undertaken in the author's laboratory that was included in this review was supported by grants from Fundação Carlos Chagas Filho de Amparo à Pesquisa do Estado do Rio de Janeiro (FAPERJ), Coordenação de Aperfeiçoamento de Pessoal de Nível Superior (CAPES), and Ministério da Ciência e da Tecnologia (MCT)/CNPq.

Conflicts of Interest

The authors declare no conflicts of interest.

References

1. Mosmann, T.R., H. Cherwinski, *et al.* 1986. Two types of murine helper T cell clone. 1. Definition according to profiles of lymphokine activities and secreted proteins. *J. Immunol.* **136:** 2348–2357.
2. Szelényi, J. 2001. Cytokines and the central nervous system. *Brain Res. Bull.* **54:** 329–338.
3. Paul, W.E. 1997. Interleukin 4: signaling mechanisms and control of T cell differentiation. *Ciba Found Symp.* **204:** 208–216.
4. Laporte, S.L., C.M. Forsyth, *et al.* 2005. De novo design of an IL-4 antagonist and its structure at 1.9 A. *Proc. Natl. Acad. Sci. USA* **102:** 1889–1894.
5. Müeller, T.D., J. Zhang, *et al.* 2002. Structure, binding, and antagonists in the IL-4/IL-13 receptor system. *Bioch. Biophys. Acta.* **1592:** 237–250.
6. Nelms, K., A.D. Keegan, *et al.* 1999. The IL-4 receptor: signaling mechanisms and biologic functions. *Annu. Rev. Immunol.* **17:** 701–738.
7. Murata, T., N. Obiri, *et al.* 1998. Structure of and signal transduction through interleukin-4 and interleukin-13 receptors. *Int. J. Mol. Med.* **1:** 551–557.
8. Wells, J.A. & A.M. De Vos. 1996. Hematopoietic receptor complexes. *Annu. Rev. Biochem.* **65:** 609–634.
9. Hinton, H.J. & M.J. Welham. 1999. Cytokine-induced protein kinase B activation and Bad phosphorylation do not correlate with cell survival of hemopoietic cells. *J. Immunol.* **162:** 7002–7009.
10. Galizzi, J.P., C.E. Zuber, *et al.* 1990. Molecular cloning of a cDNA encoding the human interleukin-4 receptor. *Int. Immunol.* **2:** 669–675.
11. Russell, S.M., A.D. Keegab, *et al.* 1993. Interleukin-2 receptor gamma chain: a functional component of the interleukin-4 receptor. *Science* **262:** 1880–1883.
12. Kelly-Welch, A.E., E.M. Hanson, *et al.* 2003. Interleukin-4 and interleukin-13 signaling connections maps. *Science* **300:** 1527–1528.
13. Finney, M., G.R. Guy, *et al.* 1990. Interleukin 4 activates human B lymphocytes via transient inositol lipid hydrolysis and delayed cyclic adenosine monophosphate generation. *Eur. J. Immunol.* **20:** 151–156.
14. Ikizawa, K., K. Kajiwara, *et al.* 1996. Evidence for a role of phosphatidylinositol 3-kinase in IL-4-induced germline C epsilon transcription. *Cell Immunol.* **170:** 134–140.
15. Silva, A.G.L.S., P. Campello-Costa, *et al.* 2008. Interleukin-4 blocks proliferation of retinal progenitor cells and increases rod photoreceptor differentiation through distinct signaling pathways. *J. Neuroimmunol.* **196:** 82–93.
16. Sholl-Franco, A., P.M.B. Marques, *et al.* 2001. Antagonistic and synergistic effects of combined treatment with interleukin-2 and interleukin-4 on mixed retinal cell cultures. *J. Neuroimmunol.* **113:** 40–48.
17. Sholl-Franco, A., C.M. Figueiredo, *et al.* 2002. Interleukin-4 increases the GABAergic phenotype in rat retinal cell cultures: involvement of muscarinic receptors and protein kinase C. *J. Neuroimmunol.* **133:** 20–29.
18. Butovsky, O., Y. Ziv, *et al.* 2006. Microglia activated by IL-4 or IFN-γ differentially induce neurogenesis and oligodendrogenesis from adult stem/progenitor cells. *Mol. Cell. Neurosci.* **3:** 149–160.
19. Eriksson, P.S., E. Perfilieva, *et al.* 1998. Neurogenesis in the adult human hippocampus. *Nat. Med.* **4:** 1313–1317.
20. Butovsky, O., A.E. Talpalar, *et al.* 2005. Activation of microglia by aggregated β-amyloid or lipopolysaccharide impairs MHC-II expression and renders them cytotoxic whereas IFN-γ and IL-4 render them protective. *Nat. Med.* **29:** 381–393.
21. Brodie, C., N. Goldreich, *et al.* 1998. Functional IL-4 receptors on mouse astrocytes: IL-4 inhibits astrocyte activation and induces NGF secretion. *J. Immunol.* **81:** 20–30.

22. Scully, I.L. & U. Otten. 1995. NGF: Not just neurons. *Cell Biol. Inst.* **19:** 459–469.

23. Varon, S. & J.M. Connor. 1994. Nerve growth factor in CNS repair. *J. Neurotrauma* **11:** 473–486.

24. Araujo, D.M. & C.W. Cotman. 1993. Trophic effects of interleukin-4,-7 and -8 on hippocampal neuronal cultures: potential involvement of glial-derived factors. *Brain Res.* **600:** 49–55.

25. Eddleston, M. & L. Mucke. 1993. Molecular profile of reactive astrocytes—implications for their role in neurologic disease. *Neuroscience* **54:** 15–36.

26. Giulian, D. & L.B. Lachman. 1985. Interleukin-1 stimulation of astroglial proliferation after brain injury. *Science* **228:** 497–499.

27. Suzumura, A., M. Sawada, *et al*. 1994. Interleukin-4 induces proliferation and activation of microglia but suppresses their induction of class II major histocompatability complex antigen expression. *J. Neuroimmunol.* **53:** 209–218.

28. Simmons, M. & S. Murphy. 1993. Cytokines regulate L-arginine-dependent cyclic GMP production in rat glial cells. *Eur. J. Neurosci.* **5:** 825–831.

29. Chao, C.C., T.W. Molitor, *et al*. 1993. Neuroprotective role of IL-4 against activated microglia. *J. Immunol.* **151:** 1473–1481.

30. Sholl-Franco, A., K.G.A. Figueiredo, *et al*. 2001. Interleukin-2 and interleukin-4 increase the survival of retinal ganglion cells in culture. *NeuroReport* **12:** 109–112.

31. Koeberle P.D., J. Gauldie, *et al*. 2004. Effects of adenoviral-mediated gene transfer of interleukin-10, interleukin-4, and transforming growth factor-beta on the survival of axotomized retinal ganglion cells. *Neuroscience* **125:** 903–920.

32. van Soest, S., A. Westerveld, *et al*. 1999. Retinitis pigmentosa: defined from a molecular point of view. *Surv. Ophthalmol.* **43:** 321–334.

33. Adão-Novaes, J. 2007. Regulação *in vitro* da morte celular de fotorreceptores induzida por ácido ocadáico e tapsigargina: efeito neuroprotetor de citocinas. Ms thesis, Universidade Federal do Rio de Janeiro, Rio de Janeiro.

34. Nolan, Y., O.F. Mahert, *et al*. 2005. Role of interleukin-4 in regulation of age-related inflammatory changes in the hippocampus. *J. Biol. Chem.* **280:** 9354–9362.

35. Maher, F.O., Y. Nolan, *et al*. 2005. Downregulation of IL-4-induced signalling in hippocampus contributes to deficits in LTP in the aged rat. *Neurobiol. Aging* **26:** 717–728.

36. Pousset, F., S. Cremona, *et al*. 1999. Interleukin-4 and interleukin-10 regulate IL1-β induced mouse primary astrocyte activation: a comparative study. *Glia* **26:** 12–21.

37. Sawada, M., Y. Itoh, *et al*. 1993. Expression of cytokine receptors in cultured neuronal and glial cells. *Neurosci. Lett.* **160:** 131–134.

38. Barton, K., M.T. McLauchlan, *et al*. 1995. The kinetics of cytokine mRNA expression in the retina during experimental autoimmune uveoretinitis. *Cell Immunol.* **164:** 133–140.

39. Zheng, M. & S.S. Atherton. 2005. Cytokine profiles and inflammatory cells during HSV-1-induced acute retinal necrosis Invest. *Ophthalmol. Vis. Sci.* **46:** 1356–1363.

40. Safieh-Garabedian B., J.J. Haddad, *et al*. 2004. Cytokines in the central nervous system: targets for therapeutic intervention. *Curr. Drug Targets CNS Neurol. Disord.* **3:** 271–280.

41. Weisman, D., E. Hakimian, *et al*. 2006. Interleukins, inflammation, and mechanisms of Alzheimer's disease. *Vitamins Hormones* **74:** 505–530.

42. Aloisi, F. 2001. Immune function of microglia. *Glia* **36:** 165–179.

43. Kim, W.G., R.P. Mohney, *et al*. 2000. Regional difference in susceptibility to liplpolysaccharide-induced neurotoxicity in the rat brain: role of microglia. *J. Neurosci.* **20:** 6309–6316.

44. Skaper, S.D. 2007. The brain as a target for inflammatory processes and neuroprotective strategies. *Ann. N. Y. Acad. Sci.* **1122:** 23–34.

45. Benveniste, E.N., V.T. Nguyen, *et al*. 2001. Immunological aspecsts of microglia: relevance to Alzheimer's disease. *Neurochem. Int.* **39:** 381–391.

46. Park, K.W., D.Y. Lee, *et al*. 2005. Neuroprotective role of microglia expressing interleusin-4. *J. Neurosci. Res.* **21:** 397–402.

47. Niinobu, T., K. Fukuo, *et al*. 2000. Negative feedback regulation of activated macrophages via Fas-mediated apoptosis. *Am. J. Physiol. Cell Physiol.* **279:** 504–509.

48. Yadav, M.C., E.M. Burudi, *et al*. 2007. IFN-gamma-induced IDO and WRS expression in microglia is differentially regulated by IL-4. *Glia* **55:** 1385–1396.

49. Furlan, R., A. Bergami, *et al*. 2000. Interferon-beta treatment in multiple sclerosis patients decreases the number of circulanting T cells producing interferon-gamma and interleukin-4. *J. Neuroimmunol.* **111:** 86–92.

50. Cannella, B. & C.S. Raine. 2004. Multiple sclerosis: cytokine receptors on oligodendrocytes predict innate regulation. *Ann. Neurol.* **55:** 46–57.

51. Butovsky, O., G. Landa, *et al*. 2006. Induction and blockage of oligodendrogenesis by differently activated microglia in an animal model of multiple sclerosis. *J. Clin. Invest.* **116:** 905–915.

52. Zubenko, G.S. 1997. Molecular neurobiology of Alzheimer's disease (syndrome?). *Harvard Rev. Psychiatry* **5:** 177–213.

53. Walker, D.G., S.U. Kim, *et al*. 1995. Complement and cytokine gene expression in cultured microglia derived from postmortem human brains. *J. Neurosci. Res.* **40:** 478–493.

54. Araujo, D.M. & C.W. Cotman. 1992. β-Amyloid stimulates glial cells in vitro to produce growth factors that accumulate in senile plaques in Alzheimer's disease. *Brain Res.* **569:** 141–151.

55. Klegeris, A. & P.L. McGeer. 1997. β-amyloid protein enhances macrophage production of oxygen free radical and glutamate. *J. Neurosci. Res.* **49:** 229–235.

56. Szczepanik, A.M., S. Funes, *et al*. 2001. IL-4, IL-10 and IL-13 modulate Aβ(1–42)-induced cytokine and chemokine production in primary murine microglia a human monocyte cell line. *J. Neuroimmunol.* **113:** 49–62.

57. Chao, C.C., S. Hu, *et al*. 1994. Transforming growth factor-β protects human neuron against β-amyloid-induced injury. *Mol. Chem. Neuropathol.* **23:** 159–178.

58. Iribarren, P., K. Chen, *et al*. 2005. IL-4 inhibits the expression of mouse formyl peptide receptor 2, a receptor for amyloid β1–42, in TNFα-activated microglia. *J. Immunol.* **175:** 6100–6106.

59. Weintraub D., C.L. Comella, *et al*. 2008. Parkinson's disease—Part 1: pathophysiology, symptoms, burden, diagnosis, and assessment. *Am. J. Manag. Care* **14:** S40–S48.

60. Chen, L.W., K.L. Yung, *et al*. 2005. Reactive astrocytes as potential manipulation targets in novel cell replacement therapy of Parkinson's disease. *Curr. Drug Targets* **6:** 821–833.

61. Nagatsu, T., M. Mogi, *et al*. 2000. Changes in cytokines and neurotrophins in Parkinson's disease. *J. Neural Transm. Suppl.* **60:** 277–290.

62. Nagatsu, T., M. Mogi, *et al*. 2000. Cytokines in Parkinson's disease. *J. Neural Transm. Suppl.* **58:** 143–151.

63. Alexander, G.M., M.J. Perreault, *et al*. 2007. Changes in immune and glial markers in the CSF of patients with Complex Regional Pain Syndrome. *Brain Behav. Immunity* **21:** 668–676.

64. Stoeck, K., B. Bodemer, *et al*. 2005. Interleukin-4 and interleukin-10 levels are elevated in the cerebrospinal fluid of patients with Creutzfeld-Jakob disease. *Arch. Neurol.* **62:** 1591–1594.

65. Navikas, V. & H. Link. 1996. Review: cytokines and the pathogenesis of multiple sclerosis. *J. Neurosci. Res.* **45:** 322–333.

66. Söderström, M., J. Hillert, *et al*. 1995. Expression of IFN-gamma, IL-4, and TGF-beta in multiple sclerosis in relation to HLA-Dw2 phenotype and stage of disease. *Mult. Scler.* **1:** 173–180.

67. Link, J., M. Söderström, *et al*. 1994. Increased transforming growth factor-beta, interleukin-4, and interferon-gamma in multiple sclerosis. *Ann. Neurol.* **36:** 379–386.

68. Bartosik-Psujek, H. & Z. Stelmasik. 2005. Correlations between IL-4, IL-12 levels and CCL2, CCL5 levels in serum and cerebrospinal fluid of multiple sclerosis patients. *J. Neural Transm.* **112:** 797–803.

69. Widhe, M., B.H. Skogman, *et al*. 2005. Upregulation of Borrelia-specific IL-4- and IFN-γ-secreting cells in cerebrospinal fluid from children with Lyme neuroborreliosis. *Int. Immunol.* **17:** 1283–1291.

70. Nagatsu, T. & M. Sawada. 2005. Inflammatory process in Parkinson's disease: role for cytokines. *Curr. Pharm. Des.* **11:** 999–1016.

71. Weber, F. 2002. Effects of autoreactive T cells and cytokines in the pathogenesis of multiple sclerosis. *Int. MS J.* **9:** 29–35.

72. Holmøy, T. 2007. Immunopathogenesis of multiple sclerosis: concepts and controversies. *Acta Neurol. Scand.* **115:** 39–45.

73. Lu, C.Z., M.A. Jensen, *et al*. 1993. Interferon gamma- and interleukin-4-secreting cells in multiple sclerosis. *J. Neuroimmunol.* **46:** 123–128.

74. Cannella, B. & C.S. Raine. 1995. The adhesion molecule and cytokine profile of multiple sclerosis lesions. *Ann. Neurol.* **37:** 424–435.

75. Hulshof, S., L. Montagne, *et al*. 2002. Cellular localization and expression patterns of interleukin-10, interleukin-4, and their receptors in multiple sclerosis lesions. *Glia* **38:** 24–35.

76. Kuchroo, V.K., M.P. Das, *et al*. 1995. B7–1 and B7–2 costimulatory molecules activate differentially the Th1/Th2 developmental pathways: application to autoimmune disease therapy. *Cell* **80:** 707–718.

77. Racke, M.K., A. Bonomo, *et al*. 1994. Cytokine-induced immune deviation as a therapy for inflammatory autoimmune disease. *J. Exp. Med.* **180:** 1961–1966.

78. Furlan, R., P.L. Poliani, *et al*. 1998. Central nervous system delivery of interleukin 4 by a nonreplicative herpes simplex type 1 viral vector ameliorates autoimmune demyelination. *Human Gene Ther.* **9:** 2605–2617.

79. Furlan, R., P.L. Poliani, *et al*. 2001. Central nervous system gene therapy with interleukin-4 inhibits progression of ongoing relapsing-remitting autoimmune encephalomyelitis in Biozzi AB/H mice. *Gene Ther.* **8:** 13–19.

80. Croxford, J.L., K. Triantaphyllopoulos, *et al*. 1998. Cytokine gene therapy in experimental allergic encephalomyelitis by injection of plasmid DNA-cationic liposome complex into the central nervous system. *J. Immunol.* **160:** 5181–5187.

81. Martino, G., P.L. Poliani, *et al*. 2000. Cytokine therapy in immune-mediated demyelinating diseases of

the central nervous system: a novel gene therapy approach. *J. Neuroimmunol.* **107:** 184–190.

82. Cunha, F.Q., S. Poole, *et al*. 1999. Cytokine-mediated inflammatory hyperalgesia limited by interleukin-4. *Br. J. Pharmacol.* **126:** 45–50.

83. Vale, M.L., J.B. Marques, *et al*. 2003. Antinociceptive effects of interleukin-4, -10, and -13 on the writhing response in mice and zymosan induced knee joint incapacitation in rats. *J. Pharmacol. Exp. Ther.* **304:** 102–108.

84. Hao, S., M. Mata, *et al*. 2006. HSV-mediated expression of interleukin-4 in dorsal root ganglion neurons reduces neuropathic pain. *Mol. Pain* **2:** 6.

85. Mijatovic, T., V. Kruys, *et al*. 1997. Interleukin-4 and -13 inhibit tumor necrosis factor-alpha mRNA translational activation in lipopolysaccharide-induced mouse macrophages. *J. Biol. Chem.* **272:** 14394–14398.

86. Te Velde, A.A., R.J. Huijbens, *et al*. 1990. Interleukin-4 (IL-4) inhibits secretion of IL-1 beta, tumor necrosis factor alpha, and IL-6 by human monocytes. *Blood* **76:** 1392–1397.

87. Kraus, J., C. Borner, *et al*. 2001. Regulation of mu-opioid receptor gene transcription by interleukin-4 and influence of an allelic variation within a STAT6 transcription factor binding site. *J. Biol. Chem.* **276:** 43901–43908.

88. Kraus, J., C. Börner, *et al*. 2006. Interferon-γ downregulates transcription of the mu-opioid receptor gene in neuronal and immune cells. *J. Neuroimmunol.* **181:** 13–18.

89. Gölz, G., L. Uhlmann, *et al*. 2006. The cytokine/neurotrophin axis in peripheral axon outgrowth. *Eur. J. Neurosci.* **24:** 2721–2730.

90. Deretzi, G., S.H. Pelidou, *et al*. 2000. High inflammation and mild demyelination in the peripheral nervous system induced by an intraneural injection of RR interleukin-4. *Cytokine* **12:** 808–810.

91. Deboy, C.A., J. Xin, *et al*. 2006. Immune-mediated neuroprotection of axotomized mouse facial motoneurons is dependent on the IL-4/STAT6 signaling pathway in CD4+ T cells. *Exp. Neurol.* **201:** 212–224.

92. Zhu, J., E. Mix, *et al*. 1996. Dynamics of mRNA expression of interferon-γ, interleukin 4 and transforming growth factor β1 in sciatic nerves and lymphoid organs in experimental allergic neuritis. *Eur. J. Neurol.* **3:** 232–240.

93. Abbas, N., L.P. Zou, *et al*. 2000. Protective effect of rolipram in experimental autoimmune neuritis: protection is associated with down-regulation of IFN-γ and inflammatory chemokines as well as up-regulation of IL-4 in peripheral nervous system. *Autoimmunity* **32:** 93–99.

94. Spina, D. & C.P. Page. 2002. Asthma—a need for a rethink? *Trends Pharmacol. Sci.* **23:** 311–315.

95. Collins, S.M. 1996. Similarities and dissimilarities between asthma and inflammatory bowel diseases. *Alimentary Pharmacol. Ther. Suppl.* **10:** 25–31.

96. Fryer, A.D., L.H. Stein, *et al*. 2006. Neuronal eotaxin and the effects of CCR3 antagonist on airway hyperreactivity and M2 receptor dysfunction. *J. Clin. Invest.* **116:** 228–236.

97. Nassenstein, C., D. Dawbarn, *et al*. 2006. Pulmonary distribution, regulation, and functional role of Trk receptors in a murine model of asthma. *J. Allergy Clin. Immunol.* **118:** 597–605.

98. Mawe, G.M., S.M. Collins, *et al*. 2004. Changes in enteric neural circuitry and smooth muscle in the inflamed and infected gut. *Neurogastroenterol. Motil.* **16:** 133–136.

99. Shea-Donohue, T., C. Sullivan, *et al*. 2001. The role of IL-4 in *Heligmosomoides polygyrus*-induced alterations in murine intestinal epithelial cell function. *J. Immunol.* **167:** 2234–2239.

100. von Boyen, G.B.T., M. Steinkamp, *et al*. 2004. Proinflammatory cytokines increase glial fibrillary acidic protein expression in enteric glia. *Gut* **53:** 222–228.

101. Besser, M. & R. Wank. 1999. Cutting edge: clonally restricted production of the neurotrophins brain-derived neurotrophic factor and neurotrophin-3 mRNA by human immune cells and Th1/Th2-polarized expression of their receptors. *J. Immunol.* **162:** 6303–6306.

Cytokine-induced Suppression of Medial Preoptic Neurons

Mechanisms and Neuroimmunomodulatory Effects

Toshihiko Katafuchi,[a] Shumin Duan,[a,b] Sachiko Take,[a] and Megumu Yoshimura[a]

[a]*Department of Integrative Physiology, Graduate School of Medical Sciences, Kyushu University, Fukuoka, Japan*

[b]*Institute of Neuroscience, Chinese Academy of Sciences, Shanghai, China*

We have shown that the medial preoptic area (MPO) in the hypothalamus is a major site where interferon (IFN)-α acts to induce suppression of splenic natural killer (NK) cell activity through an activation of sympathetic nervous system (SNS) in rats. Here, we discuss the hypothalamic mechanisms of the cytokine action using *in vivo* and *in vitro* preparations in rats. Lesion of the MPO activated the SNS and suppressed splenic NK cell activity in anesthetized rats, suggesting that the MPO had an inhibitory influence on nerve activity. Since both IFN-α and interleukin (IL)-1β are known to suppress MPO neuron activity, it is suggested that the suppression/loss of the MPO caused by cytokine actions/lesions disinhibits the hypothalamic–sympathetic pathway, thereby resulting in an increase in the splenic SNS and reduction of NK activity. To explore the cellular mechanisms of the suppression of MPO neurons, the effects of Prostaglandin E$_2$ (PGE$_2$), one of the major mediators of cytokine action in the brain, on the glutamate-induced membrane currents were examined using the perforated patch-clamp method in mechanically dissociated MPO neurons. Patch-clamp analysis revealed that PGE$_2$ potentiated the Ca^{2+}-dependent K$^+$ current (KCa) stimulated by Ca^{2+} entry through N-methyl-D-aspartate channels. We suggest that the cytokine-induced decrease in the firing rates of MPO neurons may be a result of an increase in interspike intervals caused by PGE$_2$-induced enhancement of KCa in the presence of glutamatergic inputs.

Key words: medial preoptic area; natural killer cell; splenic sympathetic nerve; patch clamp; NMDA; calcium-activated K$^+$ channel

Introduction

It is known that central administration of interferon (IFN)-α[1] and interleukin (IL)-1β,[2] but not IL-2, IL-6, or tumor necrosis factor α,[3] suppress peripheral cellular immunity, such as natural killer (NK) cell activity through the activation of the sympathetic nervous system (SNS) and/or the hypothalamic–pituitary–adrenal (HPA) axis. The reduction of NK activity induced by central IFN-α is shown to be exclusively mediated by the SNS, while the IL-1-induced suppression is dependent on both the SNS and the HPA axis.[4] We have demonstrated that the medial preoptic area (MPO) in the hypothalamus, which is known to be a region where pro-inflammatory cytokines and their major secondary mediators (i.e., prostaglandins) act to induce fever,[5,6] is also an action site of IFN-α to induce suppression of splenic NK cell activity through activation of the SNS in rats.[7,8]

Glutamate is a major excitatory neurotransmitter in the hypothalamus, including the MPO, and an activation of glutamate

Address for correspondence: Toshihiko Katafuchi, M.D., Ph.D., Department of Integrative Physiology, Graduate School of Medical Sciences, Kyushu University, Fukuoka 812-8582, Japan. Voice: +81-92-642-6087; fax: +81-92-642-6093. kataf@physiol.med.kyushu-u.ac.jp

Neuroimmunomodulation: Ann. N.Y. Acad. Sci. 1153: 76–81 (2009).
doi: 10.1111/j.1749-6632.2008.03963.x © 2009 New York Academy of Sciences.

receptors (GluRs) in the MPO has been reported to modulate various physiological functions, such as neuroendocrine, reproduction, body temperature, and vigilance state.[9–11] There is compelling evidence that pro-inflammatory cytokines and Prostaglandin E_2 (PGE_2), which is designated as a second mediator of cytokine action, are involved in the GluR-mediated physiological and pathological processes,[6,12–14] although underlying mechanisms are not clear.

In this review article, we discuss the hypothalamic mechanisms of the cytokine-induced suppression of splenic NK cell activity and investigate the cellular mechanisms of the actions of IFN-α and PGE_2 on MPO neurons by electrophysiological techniques.

Pathophysiological Significance of Immunomodulation Induced by Brain Cytokines

Cytokines produced in the brain as well as in the peripheral immune system evoke a variety of acute-phase responses, such as fever, anorexia, slow-wave sleep, and activation of the SNS and the HPA axis. These responses are considered to be part of the biological defense system and have adaptive values for the infected host.[6,15] It is debatable whether the central cytokine-induced immunosuppression is also included in the adaptive responses. However, it has been proposed, for example, that activation of the HPA axis raises plasma levels of glucocorticoids, which, in turn, inhibit a broad spectrum of immunological and inflammatory responses to limit overreaction of the biological defense system, thereby forming a negative feedback.[15] Therefore, central IFN-α- and IL-1β-induced immunomodulation may also be regarded as a part of the negative feedback loop. Furthermore, the activation of the HPA axis and SNS may not solely suppress the cellular immunity but may alter the helper T (TH)1/TH2 balance to TH2 dominance through the actions of glucocorticoids and catecholamines.[16]

IFN-α-induced Suppression of NK Cell Activity

An intracerebroventricular (i.c.v.) injection of IFN-α suppresses splenic NK activity in mice and rats, and the IFN-α-induced reduction of NK activity is completely blocked by the denervation of the splenic sympathetic nerve but not by adrenalectomy.[1,17] On the other hand, suppression of NK cell activity induced by i.c.v. IL-1β is mediated by both the activation of the HPA axis and the SNS as both chemical[2] or surgical[18] sympathectomy as well as adrenalectomy[19] only partially blocks the immunosuppression. Therefore, we conclude that the reduction of NK activity induced by central IFN-α is exclusively mediated by the SNS, while the IL-1-induced suppression is dependent on both the SNS and the HPA axis. In fact, i.c.v. injection of IFN-α as well as IL-1β enhances electrical activity of the splenic sympathetic nerve in anesthetized rats.[20,21] Since the electrical stimulation of the splenic sympathetic nerve suppresses the splenic NK activity through a β-adrenergic receptor-mediated process,[20] the enhancement of the splenic nerve activity following central administration of the cytokines plays a role, at least in part, in the cytokine-induced immunosuppression.

Microinjection studies have revealed that a site of action for IFN-α in the brain is the MPO. The microinjection of IFN-α into the lateral preoptic area, the lateral hypothalamus, the ventromedial hypothalamus, and the paraventricular nucleus (PVN) caused no changes in NK activity.[7] As was expected, microinjection of IFN-α into the MPO but not PVN increased the splenic sympathetic nerve activity in the rat.[8] When the MPO neurons were activated chemically by microinjection of an excitatory amino acid (glutamate) or electrically by current stimulation, the splenic sympathetic nerve activity was suppressed, and the suppression/loss of the MPO neurons by electrical lesion resulted in an enhancement of the nerve activity in anesthetized rats,[8] suggesting that the MPO had an inhibitory

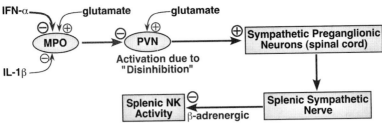

Figure 1. Hypothalamic modulation of splenic natural killer (NK) cell activity. A majority of medial preoptic area (MPO) neurons are suppressed by direct applications of interferon (IFN)-α and interleukin (IL)-1β. The paraventricular nucleus (PVN) but not the MPO has direct excitatory projection to the sympathetic pregangalionic neurons in the spinal cord. Since MPO has an inhibitory pathway to the PVN, suppression of the MPO results in the activation of the splenic sympathetic nerve from "disinhibition" of the PVN, which, in turn, suppresses splenic NK cell activity through a β-adrenergic receptor-mediated process. In accordance with this, excitation of MPO neurons by glutamate application reduces the splenic sympathetic nerve activity, while glutamate injection into the PVN enhances the nerve activity.

influence on the sympathetic nerve. Although IFN-α was without effect, microinjection of glutamate into the PVN enhanced the nerve activity. It is known that the MPO neurons scarcely project to the outside of the hypothalamus, while the PVN has an excitatory influence on the SNS by their direct projections to the sympathetic preganlionic neurons in the intermediolateral cell column of the spinal cord.

It has been reported that a majority of MPO neurons decrease their firing rate by the direct applications of IFN-α and IL-1β, probably through an action of PGE$_2$ as a second mediator.[5,15] Since the MPO neurons send an inhibitory projection to the PVN, it is suggested that suppression of the MPO neurons induced by IFN-α and/or lesion may cause a disinhibition of the PVN, which, in turn, activates PVN neurons, resulting in enhancement of nerve activity through direct projection to the preganglionic neurons in the spinal cord (Fig. 1). In accordance with this, electrical lesion of the MPO increased the splenic sympathetic nerve activity, resulting in the suppression of splenic NK cell activity, which was completely blocked by denervation.[8]

Effects of IFN-α on MPO Neurons

The cellular mechanisms of IFN-α-induced suppression of MPO neuronal activity were investigated by means of the whole-cell slice-patch method.[22] Slices including MPO (120 μm in thickness) were prepared from 10- to 20-day-old male Wistar rats. Whole-cell recordings were made from MPO neurons visually identified under Nomarski optics at the holding potential of −60 mV. Bath application of human recombinant IFN-α (100 U/mL) for 2 min attenuated the inward currents induced by glutamate and/or *N*-methyl-D-aspartate (NMDA), which were applied by pressure ejection through a glass micropipet without changing the resting membrane current. The peak amplitude of the glutamate-induced responses was suppressed to about 50% of the pre-infusion level of control responses within a few minutes, and this lasted for more than 1 h.

Since IFN-α stimulated PGE$_2$ release from rabbit hypothalamic tissue *in vitro*,[23] an involvement of PGE$_2$ as a mediator of the IFN-α-induced suppression of glutamate/NMDA responses was examined. An inhibitor of cyclooxygenase, sodium salicylate (SALC) applied immediately after administration of IFN-α partially restored the suppression of glutamate/NMDA responses. The suppression of the glutamate-induced inward current by IFN-α was still restored even when SALC was applied 40 min after IFN-α. These findings suggest that the attenuation of the glutamate/NMDA-induced current by IFN-α is at least partly mediated by the local synthesis of prostaglandins.

Modulation of Glutamate-induced Outward Currents by PGE₂

The modulatory effects of PGE_2 on the glutamate-induced membrane currents were further examined by the perforated patch-clamp method in mechanically dissociated MPO neurons.[24] In about half of MPO neurons tested, application of glutamate or NMDA evoked an outward current that followed and merged with the fast inward current at the holding potential of -30 mV. The outward current was accompanied by an increased membrane conductance and inhibited by K^+ channel blockers, tetraethylammonium and apamin. Since the outward current was abolished in the Ca^{2+}-free external solution, we suggested that the current was induced by opening K^+-activated Ca^{2+} (KCa) channels. The KCa was not a result of an inadequate space clamp and subsequent activation of voltage-gated Ca^{2+} channels because kainic acid (KA) evoked a larger inward current than NMDA but did not activate KCa. Alternatively the glutamate-induced K^+ conductance in MPO neurons was activated by Ca^{2+} entry through NMDA channels because the outward current was completely blocked by an NMDA antagonist, DL-2-amino-5-phosphonopentanoic acid. In addition, the outward current was also induced by NMDA but not KA or *trans*-(1S,3R)-1-amino-1,3-cyclopentanedicarboxylic acid.

We then examined the effects of PGE_2 on the NMDA-induced inward/outward current. Although the inward current was not affected by bath application of PGE_2, the NMDA receptor-mediated KCa current was dose-dependently enhanced by PGE_2.[24] The possible sites of PGE_2 modulation may include NMDA channel molecules, intracellular Ca^{2+} stores, and KCa channels. If PGE_2 modulates NMDA channel directly in MPO neurons, both

NMDA-induced inward current and outward current should be affected by PGE_2. This was contrary to our observation that the peak of the NMDA-induced inward current was not affected by PGE_2. Since PGE_2 alone failed to evoke the outward current, PGE_2 could not increase intracellular Ca^{2+} enough to activate KCa. It is thus most likely that PGE_2 modulates KCa, which is specifically induced by an activation of NMDA receptors directly or indirectly through second/third messengers. The PGE_2 receptors are classified into four subtypes, EP1 though EP4, with different signal transduction mechanisms, including activation of phospholipase C and stimulation and inhibition of adenylate cyclase.[25] Because it has been reported that KCa is potentiated by PGE_2[26] and protein kinase A-like protein,[27] it is possible that EP2/4 receptor subtypes, which are shown to stimulate adenylate cyclase,[25] may be involved in the PGE_2-induced potentiation of KCa. It is known that apamin-sensitive KCa plays an important role in slow afterhyperpolarization following action potentials, which determines interspike intervals. Thus it is possible that the potentiation of KCa by PGE_2 increases interspike intervals, resulting in the decrease in the firing rate of the MPO neurons in the presence of glutaminergic inputs (Fig. 2)

Conclusion

Cytokines in the brain have been shown to evoke fever, anorexia, slow-wave sleep, and activation of the SNS and the HPA axis, which are part of the biological defense system. The central IFN-α/IL-1β-induced suppression of cellular immunity is considered to be a part of the negative feedback loop between the nervous and immune systems. This system works during stress-induced immunosuppression.[4] We have shown that IFN-α suppresses splenic NK activity by its action on the MPO. Because most of the MPO neurons are suppressed by IFN-α, the PVN, which has a direct excitatory projection to the SNS, is activated by disinhibition of the inhibitory pathway from the MPO to the PVN.

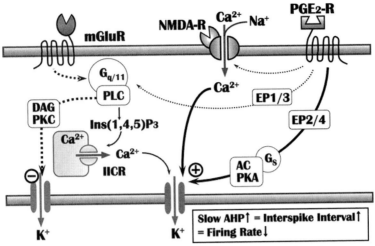

Figure 2. Possible mechanisms of Prostaglandin E_2 (PGE$_2$)-induced potentiation of the Ca^{2+}-dependent K^+ current (KCa). It is likely that PGE$_2$ enhances the N-methyl-D-aspartate (NMDA) receptor-activated KCa probably through EP2/4 receptors but not EP1/3 or metabotropic glutamate receptors. The potentiation of apamin-sensitive KCa increases interspike intervals by enhancing slow afterhyperpolarization, resulting in a decrease in the firing rate of MPO neurons in the presence of glutamatergic inputs. For details, see text. Abbreviations: Gs, G$_{q111}$, G-proteins; Ins(1,4,5)P$_3$, Inositol(1,4,5) triphosphate; mGluR, metabotropic glutamate receptors; NMDA-R, NMDA receptors; PGE$_2$-R, PGE$_2$ receptors; PLC, phospholipase C; DAG, diacyl glycerol; PKC, protein kinase C; AC, adenylate cylase; PKA, protein kinase A; AHP, afterhyperpolarization; IICR, inositol-induced Ca^{2+} release.

One of the possible mechanisms of the IFN-α-induced suppression of MPO neurons is the potentiation of the NMDA receptor-mediated outward current by PGE$_2$, which is a major second mediator of cytokine actions. It has been demonstrated that cytokines, such as IFN-α and IL-1β, reduce the firing rates of MPO neurons in an appropriate way to explain fever, hyperalgesia, and immunosuppression through a mediation of, at least in part, local production of PGE$_2$ by these cytokines.[15]

Acknowledgments

This study was supported by Grants-in-Aid for Scientific Research (19603004) to T.K. from the Ministry of Education, Culture, Sports, Science and Technology, the Japanese Government.

Conflicts of Interest

The authors declare no conflicts of interest.

References

1. Take, S. *et al.* 1993. Central interferon-α inhibits natural killer cytotoxicity through sympathetic innervation. *Am. J. Physiol.* **265:** R453–R459.
2. Sundar, S.K. *et al.* 1990. Brain IL-1-induced immunosuppression occurs through activation of both pituitary-adrenal axis and sympathetic nervous system by corticotropin-releasing factor. *J. Neurosci.* **10:** 3701–3706.
3. Connor, T.J. *et al.* 1998. An assessment of the effects of central interleukin-1β, -2, -6, and tumor necrosis factor-α administration on some behavioural, neurochemical, endocrine and immune parameters in the rat. *Neuroscience* **84:** 923–933.
4. Katafuchi, T. 2008. Involvement of brain cytokines in stress-induced immunosuppression. In *Cytokines and the Brain.* C. Phelps & E. Korneva, Eds.: 391–401. Elsevier Sci. Publ. Amsterdam.
5. Hori, T. *et al.* 1991. Immune cytokines and regulation of body temperature, food intake and cellular immunity. *Brain Res. Bull.* **27:** 309–313.
6. Rothwell, N.J. & S.J. Hopkins. 1995. Cytokines and the nervous system II: Actions and mechanisms of action. *Trends Neurosci.* **18:** 130–136.

7. Take, S. *et al.* 1995. Interferon-a acts at the preoptic hypothalamus to reduce natural killer cytotoxicity in rats. *Am. J. Physiol.* **268:** R1406–R1410.

8. Katafuchi, T. *et al.* 1993. Hypothalamic modulation of splenic natural killer cell activity in rats. *J. Physiol. (Lond.)* **471:** 209–221.

9. Azuma, S. *et al.* 1996. State-dependent changes of extracellular glutamate in the medial preoptic area in freely behaving rats. *Neurosci. Lett.* **214:** 179–182.

10. Brann, D.W. 1995. Glutamate: a major excitatory transmitter in neuroendocrine regulation. *Neuroendocrinology* **61:** 213–225.

11. Zhang, Y.H. *et al.* 1995. Warm and cold signals from the preoptic area: which contribute more to the control of shivering in rats? *J. Physiol. (Lond.)* **485:** 195–202.

12. Akaike, A. *et al.* 1994. Prostaglandin E$_2$ protects cultured cortical neurons against N-methyl-D-aspartate receptor-mediated glutamate cytotoxicity. *Brain Res.* **663:** 237–243.

13. Cazevieille, C. *et al.* 1994. Protection by prostaglandins from glutamate toxicity in cortical neurons. *Neurochem. Int.* **24:** 395–398.

14. Strijbos, P.J. & N.J. Rothwell. 1995. Interleukin-1β attenuates excitatory amino acid-induced neurodegeneration in vitro: involvement of nerve growth factor. *J. Neurosci.* **15:** 3468–3474.

15. Hori, T., T. Katafuchi & T. Oka. 2001. Central cytokines: effects on peripheral immunity, inflammation and nociception. In *Psychoneuroimmunology*, Vol. 1. R. Ader, D.L. Felten & N. Cohen, Eds.: 517–545. Academic Press. San Diego.

16. Elenkov, I.J. *et al.* 1996. Modulatory effects of glucocorticoids and catecholamines on human interleukin-12 and interleukin-10 production: clinical implications. *Proc. Assoc. Am. Physicians* **108:** 374–381.

17. Take, S. *et al.* 1992. Central interferon-α suppresses the cytotoxic activity of natural killer cells in the mouse spleen. *Ann. N. Y. Acad. Sci.* **650:** 46–50.

18. Brown, R. *et al.* 1991. Suppression of splenic macrophage interleukin-1 secretion following intracerebroventricular injection of interleukin-1β: evidence for pituitary-adrenal and sympathetic control. *Cell. Immunol.* **132:** 84–93.

19. Sundar, S.K. *et al.* 1989. Intracerebroventricular infusion of interleukin 1 rapidly decreases peripheral cellular immune responses. *Proc. Natl. Acad. Sci. USA* **86:** 6398–6402.

20. Katafuchi, T., S. Take & T. Hori. 1993. Roles of sympathetic nervous system in the suppression of cytotoxicity of splenic natural killer cells in the rat. *J. Physiol. (Lond.)* **465:** 343–357.

21. Ichijo, T., T. Katafuchi & T. Hori. 1994. Central interleukin-1β enhances splenic sympathetic nerve activity in rats. *Brain Res. Bull.* **34:** 547–553.

22. Katafuchi, T., S. Take & T. Hori. 1995. Roles of cytokines in the neural-immune interactions: modulation of NMDA responses by IFN-α. *Neurobiology (Budapest)* **3:** 319–327.

23. Dinarello, C.A. *et al.* 1984. Mechanisms of fever induced by recombinant human interferon. *J. Clin. Invest.* **74:** 906–913.

24. Katafuchi, T. *et al.* 2005. Modulation of glutamate-induced outward current by prostaglandin E$_2$ in rat dissociated preoptic neurons. *Brain Res.* **1037:** 180–186.

25. Narumiya, S. & G.A. FitzGerald. 2001. Genetic and pharmacological analysis of prostanoid receptor function. *J. Clin. Invest.* **108:** 25–30.

26. Li, Q. *et al.* 1996. Prostaglandin E$_2$ stimulates a Ca^{2+}-dependent K$^+$ channel in human erythrocytes and alters cell volume and filterability. *J. Biol. Chem.* **271:** 18651–18656.

27. Gong, L.W. *et al.* 2002. ATP modulation of large conductance Ca^{2+}-activated K$^+$ channels via a functionally associated protein kinase A in CA1 pyramidal neurons from rat hippocampus. *Brain Res.* **951:** 130–134.

Interleukin-1β and Insulin Elicit Different Neuroendocrine Responses to Hypoglycemia

Kazuki Ota, Johannes Wildmann, Taeko Ota, Hugo O. Besedovsky, and Adriana del Rey

Department of Immunophysiology, Institute of Physiology and Pathophysiology, Medical Faculty, Philipps University, Marburg, Germany

Interleukin (IL)-1β induces a prolonged hypoglycemia in mice that is not caused by a reduction in food intake and is dissociable from insulin effects. There is a peripheral component in the hypoglycemia that the cytokine induces resulting from an increased glucose uptake, an effect that can be exerted in a paracrine fashion at the site where IL-1 is locally produced. However, the maintenance of hypoglycemia is controlled at brain levels because the blockade of IL-1 receptors in the central nervous system inhibits this effect to a large extent. Furthermore, there is evidence that the cytokine interferes with counter regulation to hypoglycemia. Here we report that administration of IL-1 or long-lasting insulin results in different changes in food intake and in neuroendocrine mechanisms 8 h following induction of the same degree of hypoglycemia (40–45% decrease in glucose blood levels). Insulin, but not IL-1, caused an increase in food intake and an endocrine response that tends to reestablish euglycemia. Conversely, a decrease in noradrenergic and an increase in serotonergic activity in the hypothalamus occur in parallel with a reduction of glucose blood levels only in IL-1-treated mice, effects that can contribute to the maintenance of hypoglycemia. These results are compatible with the proposal that IL-1 acting in the brain can reset glucose homeostasis at a lower level. The biologic significance of this effect is discussed.

Key words: IL-1; insulin; glucose; counter regulation; hypoglycemia; hypothalamus; neurotransmitters; corticosterone; noradrenaline; food consumption

Introduction

Interleukin (IL)-1β induces a profound and long-lasting hypoglycemia in mice, an effect that is not mediated by insulin because it is observed in insulin-resistant diabetic mice and rats. Such hypoglycemia is not caused by glucose loss and is independent of the anorexic effect of the cytokine.[1–7] IL-1 stimulates glucose uptake *in vitro* in a variety of tissues.[8–14] Studies *in vivo* also show that overproduction of IL-1 results in increased 2-deoxyglucose uptake in all tissues tested, including lymphoid organs and the brain.[15] Several of the *in vitro* studies have been performed using human cells, and injection of very low doses of recombinant IL-1β to patients with cancer induces a transient hypoglycemia.[16] IL-1β-stimulated glucose transport is protein kinase C- and p38 mitogen-activated protein activation dependent and is accompanied by increased expression and membrane incorporation of different glucose transporters.[17] The type of transporter affected depends on the tissue, for example, GLUT3 in the liver and brain and GLUT1 in chondrocytes.[17] Furthermore, IL-1 inhibits gluconeogenesis by inhibiting the activity of phosphoenolpyruvate carboxykinase and also mediates a reduction in hepatic glycogen content.[7,15]

Besides these peripheral actions, there are indications that IL-1 can affect glucose homeostasis by acting at brain levels. Indeed, IL-1-mediated hypoglycemia develops

Address for correspondence: Adriana del Rey, Department of Immunophysiology, Institute of Physiology and Pathophysiology, Medical Faculty, Deutschhausstrasse 2, 35037 Marburg, Germany. Voice: +49 6421 2862175; fax: +49 6421 2868925. delrey@mailer.uni-marburg.de

Neuroimmunomodulation: Ann. N.Y. Acad. Sci. 1153: 82–88 (2009).
doi: 10.1111/j.1749-6632.2008.03981.x © 2009 New York Academy of Sciences.

against an initial enhanced output of counter-regulatory hormones, such as glucocorticoids, catecholamines, and glucagon.[1,4] However, this counter regulation is extinguished 4 h after administration of the cytokine, and the hypoglycemia persists for a long time (more than 12 h). Such prolonged hypoglycemia is surprising because the regulation of glucose levels in blood is one of the homeostatic mechanisms under the most tight feedback control at the level of the central nervous system (CNS). Previous studies have shown that injection of picogram amounts of IL-1 into the lateral brain ventricle induces hypoglycemia[5,7] and that peripheral administration of the cytokine induces the expression of its own gene in the hypothalamus. There is also evidence for physiologic actions of IL-1 in the CNS,[18,19] including the control of glucose homeostasis. We have recently demonstrated that blockade of IL-1 receptors in the brain interferes with the hypoglycemia induced by the cytokine. Furthermore, we have obtained evidence that the lack of an extended counter regulation to IL-1-induced hypoglycemia is related to a change in the set point for glucoregulation integrated at brain level.[20]

These facts, together with the known effects of IL-1 on the concentration and turnover rate of monoaminergic neurotransmitters,[21,22] led us to hypothesize that such effects can contribute to interference with counter-regulatory mechanisms, thus allowing the maintenance of IL-1-induced hypoglycemia. Here we report that the pattern of changes in neurotransmitters in the hypothalamus of IL-1-treated mice is different from that of insulin, a hormone known to trigger an effective counter regulation.

Materials and Methods

Animals

C57Bl/6J male mice (7–8 week-old, $n = 8$ per group) were caged individually for 7 days before the experiments were started and maintained in temperature-controlled rooms (12 h light:dark cycles). Food was provided *ad libitum*.

IL-1 and insulin administration: Recombinant human IL-1β (0.1 μg/mouse diluted in endotoxin free 0.15 mol/L NaCl containing 0.01% human serum albumin) was administered i.p., and long-acting insulin (4 U/kg; Detemir, Novo Nordisk Pharma, Bagsvaerd, Danemark) was injected s.c. To control for the effect of the different routes, mice receiving IL-1 injected i.p. also received the vehicle injected s.c., and those that received insulin s.c. were also injected with vehicle i.p. Control mice received the vehicle alone, injected i.p. and s.c. The same dose of insulin was again administered s.c. 4 h later to those mice that had previously received insulin. To control for the manipulation from the second insulin injection, IL-1-injected and control mice also received the vehicle injected s.c. 4 h later.

Experimental procedure: Eight hours after the first injection, animals were weighed and then immediately killed. Blood was obtained from the orbital plexus venous, and the hypothalamus was rapidly removed and frozen. Food consumption during the 8-h period after the first injection was also determined.

Plasma glucose and hormone determinations: Glucose levels were determined by an enzymatic (glucose oxidase) method, using a commercially available kit (Randox Laboratories, Crumlin, UK); insulin levels were determined by ELISA (Mouse Insulin Kit; DRG, Marburg, Germany); corticosterone levels were determined by radioimmunoassay; and catecholamines were determined by HPLC, as previously described.[1,22]

Neurotransmitter, metabolite, and precursor determinations were measured by HPLC, as previously described.[22]

Statistical Analysis

Results are expressed as mean $\pm$ SEM. Data were analyzed using one-way analysis of variance (ANOVA) followed by Fisher's test for multiple comparisons.

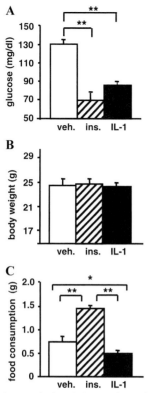

Figure 1. Interleukin (IL)-1 and insulin induce a comparable decrease in glucose blood levels but have different effects on food consumption. Mice (eight per group) received recombinant human IL-1β (0.1 µg/mouse) injected i.p. and the vehicle injected s.c. (IL-1); or long-lasting insulin (4 U/kg) injected s.c. and vehicle injected i.p. (ins.); or the vehicle alone, injected i.p. and s.c. (veh.). Four hours later, the mice that were injected with insulin received a second s.c. injection of insulin (4 U/kg). The other two groups received the vehicle injected s.c. Four hours after the second injection, mice were weighed (**B**) and immediately killed. Blood was collected and glucose levels in plasma (**A**) were determined. Food consumption during the 8-h period (**C**) was recorded. Data are expressed as mean ± SEM; *$P < 0.05$, **$P < 0.01$ between the groups indicated by the horizontal lines.

Results and Discussion

Glucose Concentration in Plasma after IL-1β or Insulin Administration

Preliminary experiments were performed to define doses of IL-1 and insulin that resulted in a comparable hypoglycemia. As can be seen in Figure 1A, administration of IL-1 at

0.1 µg/mouse or of long-lasting insulin at 4 U/kg resulted in 40–45% reduction in glucose blood levels. However, insulin had to be injected twice, 4 h apart, so that these hypoglycemic levels were of a duration comparable to that induced by one single injection of 0.1 µg of IL-1 (at least 12 h).

Body Weight and Food Intake following Administration of IL-1 or Insulin

At the doses administered and during the period studied (8 h), neither IL-1 nor insulin influenced body weight (Fig. 1B). However, insulin significantly increased while IL-1 decreased food consumption (Fig. 1C). It is well known that hypoglycemia is one of the main physiologic stimuli that leads to increased food consumption as part of the brain-integrated mechanisms that operate to counter regulate a decrease in glucose blood levels. However, it was clear that while animals actively searched for food after receiving insulin, this was not the case of the mice inoculated with the cytokine. The orexigenic effects of insulin and the evidence that IL-1 can induce anorexia are well documented.[23] However, the fact that both mediators had opposite effects in feeding behavior at the same level of hypoglycemia is remarkable since it indicates that IL-1-injected mice cannot sense or respond to a reduction in glucose levels. The control of food intake is a mechanism integrated by a complex neuronal brain network. Thus, the lack of stimulation of food intake during the prolonged hypoglycemia induced by IL-1 already indicates that the cytokine interferes with the activity of this central mechanism.

Effect of IL-1 or Insulin Administration on Insulin, Noradrenaline, Adrenaline, and Corticosterone Blood Levels

As expected, insulin blood levels are increased in insulin-treated animals (Fig. 2A). IL-1 did not affect the level of this hormone, confirming that the hypoglycemic effect of the

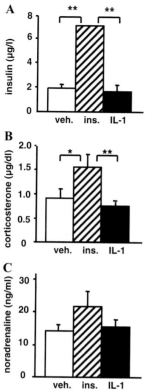

Figure 2. Changes in hormonal levels 8 h after injection of IL-1 or insulin. (**A**) Insulin, (**B**) corticosterone, and (**C**) noradrenaline levels were determined in plasma of the same mice used above. Data are expressed as mean ± SEM; *$P < 0.05$, **$P < 0.01$ between the groups indicated by the horizontal lines.

cytokine does not depend on an increased insulin release.[3] A reduction in insulin blood levels is an important component of the counter regulation to hypoglycemia, and administration of this hormone results in a decreased release of endogenous insulin by pancreatic β cells.[24] Thus, the fact that insulin blood levels were not reduced in IL-1-treated mice indicates that the cytokine interfered with a counter regulation. In addition, the levels of corticosterone, a hormone that also induces an increase in glucose blood levels, were increased in insulin, but not in IL-1-treated animals 8 h after administration (Fig. 2B). Although not statistically significant, there was also a tendency for levels of noradrenaline (NA) to increase in insulin-treated mice (Fig. 2C). Most

interestingly, IL-1 is known to stimulate the hypothalamus–pituitary–adrenal axis and the sympathetic nervous system. However, it seems that these centrally integrated effects, which are observed soon after IL-1 administration, are restricted in time and are later interfered with by the cytokine because an increase in corticosterone and catecholamines levels is expected to occur as a consequence of hypoglycemia.

Hypothalamic Concentration of Monoaminergic Neurotransmitters and Their Precursors and Metabolites following Administration of IL-1 or Insulin

No significant changes in the concentration of NA, its precursor tyrosine, and its metabolite 3-methoxy-4-hydroxyphenylethylene glycol (MHPG) or in the ratio MHPG/NA were detected in the hypothalamus of mice 8 h after receiving insulin when compared to control mice (Fig. 3A–C). In contrast, a clear decrease in NA and tyrosine concentration was observed in the hypothalamus of mice injected with IL-1 (Fig. 3A and C). This decrease was not paralleled by changes in the MHPG/NA and tyrosine/NA ratios, indicating that IL-1 induces a proportional reduction in the production and use of this catecholamine in the hypothalamus. The concentrations of serotonin (5-HT) and its metabolite 5-hydroxyindole acetic acid (5-HIAA) in the hypothalamus of insulin-injected mice were not different from those of control mice, although the concentration of tryptophan, the amino acid precursor of 5-HT, was increased (Fig. 3D–F). In contrast, a clear increase in 5-HT, 5-HIAA, and tryptophan was detected in the hypothalamus of IL-1-treated mice (Fig. 3D–F). The increase in tryptophan concentration was significantly higher in IL-1-treated mice than in animals treated with insulin. The ratio 5-HIAA/5-HT was unchanged in IL-1-treated mice, indicating a proportional increased synthesis and utilization of 5-HT in the hypothalamus. We and others have previously reported that an increase

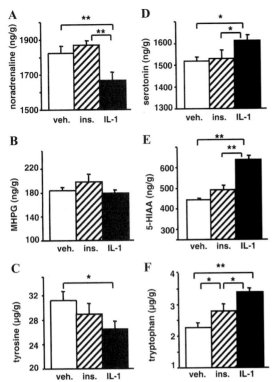

Figure 3. IL-1 and insulin induce a different pattern of changes in neurotransmitter concentration in the hypothalamus. Immediately after collecting the blood, the hypothalamus of the mice used for glucose and hormonal determinations (Figs. 1 and 2) was dissected and used to evaluate the concentration of the neurotransmitters noradrenaline (**A**) and serotonin (**D**), their metabolites MHPG (**B**) and 5-HIAA (**E**), and their precursors tyrosine (**C**) and tryptophan (**F**), respectively. Results are expressed as mean ± SEM; *$P < 0.05$, **$P < 0.01$ between the groups indicated by the horizontal lines.

in NA and 5-HT metabolism is observed in the hypothalamus 2–4 h after IL-1 administration.[25] In contrast, our present results indicate that while the increase in 5-HT metabolism is maintained and is even higher 8 h after injection of IL-1, NA metabolism clearly decreases at this time in parallel with the hypoglycemia that the cytokine induced. It is known that catecholaminergic neurons stimulate multiple glucoregulatory responses, including increased food intake and adrenal medullary and corticosterone secretion.[26-28] Thus, the decreased brain NA metabolism, which reflects

a reduction in noradrenergic brain activity, is likely to underlie the decrease in neuroendocrine counter-regulatory mechanisms that characterizes the later stage of IL-1-induced hypoglycemia. In addition, the IL-1- induced increase in serotonergic activity in the hypothalamus may induce hypophagia because depletion of central 5-HT using selective neurotoxins results in hyperphagia and obesity[29,30] whereas increased 5-HT bioavailability potently inhibits feeding and reduces body weight.[31-33] Thus, the stimulatory effect of IL-1 on brain 5-HT is likely to underlie the paradoxical reduction of food consumption during the hypoglycemia induced by the cytokine. As illustrated by the results obtained following injection of insulin, a usual behavioral counter-regulatory mechanism to hypoglycemia is an increase in food intake.

Conclusions

Glucoregulation is at the center of homeostasis because it is essential for the distribution and control of fuel supply to different body compartments. It is well known that in healthy individuals hypoglycemic counter regulation, for example, as a consequence of fasting or following insulin administration, is a multifactorial redundant process that involves reduction of insulin secretion and increased glucagon, growth hormone, and glucocorticoid secretion and adrenergic activation. Metabolically, these responses lead to increased glucose levels, initially from glycogenolysis and later from gluconeogenesis, decreased muscle glucose oxidation and storage, and increased release and use of alternative fuels, primarily free fatty acids. A prolonged hypoglycemia also leads to neurologic symptoms and hunger, which in turn stimulate food intake. Several brain mechanisms, including glucose-sensing neurons and brain neurotransmitters, coordinate this process and the maintenance of blood glucose at a predefined set point.

Our data indicate that IL-1 interferes with counter-regulatory mechanisms, such as those triggered by insulin-induced hypoglycemia. Indeed, although IL-1 and insulin induced hypoglycemia of comparable magnitude and duration, food consumption and plasma corticosterone levels were increased only in insulin-treated mice and brain neurotransmitters known to affect glucose homeostasis are affected only in IL-1β-injected animals. These data indicate that while insulin triggers the well-known counter-regulatory mechanisms to hypoglycemia, IL-1β tends to inhibit them. The fact that a decrease in noradrenergic and an increase in serotonergic neuronal activity were observed in the hypothalamus when glucose blood levels were reduced by 50% during the 8 h following IL-1 administration indicates a pattern that, as mentioned, should favor the maintenance of blood glucose levels below the "physiologic" set point.

These results are in line with our previous studies showing that IL-1 acting in the brain can change the set point of glucoregulation to a lower level. Furthermore, our results indicate that, as a result of the known capacity of IL-1 to induce its own production in the brain,[20,34] the described effects on monoaminergic neurons can be exerted by brain-borne IL-1. In addition, it is also possible that the cytokine directly or indirectly protects the brain from the hypoglycemia that it induces. Since the positive feedback by which IL-1 induces more IL-1 production is also expressed in lymphoid and inflamed tissues,[35,36] IL-1 acting in a paracrine fashion could deviate glucose to activated immune cells, which are highly demanding in terms of energy. This mechanism would represent another way by which IL-1 could contribute to immunoregulation.

Acknowledgments

This work was supported by the German Research Council (DFG).

Conflicts of Interest

The authors declare no conflicts of interest.

References

1. del Rey, A. & H. Besedovsky. 1987. Interleukin 1 affects glucose homeostasis. *Am. J. Physiol.* **253:** R794–798.
2. Besedovsky, H. & A. del Rey. 1987. Neuroendocrine and metabolic responses induced by interleukin-1. *J. Neurosci. Res.* **18:** 172–178.
3. del Rey, A. & H. Besedovsky. 1989. Antidiabetic effects of interleukin 1. *Proc. Natl. Acad. Sci. USA* **86:** 5943–5947.
4. Berkenbosch, F., D.E. de Goeij, A. del Rey, *et al.* 1989. Neuroendocrine, sympathetic and metabolic responses induced by interleukin-1. *Neuroendocrinology* **50:** 570–576.
5. del Rey, A. & H.O. Besedovsky. 1992. Metabolic and neuroendocrine effects of pro-inflammatory cytokines. *Eur. J. Clin. Invest.* **22**(Suppl 1): 10–15.
6. del Rey, A., G. Monge-Arditi, I. Klusman, *et al.* 1996. Metabolic and endocrine effects of interleukin-1 in obese, diabetic Zucker fa/fa rats. *Exp. Clin. Endocrinol. Diabetes* **104:** 317–326.
7. del Rey, A., G. Monge-Arditi & H.O. Besedovsky. 1998. Central and peripheral mechanisms contribute to the hypoglycemia induced by interleukin-1. *Ann. N. Y. Acad. Sci.* **840:** 153–161.
8. Garcia-Welsh, A., J.S. Schneiderman & D.L. Baly. 1990. Interleukin-1 stimulates glucose transport in rat adipose cells. Evidence for receptor discrimination between IL-1 beta and IL-1 alpha. *FEBS Lett.* **269:** 421–424.
9. Bird, T.A., A. Davies, S.A. Baldwin, *et al.* 1990. Interleukin 1 stimulates hexose transport in fibroblasts by increasing the expression of glucose transporters. *J. Biol. Chem.* **265:** 13578–13583.
10. Shikhman, A.R., D.C. Brinson, J. Valbracht, *et al.* 2001. Cytokine regulation of facilitated glucose transport in human articular chondrocytes. *J. Immunol.* **167:** 7001–7008.
11. Gould, G.W., A. Cuenda, F.J. Thomson, *et al.* 1995. The activation of distinct mitogen-activated protein kinase cascades is required for the stimulation of 2-deoxyglucose uptake by interleukin-1 and insulin-like growth factor-1 in KB cells. *Biochem. J.* **311**(Pt 3): 735–738.
12. Fukuzumi, M., H. Shinomiya, Y. Shimizu, *et al.* 1996. Endotoxin-induced enhancement of glucose influx into murine peritoneal macrophages via GLUT1. *Infect. Immun.* **64:** 108–112.
13. Fischereder, M., B. Schroppel, P. Wiese, *et al.* 2003. Regulation of glucose transporters in human peritoneal mesothelial cells. *J. Nephrol.* **16:** 103–109.
14. Vega, C., L. Pellerin, R. Dantzer, *et al.* 2002. Long-term modulation of glucose utilization by IL-1 alpha

and TNF-alpha in astrocytes: Na+ pump activity as a potential target via distinct signaling mechanisms. *Glia* **39:** 10–18.

15. Metzger, S., S. Nusair, D. Planer, *et al.* 2004. Inhibition of hepatic gluconeogenesis and enhanced glucose uptake contribute to the development of hypoglycemia in mice bearing interleukin-1beta- secreting tumor. *Endocrinology* **145:** 5150–5156.

16. Crown, J., A. Jakubowski, N. Kemeny, *et al.* 1991. A phase I trial of recombinant human interleukin-1 beta alone and in combination with myelosuppressive doses of 5-fluorouracil in patients with gastrointestinal cancer. *Blood* **78:** 1420–1427.

17. Shikhman, A.R., D.C. Brinson & M.K. Lotz. 2004. Distinct pathways regulate facilitated glucose transport in human articular chondrocytes during anabolic and catabolic responses. *Am. J. Physiol. Endocrinol. Metab.* **286:** E980–985.

18. Rettori, V., W.L. Dees, J.K. Hiney, *et al.* 1994. An interleukin-1-alpha-like neuronal system in the preoptic-hypothalamic region and its induction by bacterial lipopolysaccharide in concentrations which alter pituitary hormone release. *Neuroimmunomodulation* **1:** 251–258.

19. Wong, M.L., P.B. Bongiorno, V. Rettori, *et al.* 1997. Interleukin (IL) 1beta, IL-1 receptor antagonist, IL-10, and IL-13 gene expression in the central nervous system and anterior pituitary during systemic inflammation: pathophysiological implications. *Proc. Natl. Acad. Sci. USA* **94:** 227–232.

20. del Rey, A., E. Roggero, A. Randolf, *et al.* 2006. IL-1 resets glucose homeostasis at central levels. *Proc. Natl. Acad. Sci. USA* **103:** 16039–16044.

21. Dunn, A.J. 1988. Systemic interleukin-1 administration stimulates hypothalamic norepinephrine metabolism parallelling the increased plasma corticosterone. *Life Sci.* **43:** 429–435.

22. Kabiersch, A., A. del Rey, C.G. Honegger, *et al.* 1988. Interleukin-1 induces changes in norepinephrine metabolism in the rat brain. *Brain Behav. Immun.* **2:** 267–274.

23. Gayle, D., S.E. Ilyin & C.R. Plata-Salaman. 1997. Central nervous system IL-1 beta system and neuropeptide Y mRNAs during IL-1 beta-induced anorexia in rats. *Brain Res. Bull.* **44:** 311–317.

24. Waldhausl, W.K., S. Gasic, P. Bratusch-Marrain, *et al.* 1982. Feedback inhibition by biosynthetic human insulin of insulin release in healthy human subjects. *Am. J. Physiol.* **243:** E476–482.

25. Dunn, A.J. 2008. Effects of the immune system on brain neurochemistry. In *Handbook of Neurochemistry and Molecular Neurobiology.* A. Lajtha, Ed.: 37–59. Springer. New York.

26. Leibowitz, S.F. 1988. Hypothalamic paraventricular nucleus: interaction between alpha 2-noradrenergic system and circulating hormones and nutrients in relation to energy balance. *Neurosci. Biobehav. Rev.* **12:** 101–109.

27. Foscolo, R.B., M.G. de Castro, U. Marubayashi, *et al.* 2003. Medial preoptic area adrenergic receptors modulate glycemia and insulinemia in freely moving rats. *Brain Res.* **985:** 56–64.

28. Ritter, S., T.T. Dinh & A.J. Li. 2006. Hindbrain catecholamine neurons control multiple glucoregulatory responses. *Physiol. Behav.* **89:** 490–500.

29. Breisch, S.T., F.P. Zemlan & B.G. Hoebel. 1976. Hyperphagia and obesity following serotonin depletion by intraventricular p-chlorophenylalanine. *Science* **192:** 382–385.

30. Saller, C.F. & E.M. Stricker. 1976. Hyperphagia and increased growth in rats after intraventricular injection of 5,7-dihydroxytryptamine. *Science* **192:** 385–387.

31. Levine, L.R., S. Rosenblatt & J. Bosomworth. 1987. Use of a serotonin re-uptake inhibitor, fluoxetine, in the treatment of obesity. *Int. J. Obes.* **11**(Suppl 3): 185–190.

32. Guy-Grand, B. 1995. Clinical studies with dexfenfluramine: from past to future. *Obes. Res.* **3**(Suppl 4): 491S–496S.

33. Heal, D.J., S.C. Cheetham, M.R. Prow, *et al.* 1998. A comparison of the effects on central 5-HT function of sibutramine hydrochloride and other weight-modifying agents. *Br. J. Pharmacol.* **125:** 301–308.

34. Hansen, M.K., P. Taishi, Z. Chen, *et al.* 1998. Vagotomy blocks the induction of interleukin-1beta (IL-1beta) mRNA in the brain of rats in response to systemic IL-1beta. *J. Neurosci.* **18:** 2247–2253.

35. Dinarello, C.A., T. Ikejima, S.J. Warner, *et al.* 1987. Interleukin 1 induces interleukin 1. I. Induction of circulating interleukin 1 in rabbits in vivo and in human mononuclear cells in vitro. *J. Immunol.* **139:** 1902–1910.

36. Manson, J.C., J.A. Symons, F.S. Di Giovine, *et al.* 1989. Autoregulation of interleukin 1 production. *Eur. J. Immunol.* **19:** 261–265.

Intrapituitary Expression and Regulation of the gp130 Cytokine Interleukin-6 and Its Implication in Pituitary Physiology and Pathophysiology

Ulrich Renner,[a] Eliane Correa De Santana,[a] Juan Gerez,[b] Bianca Fröhlich,[a] Mariana Haedo,[b] Marcelo Paez Pereda,[a,c] Chiara Onofri,[a] Günter K. Stalla,[a] and Eduardo Arzt[b]

[a]Max Planck Institute of Psychiatry, Neuroendocrinology Group, Munich, Germany

[b]Laboratorio de Fisiologia y Biologia Molecular, Departamento de Fisiologia y Biologia Molecular e Celular, Facultad de Ciencias Exactas y Naturales, Universidad de Buenos Aires, Buenos Aires, Argentina

[c]Affectis Pharmaceuticals, Munich, Germany

Interleukin (IL)-6, a member of the gp130 cytokine family, is sometimes designated as an "endocrine" cytokine because of its strong regulatory influence on hormone production. Systemically acting IL-6 derived from immune cells is a potent stimulator of the hypothalamus–pituitary–adrenal axis and therefore plays an important role in modulating immune–neuroendocrine interactions during inflammatory or infectious processes. However, IL-6 is also produced within the anterior pituitary by so-called folliculostellate (FS) cells and is also synthesized in and released by tumor cells in pituitary adenomas. Growth factors (e.g., transforming growth factor-beta), neuropeptides (e.g., pituitary adenylate cyclase-activating polypeptide), or hormones (e.g., glucocorticoids) regulate IL-6 production both in FS and pituitary tumor cells. Interestingly, components of the innate immune system, such as toll-like receptor 4 and nucleotide-binding oligomerization domains (NODs), are expressed in FS and pituitary tumor cells. Therefore, cell-wall components of bacteria (lipopolysaccharide, muramyl dipeptide, diamino pimelic acid) stimulate IL-6 production in normal and tumoral pituitary. The intrinsic IL-6 production by FS cells in normal anterior pituitary may participate in immune–neuroendocrine interactions during inflammatory processes. In pituitary adenomas, IL-6 stimulates hormone secretion, tumor cell proliferation, and the production of angiogenic factors, such as vascular endothelial growth factor-A, suggesting an important role of IL-6 in the pathophysiology and progression of pituitary adenomas.

Key words: interleukin-6; pituitary; folliculostellate cells; pituitary tumors; toll-like receptor 4; NOD1/NOD2; lipopolysaccharide; hormone secretion; proliferation; angiogenesis

Introduction

During inflammatory or infectious processes, pathogen-induced alterations of the immune system alter the hormonal homeostasis of the endocrine system. These adaptive immune–endocrine interactions are mediated, among others, by cytokines, such as interleukin-1 (IL-1), tumor necrosis factor-α (TNF-α), and IL-6, and are important for the organism to overcome the pathogenic events in an optimal manner.[1,2] In particular, activation of the hypothalamus–pituitary–adrenal (HPA)

Address for correspondence: Dr. Ulrich Renner, Max Planck Institute of Psychiatry, Neuroendocrinology Group, Kraepelinstr. 10, D-80804 Munich, Germany. Voice: +49 89 30622 349; fax: +49 89 30622 605. renner@mpipsykl.mpg.de

Neuroimmunomodulation: Ann. N.Y. Acad. Sci. 1153: 89–97 (2009).
doi: 10.1111/j.1749-6632.2008.03970.x © 2009 New York Academy of Sciences.

axis by the above-mentioned cytokines plays a crucial role in immune–endocrine communication.[3] Enhanced circulating levels of immune cell-derived TNF-α, IL-1, and IL-6 induce a strong rise of systemic glucocorticoids by the combined stimulation of the release of hypothalamic corticotropin-releasing factor, hypophyseal adrenocorticotropic hormone (ACTH), and adrenergic glucocorticoids.[3] The elevated levels of anti-inflammatory-acting glucocorticoids prevent the organism from self-destructive mechanisms of the activated immune system, which would lead to septic shock syndrome.[2,3] In case of IL-6 there is also the possibility that intrapituitary IL-6 levels are elevated during infectious or inflammatory processes.[4] TNF-α and IL-1 strongly induce the secretion of IL-6 from a specific pituitary cell type, the so-called folliculostellate (FS) cells.[4] Paracrine-acting intrapituitary IL-6 may mediate, in concert with circulating systemically acting IL-6, the adaptive processes between the activated immune system and the endocrine system. However, in addition to the important role of IL-6 on immune–endocrine interaction, it is now well accepted that IL-6 is a trigger of the pathophysiology of pituitary tumors.[5] In the following, the regulation and role of intrahypophyseal IL-6 with a focus on its consequences for pituitary physiology and pathophysiology is discussed.

gp130 Cytokines

The so-called gp130 cytokine family is a heterogeneous group of cytokines comprising, in addition to IL-6, leukemia inhibitory factor (LIF), IL-11, ciliary neurotrophic factor (CNTF), oncostatin M (OSM), cardiotrophin-1 (CT-1), and novel neurotrophin-1/B-cell stimulating factor-3 (NNT-1/BSF-3).[6,7] All these cytokines bind to cell-surface receptors, which have no intrinsic enzymatic activities on their own but need the gp130 protein to induce intracellular signal transduction.[6,7] For some of the cytokines, such as IL-6, IL-11, and CNTF,

specific receptors exist, whereas other cytokines (LIF, OSM, CT-1) share, in part, common receptors. After ligand binding to receptor homodimers or heterodimers and after recruitment of two gp130 proteins to the ligand–receptor complex, mainly the Janus kinase-signal transducer and activator of transcription (JAK/STAT) signaling cascade is induced and Stat3 and/or Stat1 are phosphorylated and transferred to the nucleus. However, other signaling cascades, such as mitogen-activated protein (MAP) kinase pathways, have also been shown to be activated by gp130 cytokines.[6,7]

For some of the gp130 cytokines, such as OSM, CT-1, or NNT-1/BSF-3, little is known about their expression and functional role in pituitary or in pituitary tumors.[8,9] Expression of mRNA of CNTF, IL-11, and their receptors has been demonstrated in normal pituitary, pituitary adenomas, and pituitary tumor cell lines.[9–11] CNTF stimulates growth hormone (GH) and prolactin (PRL) secretion as well as pituitary tumor cell growth.[10,11] IL-11 has been reported to enhance ACTH, GH, and PRL secretion and stimulates proliferation and vascular endothelial growth factor (VEGF) production of FS cells.[10,11]

LIF was reported to be an important stimulator of proopiomelanocortin (POMC) expression and ACTH secretion through the JAK/STAT pathway and plays an important role in the activation of the HPA axis during stress and inflammation.[12,13] Transgenic mice that overexpress LIF in the pituitary have corticotroph hyperplasia and exhibit symptoms of Cushing's syndrome, whereas somatotroph and lactotroph cell development and function is disturbed.[14] However, in human corticotropinomas no overexpression of LIF has been found.[13] LIF might also play a role in prolactinoma pathophysiology because this type of pituitary tumor seems to be the only one in which LIF is not expressed. Stimulation of prolactinoma cell cultures with LIF inhibited PRL secretion,[15] suggesting that loss of this suppressive autocrine loop may participate in prolactinoma development. As demonstrated in the following, the best-studied cp130 cytokine in pituitary is IL-6.

Expression of IL-6 in Normal and Adenomatous Pituitary

As mentioned, IL-6 not only reaches the pituitary through circulation but is intrinsically expressed and released. In normal anterior pituitary the major or even exclusive source of IL-6 are the FS cells, which have a stellate-like morphology and are able to form small intrapituitary follicles.[16–18] FS cells do not produce pituitary hormones and are immunopositive for S-100 protein and glial fibrillary acidic protein.[4] FS cells represent about 5% of all anterior pituitary cells[17,18] and form an intrapituitary network with their long cellular processes.[19,20] Through gap junctions, they are connected to each other and to the endocrine cells for which they seem to have supportive and protective roles.[4,21–23] FS cells have also been shown to remove intrapituitary cell debris by performing phagocytosis.[24] The origin of FS cells is still unclear, but it has been speculated that they might derive from dendritic immune cells, from astrocytes invading the anterior pituitary after formation of the infundibulum, or from progenitor cells (which were recently detected in adult pituitary and which differentiate to both endocrine and FS cells).[25,26] FS cells are thought to play regulating and coordinative functions on endocrine cells because they contain receptors for many growth factors, cytokines, neuropeptides, and hormones and because they secrete a number of substances, among them IL-6, affecting endocrine cell functions.[4,27–30]

In pituitary adenomas, the hormone-active and -inactive tumor cells are the source of IL-6.[31–34] They have acquired during the tumoral transformation processes the ability to produce heterogeneous amounts of IL-6 by themselves. The role of FS cells as a source of intratumoral IL-6 is still a matter of debate. With the exception of the extremely rare pituitary tumors that derive by monoclonal expansion from transformed FS cells,[35,36] it has been reported that FS cells are rare or absent in the majority of pituitary adenomas.[32,36,37] However, it has also been shown, that FS cells accumulate at the border between normal and tumoral tissue,[32,36,38] suggesting the possibility that FS-cell-derived IL-6 might diffuse into the tumor tissue to affect pituitary adenoma pathophysiology and progression.

Regulation of Intrinsic IL-6 in Pituitary and Pituitary Adenomas

Studies on the regulation of intrapituitary IL-6 have mainly been performed in the FS TtT/GF mouse pituitary tumor cell line[4,39] and have then been confirmed in FS cells of primary rat or mouse pituitary cell cultures. Human pituitary adenoma cell cultures have been used to investigate the intratumoral regulation of IL-6.

In FS cells the basal IL-6 secretion was low and was strongly stimulated by TNF-α and IL-1.[4] Both basal and stimulated IL-6 secretion was nearly completely blocked by the synthetic glucocorticoid dexamethasone.[4] Pituitary adenylate cyclase-activating polypeptide (PACAP) and vasoactive intestinal peptide enhanced IL-6 secretion in TtT/GF cells by stimulating the activity of transcription factors cAMP response element binding and alkaline phosphatase (AP)-1.[4,40] The PACAP-induced IL-6 production was inhibited by estradiol through estrogen receptor-mediated suppression of AP-1 activity.[40] Interestingly, FS cells contain the toll-like receptor 4 (Tlr4),[41] a cell-surface receptor recognizing lipopolysaccharides (LPS) of bacterial cell walls.[42] FS cells also express CD14, a cell-surface protein binding the LPS–lipopolysaccharide binding protein (LPS-LBP) complex.[41,42] LPS can directly induce in FS cells, through the LPS-LBP-CD14-Tlr4 complex, the secretion of IL-6, which then could stimulate ACTH secretion in a pituitary cell-aggregate model.[41,43] The

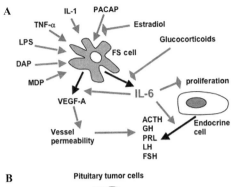

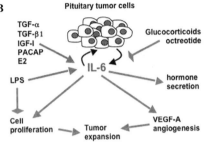

Figure 1. Overview of the regulation and role of intrapituitary interleukin (IL)-6 in normal pituitary (**A**) and in pituitary adenomas (**B**). In normal anterior pituitary (**A**), IL-6 production by folliculostellate (FS) cells is stimulated by bacterial cell-wall components [lipopolysaccharide (LPS), muramyl dipeptide (MDP), diamino pimelic acid (DAP)], tumor necrosis factor-α (TNF-α), IL-1, and pituitary adenylate cyclase-activating polypeptide (PACAP). Basic and stimulated IL-6 secretion is suppressed by glucocorticoids whereas estrogen 2 (E2) seems to inhibit only PACAP-induced IL-6. The latter blocks endocrine cell growth and stimulates the secretion of the hormones indicated. Through IL-6 stimulated vascular endothelial growth factor (VEGF)-A and subsequently increased vessel permeability, the release of hormones into the blood will be facilitated further. In pituitary adenomas (**B**), tumor cell-derived IL-6 is enhanced in varying numbers of pituitary adenomas by growth factors, PACAP, E2, and LPS. In all adenomas studied, glucocorticoids inhibited IL-6 secretion whereas the somatostatin analogue octreotide suppressed IL-6 only in a subset of tumors. IL-6 contributes to the excessive hormone secretion in endocrine-active tumors and supports tumor expansion by concomitantly stimulating tumor cell proliferation and tumor neovascularization. See text for details. (In color in *Annals* online.)

Tlr4-mediated IL-6 stimulation involved activation of the p38 MAP-kinase pathway and induction of the transcription factor nuclear factor-κB. My4 (an antibody blocking the inter-

action between LPS-LBP and CD14), the p38α MAP kinase inhibitor SB203580, and dexamethasone all strongly suppressed LPS-induced IL-6 secretion in FS cells.[41] Recently, it has been shown that FS cells express nucleotide-binding oligomerization domain (NOD)1 and NOD2,[44] which are intracellular receptors recognizing pathogen-associated molecules, such as bacterial muramyl dipeptide (MDP) and diamino pimelic acid (DAP).[45] There is first evidence that the ligands of NOD receptors can also induce IL-6 secretion in FS cells and that NOD and Tlr4 ligands synergistically activate IL-6 production (Fig. 1A).[44]

In GH-producing somatotroph pituitary tumors, transforming growth factor (TGF)-α and TGF-β1 stimulated tumoral IL-6 secretion in most adenomas whereas insulin-like growth factor-1 and PACAP only sporadically enhanced IL-6 production.[46] In a minority of somatotroph adenomas, octreotide suppressed IL-6 secretion whereas dexamethasone strongly suppressed IL-6 in all somatotroph and corticotroph pituitary adenomas studied.[46,47] Interestingly, in contrast to its inhibitory effects in FS cells, estradiol enhanced the IL-6 production in most PRL-secreting prolactinomas and PRL/GH-producing lactosomatotroph pituitary tumors,[48] which could contribute, at least in part, to the higher incidence of prolactinomas in women.[49] In about 40% of all pituitary adenoma types studied, expression of Tlr4 in subsets of the tumor cells was found and LPS strongly stimulated the IL-6 production in Tlr4-expressing tumors but had no effect in Tlr4-negative pituitary adenomas.[50] As in FS cells, dexamethasone and the p38α MAP kinase inhibitor SB203580 suppressed the LPS-induced IL-6 secretion in Tlr4-positive pituitary adenomas.[50] Interestingly, LPS did not only stimulate pituitary tumor development-supporting IL-6 but directly inhibited pituitary tumor cell growth.[50] Whether the direct antitumorigenic effect of LPS or its indirect growth-stimulatory effect through enhancing protumorigenic-acting IL-6 (see below) dominates in human pituitary adenomas during bacterial infections is not yet clear and should be clarified in future studies (Fig. 1B).

Physiological and Pathophysiological Roles of Intrapituitary IL-6

In normal anterior pituitary, the effects of intrapituitary IL-6 may mainly be linked to immune–endocrine interactions during infectious or inflammatory processes. In contrast, the constitutive IL-6 production in pituitary adenomas may contribute to the hormonal excess and progression of pituitary tumors.

IL-6 stimulates the synthesis and secretion of ACTH GH, PRL, luteinizing hormone, and follicle-stimulating hormone in normal anterior pituitary cells,[5] it suppresses the growth of normal endocrine cells,[51] and stimulates the release of VEGF-A from FS cells.[52,53] Under normal physiological conditions when the levels of systemic IL-6 and the intrapituitary production of IL-6 by FS cells are low, IL-6 may not affect hormone secretion, growth of endocrine cells, or VEGF release. During inflammatory or infectious processes, immune cell-derived TNF-α, IL-1, and IL-6 levels consecutively rise in serum. TNF-α, IL-1, and, in case of bacterial-induced infections/inflammations, bacterial cell-wall components stimulate the intrapituitary IL-6 release by FS cells.[4,42] Systemic and intrapituitary IL-6 act in concert to stimulate pituitary hormones, in particular ACTH,[3,43] which participates in inducing the HPA axis activity to produce anti-inflammatory-acting glucocorticoids. The IL-6-induced suppression of anterior pituitary cell growth[51] may serve energy that is needed for hormone synthesis and secretion during immune–endocrine interactions. The IL-6 mediated intrapituitary release of VEGF-A,[52] which is a potent stimulator of vessel permeability,[54] may locally improve the transport of hormones from endocrine cells into the blood as well as the transport of regulatory substances from the blood to the endocrine cells.

All together, the actions of IL-6 on pituitary hormone secretion, cell growth, and vessel permeability may be needed for the anterior pituitary to properly respond and to adapt to the activated immune system. It is not clear why systemically or locally produced IL-6 alone is not sufficient to mediate the intrapituitary effects. We speculate that mechanisms that are important for the survival of organisms are redundantly expressed in order to guarantee, in case of a failure in one system, the intact system will still be active. Interestingly, PACAP, an anti-inflammatory-acting peptide suppressing the production of pro-inflammatory cytokines, such as IL-6 in immune cells,[55] stimulates the intrapituitary IL-6 production by FS cells.[4] The mechanism and impact of these opposing effects of PACAP on IL-6 secretion is still not clear but may be part of the complex and still poorly understood regulatory mechanisms in immune–endocrine interactions.

In pituitary tumors, IL-6 stimulated POMC mRNA expression and ACTH secretion in human corticotroph adenomas[47] and enhanced the GH release in human somatotroph tumors.[46] In the latter, IL-6 stimulated the GH production more than growth hormone-releasing hormone (GHRH) and was active in gsp-oncogene-positive somatotropinomas in which GHRH had no stimulatory effect.[46] In addition, IL-6 was able to stimulate the PRL release in lactosomatotroph GH3 rat pituitary tumor cells.[51] Taken together, these findings clearly show that constitutively produced intratumoral IL-6 participates by autocrine/paracrine mechanisms in the excessive hormone production of endocrine-active pituitary adenomas. Interestingly, in contrast to the inhibitory action of IL-6 on the growth of normal pituitary cells,[51] IL-6 stimulates pituitary tumor cell proliferation[51,56] and differently regulates c-fos expression in pituitary adenomas.[57] The reason for these opposing effects of IL-6 on growth is not yet clear; however, IL-6 is linked through gp130 to different signaling pathways, such as the JAK/STAT pathway or the MAP kinase pathway, but gp130 also induces cytokine-signaling inhibitors, such as suppressor of cytokine signaling-3.[6] Thus, differences in the induction of activating signal pathways or stimulation of cytokine-signaling inhibitor production by the IL-6/gp130 complex may be responsible for the different mitogenic effects of IL-6 in the normal and adenomatous pituitary.

The Role of gp130 Cytokines in Pituitary Tumorigenesis

To date there is no evidence that mutations or disturbances in the expression of gp130 cytokines and their receptors play a causative role in the initiation of pituitary tumors.[49] However, their intratumoral expression and action suggests that IL-6 and other gp130 cytokines might play a role in the progression of these adenomas. This hypothesis was strongly supported by findings of pituitary tumor development in athymic nude mice.[58–60] When wild-type GH3 or MtT/S cells were injected under the skin of nude mice, these cells formed well-vascularized, large, solid tumors within 4 weeks.[59,60] However, GH3 and MtT/S cells, in which the expression of gp130 protein was downregulated by an antisense approach, formed extremely small and poorly vascularized tumors.[59,60] MtT/S cells overexpressing gp130 protein after transfecting the tumor cells with a gp130-expression plasmid also formed large tumors in which the vessel density was significantly increased in comparison to tumors generated by wild-type MtT/S cells.[60,61] From these nude-mice experiments it is evident that gp130 cytokines play a role in pituitary tumor progression, although it is not yet clear which of the different gp130 cytokines are involved in pituitary tumor progression and whether gp130 cytokines play a similar role in human pituitary adenomas. From the results of the nude-mice experiments, it seems that the gp130 cytokines stimulate tumor cell growth and intratumoral neovascularization in parallel. Regarding the latter, recently a novel protein designated as

RSUME (RWD-containing sumoylation enhancer) has been detected to be upregulated in gp130 overexpressing MtT/S cells.[61] RSUME stabilizes, through involvement in sumoylation processes, the expression of the transcription factor hypoxia-inducible factor-1α (HIF-1α),[61] which is the major inducer of angiogenesis, by stimulating the production of angiogenic factors, among them VEGF-A.[54] In future studies it needs to be determined whether gp130 cytokines can regulate the angiogenesis in human pituitary tumors through RSUME/HIF-1α and whether there are differences in these regulatory processes in microadenomas versus macroadenomas or in the different endocrine and nonendocrine types of human pituitary adenomas.

Conclusion

The gp130 cytokine IL-6 is a major regulator of immune–endocrine interactions during inflammatory or infectious processes. At the level of the pituitary, not only systemic immune-cell-derived IL-6 but also intrapituitary FS-cell-derived IL-6 affects hormone secretion, cell growth, and vascular permeability in the anterior pituitary. During transient or chronic bacterial infections, the intrapituitary IL-6 secretion is not only stimulated by circulating cytokines, such as TNF-α or IL-1, but is directly induced by bacterial cell-wall components through pathogen-recognition receptors (Tlr4, NODs) expressed in FS cells.

Regarding pituitary tumors, the intratumoral production of IL-6 contributes to excessive hormone production, growth, and neovascularization of pituitary adenomas and thus may participate considerably in adenoma pathophysiology and progression. Whether infectious or inflammatory processes and the associated rise in systemic and intratumoral IL-6 will have direct or indirect effects on pituitary adenoma progression needs to be clarified in future studies along with the probable role of gp130 cytokine-induced RSUME/HIF-1α system, which seems to be involved in pituitary tumor neovascularization. Moreover, the strong suppression of growth of gp130-deficient pituitary tumors in nude mice suggests that intratumoral receptors, signal transducers, or cell signaling components of gp130 cytokines might represent targets for the development of future pharmacological treatment concepts in pituitary adenomas.

Acknowledgments

This work was supported by a grant of the German Research Foundation (DFG: ON 79/1-1). E.A. is a member of the Consejo Nacional de Investigaciones Científicas y Técnicas, Argentina.

Conflicts of Interest

The authors declare no conflicts of interest.

References

1. Spangelo, B.L. & W.C. Gorospe. 1995. Role of the cytokines in the neuroendocrine-immune system axis. *Front. Neuroendocrinol.* **16:** 1–22.

2. Besedovsky, H.O. & A. del Rey. 1996. Immune-neuro-endocrine interactions: facts and hypotheses. *Endocr. Rev.* **17:** 64–102.

3. Chrousos, G.P. 1995. The hypothalamic-pituitary-adrenal axis and immune-mediated inflammation. *N. Engl. J. Med.* **332:** 1351–1362.

4. Renner, U., J. Gloddek, M.P. Pereda, *et al*. 1998. Regulation and role of intrapituitary IL-6 production by folliculostellate cells. *Domest. Anim. Endocrinol.* **15:** 353–362.

5. Arzt, E., M.P. Pereda, C.P. Castro, *et al*. 1999. Pathophysiological role of the cytokine network in the anterior pituitary gland. *Front. Neuroendocrinol.* **20:** 71–95.

6. Arzt, E. 2001. gp130 cytokine signalling in the pituitary gland: a paradigm for cytokine-neuroendocrine pathways. *J. Clin. Invest.* **108:** 1729–1733.

7. Graciarena, M., A. Carbia-Nagashima, C. Perez-Castro, *et al*. 2003. Pituitary gp130 cytokine networks. In *Pituitary and Periphery: Communication In and Out.* C.J. Strasburger, Ed.: 197–210. BioScientifica Ltd. Bristol, UK.

8. Vlotides, G., K. Zitzmann, S. Hengge, *et al*. 2004. Expression of novel neurotrophin-1/B-cell stimu-lating factor-3 (NNT-1/BSF-3) in murine pituitary folliculostellate TtT/GF cells: pituitary adenylate cyclase-activating polypeptide and vasoactive intestinal peptide-induced stimulation of NNT-1/BSF-3 is mediated by protein kinase A, protein kinase C, and extracellular-signal-regulated kinase 1/2 pathways. *Endocrinology* **145:** 716–727.

9. Hanisch, A., K.D. Dieterich, K. Dietzmann, *et al*. 2000. Expression of members of the interleukin-6 family of cytokines and their receptors in human pituitary and pituitary adenomas. *J. Clin. Endocrinol. Metab.* **85:** 4411–4414.

10. Perez Castro, C., A.C. Nagashima, M.P. Pereda, *et al*. 2000. The gp130 cytokines interleukin-11 and ciliary neurotropic factor regulate through specific receptors the function and growth of lactosomatotropic and folliculostellate pituitary cell lines. *Endocrinology* **141:** 1746–1753.

11. Perez Castro, C., A. Carbia Nagashima, M. Paez Pereda, *et al*. 2001. Effects of the gp130 cytokines ciliary neurotropic factor (CNTF) and interleukin-11 on pituitary cells: CNTF receptors on human pituitary adenomas and stimulation of prolactin and GH secretion in normal rat anterior pituitary aggregate cultures. *J. Endocrinol.* **169:** 539–547.

12. Auernammer, C.J. & S. Melmed. 1999. Leukemia inhibitory factor—neuroimmune modulator of endocrine function. *Endocr. Rev.* **21:** 313–345.

13. Kontogeorgos, G., H. Patralexis, A. Tran, *et al*. 2000. Expression of leukemia inhibitory factor in human pituitary adenomas: a morphologic and immunocytochemical study. *Pituitary* **2:** 245–251.

14. Yano, H., C. Readhead, M. Nakashima, *et al*. 1998. Pituitary-directed leukemia inhibitory factor transgene causes Cushing's syndrome: neuro-immune-endocrine modulation of pituitary development. *Mol. Endocrinol.* **12:** 1708–1720.

15. Ben-Shlomo, A., I. Miklovsky, S.-G. Ren, *et al*. 2003. Leukemia inhibitory factor regulates prolactin secretion in prolactinoma and lactotroph cells. *J. Clin. Endocrinol. Metab.* **88:** 858–863.

16. Rinehart, J.F. & M.G. Farquhar. 1953. Electron microscopic studies of the anterior pituitary gland. *J. Histochem. Cytochem.* **1:** 93–113

17. Inoue, K., E.F. Couch, K. Takano, *et al*. 1999. The structure and function of folliculo-stellate cells in the anterior pituitary gland. *Archiv. Histol. Cytol.* **62:** 205–218.

18. Allaerts, W. & H. Vankelecom. 2005. History and perspectives of pituitary folliculo-stellate cell research. *Eur. J. Endocrinol.* **153:** 1–12.

19. Fauquier, T., N.C. Guerineau, R.A. McKinney, *et al*. 2001. Folliculostellate cell network: a route for long-distance communication in the anterior pituitary. *Proc. Natl. Acad. Sci. USA* **98:** 8891–8896.

20. Fauquier, T., A. Lacampagne, P. Travo, *et al.* 2002. Hidden face of the anterior pituitary. *Trends Endocrinol. Metab.* **13:** 304–309.

21. Morand, I., P. Fonlupt, A. Guerrier, *et al.* 1996. Cell-to-cell communication in the anterior pituitary: evidence for gap junctions-mediated exchanges between endocrine cells and folliculostellate cells. *Endocrinology* **137:** 3356–3367.

22. Lewis, B.M., A. Pexa, K. Francis, *et al.* 2006. Adenosine stimulates connexin 43 expression and gap junctional communication in pituitary folliculostellate cells. *FASEB J.* **20:** 2585–2587.

23. Meilleur, M.A., C.D. Akpovi, R.M. Pelletier, *et al.* 2007. Tumor necrosis factor-alpha-induced anterior pituitary folliculostellate TtT/GF cell uncoupling is mediated by connexin 43 dephosphorylation. *Endocrinology* **148:** 5913–5924.

24. Aoki, A., E.O. de Gaisan, H.A. Pasolli, *et al.* 1996. Disposal of cell debris from surplus lactotrophs of pituitary gland. *Exp. Clin. Endocrinol. Diabetes* **104:** 256–262.

25. Allaerts, W., P.H.M. Jeucken, R. Debets, *et al.* 1997. Heterogeneity of pituitary folliculo-stellate cells: implications for IL-6 production and accessory function in vitro. *J. Neuroendocrinol.* **9:** 43–53.

26. Fauquier, T., K. Rizzoti, M. Dattani, *et al.* 2008. SOX2-expressing progenitor cells generate all of the major cell types in the adult mouse pituitary gland. *Proc. Natl. Acad. Sci. USA* **105:** 2907–2912.

27. Vankelecom, H., P. Carmeliet, J. Van Damme, *et al.* 1989. Production of interleukin-6 by folliculo-stellate cells of the anterior pituitary gland in a histiotypic cell aggregate culture system. *Neuroendocrinology* **49:** 102–106.

28. Vankelecom, H., P. Matthys, J. Van Damme, *et al.* 1993. Immunocytochemical evidence that S-100 positive cells of the mouse anterior pituitary contain interleukin-6 immunoreactivity. *J. Histochem. Cytochem.* **41:** 151–156.

29. Prummel, M.F., L.J.S. Brokken, G. Meduri, *et al.* 2000. Expression of the thyroid-stimulating hormone receptor in the folliculo-stellate cells of the human anterior pituitary. *J. Clin. Endocrinol. Metab.* **85:** 4347–4353.

30. Herkenham, M. 2005. Folliculo-stellate (FS) cells of the anterior pituitary mediate interactions between the endocrine and immune systems. *Endocrinology* **146:** 33–34.

31. Ueta, Y., A. Levy, H.S. Chowdrey, *et al.* 1995. S-100 antigen-positive folliculostellate cells are not the source of IL-6 gene expression in human pituitary adenomas. *J. Neuroendocrinol.* **7:** 467–474.

32. Marin, F., K. Kovacs, L. Stefaneanu, *et al.* 1992. S-100 protein immunopositivity in human nontu-morous hypophyses and pituitary adenomas. *Endocr. Pathol.* **3:** 28–38.

33. Jones, T.H., M. Daniels, R.A. James, *et al.* 1994. Production of bioactive and immunoreactive interleukin-6 (IL-6) and expression of IL-6 messenger ribonucleic acid by human pituitary adenomas. *J. Clin. Endocrinol. Metab.* **78:** 180–187.

34. Borg, S.A., K.E. Kerry, L. Baxter, *et al.* 2003. Expression of interleukin-6 and its effect on growth of HP75 human pituitary tumor cells. *J. Clin. Endocrinol. Metab.* **88:** 4938–4944.

35. Roncaroli, F., B.W. Scheithauer, G. Cenacchi, *et al.* 2002. "Spindle cell oncocytoma" of the adenohypophysis: a tumor of folliculostellate cells? *Am. J. Surg. Pathol.* **26:** 1048–1055.

36. Höfler, H., G.F. Walter & H. Denk. 1984. Immunohistochemistry of folliculo-stellate cells in normal human adenohypophyses and in pituitary adenomas. *Acta Neuropathol.* **65:** 35–40.

37. Yamashita, M., Z.R. Quia, T. Sano, *et al.* 2005. Immunohistochemical study on so-called follicular cells and folliculostellate cells in the human adenohypophysis. *Pathol. Int.* **55:** 244–247.

38. Farnoud, M.R., M. Kujas, P. Derome, *et al.* 1994. Interactions between normal and tumoral tissues at the boundary of human pituitary adenomas. *Virch. Arch.* **424:** 75–82.

39. Inoue, K., H. Matsumoto, C. Koyama, *et al.* 1992. Establishment of a folliculostellate-like cell line from a murine thyrotropic pituitary tumor. *Endocrinology* **131:** 3110–3116.

40. Carbia Nagashima, A., D. Giacomini, C. Perez Castro, *et al.* 2003. Transcriptional regulation of interleukin-6 in pituitary folliculo-stellate TtT/GF cells. *Mol. Cell. Endocrinol.* **201:** 47–56.

41. Lohrer, P., J. Gloddek, A.C. Nagashima, *et al.* 2000. Lipopolysaccharide directly stimulates the intrapituitary interleukin-6 production by folliculostellate cells via specific receptors and the p38alpha mitogen-activated protein kinase/nuclear factor-kappaB pathway. *Endocrinology* **141:** 4457–4465.

42. Akira, S., K. Takeda & T. Kaisho. 2001. Toll-like receptors: critical proteins linking innate and acquired immunity. *Nat. Immunol.* **2:** 675–680.

43. Gloddek, J., P. Lohrer, J. Stalla, *et al.* 2001. The intrapituitary stimulatory effect of lipopolysaccharide on ACTH secretion is mediated by paracrine-acting IL-6. *Exp. Clin. Endocrinol. Diabetes* **109:** 410–415.

44. Correa-de-Santana, E., M. Theodoropoulou, M. Paez-Pereda, *et al.* 2007. Expression and functionality of NOD molecules in the adenopituitary folliculostellate cells. *Exp. Clin. Endocrinol. Diabetes* **115:** 548.

45. Fritz, J.H., R.L. Ferrero, D.J. Philpott, *et al*. 2006. Nod-like proteins in immunity, inflammation and disease. *Nat. Immunol.* **7:** 1250–1257.

46. Thiele, J.-O., P. Lohrer, L. Schaaf, *et al*. 2003. Functional in vitro studies on the role and regulation of interleukin-6 in human somatotroph pituitary adenomas. *Eur. J. Endocrinol.* **149:** 455–461.

47. Paez Pereda, M., P. Lohrer, D. Kovalovsky, *et al*. 2000. Interleukin-6 is inhibited by glucocorticoids and stimulates ACTH secretion and POMC expression in human corticotroph pituitary adenomas. *Exp. Clin. Endocrinol. Diabetes* **108:** 202–207.

48. Onofri, C., A. Carbia Nagashima, L. Schaaf, *et al*. 2004. Estradiol stimulates vascular endothelial growth factor and interleukin-6 in human lactotroph and lactosomatotroph pituitary adenomas. *Exp. Clin. Endocrinol. Diabetes* **112:** 18–23.

49. Asa, S.L. & S. Ezzat. 1998. The cytogenesis and pathogenesis of pituitary adenomas. *Endocr. Rev.* **19:** 798–827.

50. Tichomirowa, M., M. Theodoropoulou, P. Lohrer, *et al*. 2005. Bacterial endotoxin (lipopolysaccharide) stimulates interleukin-6 production and inhibits growth of pituitary tumour cells expressing the Toll-like receptor 4. *J. Neuroendocrinol.* **17:** 152–160.

51. Arzt, E., R. Buric, G. Stelzer, *et al*. 1993. Interleukin involvement in anterior pituitary cell growth regulation: effects of interleukin-2 (IL-2) and IL-6. *Endocrinology* **132:** 459–467.

52. Gloddek, J., U. Pagotto, M. Paez Pereda, *et al*. 1999. Pituitary adenylate cyclase-activating polypeptide, interleukin-6 and glucocorticoids regulate the release of vascular endothelial growth factor in pituitary folliculostellate cells. *J. Endocrinol.* **160:** 483–490.

53. Lohrer, P., J. Gloddek, U. Hopfner, *et al*. 2001. Vascular endothelial growth factor production and regulation in rodent and human pituitary tumor cells in vitro. *Neuroendocrinology* **74:** 95–105.

54. Ferrara, N. 2004. Vascular endothelial growth factor: basic science and clinical progress. *Endocr. Rev.* **25:** 581–611.

55. Gomariz, R.P., Y. Juarranz, C. Abad, *et al*. 2006. VIP-PACAP system in immunity: new insights for multitarget therapy. *Ann. N. Y. Acad. Sci.* **1070:** 51–74.

56. Sawada, T., K. Koike, Y. Kanda, *et al*. 1995. IL-6 stimulates cell proliferation of rat anterior pituitary clonal cell lines in vitro. *J. Endocrinol. Invest.* **18:** 83–90.

57. Paez Pereda, M., V. Goldberg, A. Chervin, *et al*. 1996. Interleukin-2 (IL-2) and IL-6 regulate c-fos protooncogene expression in human pituitary adenoma explants. *Mol. Cell. Endocrinol.* **124:** 33–42.

58. Koyama, C., H. Matsumoto, T. Sakai, *et al*. 1995. Pituitary folliculo-stellate-like cells stimulate somatotropic pituitary growth in nude mice. *Endocr. Pathol.* **6:** 67–75.

59. Castro, C.P., D. Giacomini, A.C. Nagashima, *et al*. 2003. Reduced expression of the cytokine transducer gp130 inhibits hormone secretion, cell growth, and tumor development in pituitary lactosomatotrophic GH3 cells. *Endocrinology* **144:** 693–700.

60. Graciarena, M., A. Carbia-Nagashima, C. Onofri, *et al*. 2004. Involvement of the gp130 cytokine transducer in MtT/S somatotroph tumour development in an autocrine-paracrine model. *Eur. J. Endocrinol.* **151:**595–604.

61. Carbia-Nagashima, A., J. Gerez, C. Perez-Castro, *et al*. 2007. RSUME, a small RWD-containing protein, enhances SUMO conjugation and stabilizes HIF-1a during hypoxia. *Cell* **131:** 309–323.

The Thymus–Neuroendocrine Axis

Physiology, Molecular Biology, and Therapeutic Potential of the Thymic Peptide Thymulin

Paula C. Reggiani,[a,b,]* Gustavo R. Morel,[a,b,]*
Gloria M. Cónsole,[b] Claudio G. Barbeito,[c]
Silvia S. Rodriguez,[a,b] Oscar A. Brown,[a,b] Maria Jose Bellini,[a,b]
Jean-Marie Pléau,[d] Mireille Dardenne,[d] and Rodolfo G. Goya[a,b]

[a]Institute for Biochemical Research, Faculty of Medicine, CONICET, National University of La Plata, La Plata, Argentina

[b]Histology B- Scientific Research Commission of the Province of Buenos Aires, Faculty of Medicine, National University of La Plata, La Plata, Argentina

[c]Faculty of Veterinary Medicine, National University of La Plata, La Plata, Argentina

[d]Centre National de la Recherche Scientifique UMR 8147, Université Paris V, Hôpital Necker, Paris, France

Thymulin is a thymic hormone exclusively produced by the thymic epithelial cells. It consists of a nonapeptide component coupled to the ion zinc, which confers biological activity to the molecule. After its discovery in the early 1970s, thymulin was characterized as a thymic hormone involved in several aspects of intrathymic and extrathymic T cell differentiation. Subsequently, it was demonstrated that thymulin production and secretion is strongly influenced by the neuroendocrine system. Conversely, a growing core of information, to be reviewed here, points to thymulin as a hypophysotropic peptide. In recent years, interest has arisen in the potential use of thymulin as a therapeutic agent. Thymulin was shown to possess anti-inflammatory and analgesic properties in the brain. Furthermore, an adenoviral vector harboring a synthetic gene for thymulin, stereotaxically injected in the rat brain, achieved a much longer expression than the adenovirally mediated expression in the brain of other genes, thus suggesting that an anti-inflammatory activity of thymulin prevents the immune system from destroying virus-transduced brain cells. Other studies suggest that thymulin gene therapy may also be a suitable therapeutic strategy to prevent some of the endocrine and metabolic alterations that typically appear in thymus-deficient animal models. The present article briefly reviews the literature on the physiology, molecular biology, and therapeutic potential of thymulin.

Key words: thymulin; neuroendocrine control; hypophysiotropic activity; artificial gene; gene therapy; anti-inflammatory; ovarian dysgenesis

Relevance of the Thymus in the Immune–Neuroendocrine Homeostatic Network

Address for correspondence: Rodolfo G. Goya, INIBIOLP, Faculty of Medicine, UNLP, CC 455, 1900 La Plata, Argentina. Voice: 54-221-425-6735; fax: 54-221-425-0924/425-8988. rgoya@netverk.com.ar (please CC to preggiani@fcm.uncu.edu.ar)

*These two authors contributed equally to this work.

The immune system is functionally linked to the nervous and endocrine systems thus constituting an integrated homeostatic network.[1] Within this network, the neuroendocrine

Neuroimmunomodulation: Ann. N.Y. Acad. Sci. 1153: 98–106 (2009).
doi: 10.1111/j.1749-6632.2008.03964.x © 2009 New York Academy of Sciences.

system monitors and controls the physical and chemical variables of the internal milieu. On its part, the immune system perceives, through antigenic recognition, an internal image of the macromolecular and cellular components of the body and reacts to alterations of this image, effectively participating in the "biological" homeostasis of the organism.

In mammals, the interaction of the thymus gland with the neuroendocrine system seems to be particularly important during perinatal life when the thymus and the neuroendocrine system influence the maturation of each other. This was initially suggested by early findings showing that in species in which neonatal thymectomy does not produce any evident impairment of immune capacity,[2] neuroendocrine functions are already highly developed at birth.[3] In mice, the importance of the thymus for proper maturation of the neuroendocrine system is revealed by the endocrine alterations caused by neonatal thymectomy or congenital absence of the thymus. In effect, congenitally athymic (nude) female mice show significantly reduced levels of circulating and pituitary gonadotropins, a fact that seems to be causally related to a number of reproductive derangements described in these mutants.[4] Thus, in homozygous (nu/nu) females the times of vaginal opening and first ovulation are delayed,[5] fertility is reduced,[4] and follicular atresia is increased such that premature ovarian failure results.[6] Similar abnormalities result from neonatal thymectomy of normal female mice.[7,8] Ovaries of athymic mice respond normally to exogenous gonadotropins, suggesting that the defect is at the level of the hypothalamic–pituitary axis.[9,10] In homozygous, adult, nude CD-1, male mice, thyrotropin (TSH), prolactin (PRL), growth hormone (GH), and gonadotropin responses to immobilization and cold stress are reduced as also are serum basal levels of the same hormones compared to the heterozygous counterparts.[11–13] A functional impairment of the hypothalamic–adrenal axis has been reported in nude mice, suggesting that humoral thymic factors may play a role in the maturation of this axis.[14]

The influence of the neuroendocrine system on thymus (and immune) function seems to continue during adult life either through a direct action of pituitary hormones or via peripheral hormones, both of which act on the thymic epithelial cells (TEC) and/or on immature thymocytes within the gland (for a review, see Ref. 15).

Thymulin

Thymulin is a thymic metallopeptide involved in several aspects of intrathymic and extrathymic T cell differentiation.[16] Thymulin, which is exclusively produced by the thymic epithelial cells,[17] consists of a biologically inactive nonapeptide component termed *FTS* (an acronym for serum thymus factor in French) coupled in an equimolecular ratio to the ion zinc,[18] which confers biological activity to the molecule.[19] The metallopeptide active form bears a specific molecular conformation that has been evidenced by nuclear magnetic resonance.[20]

Neuroendocrine Control of Thymulin Production

The control of thymulin secretion seems to be dependent on a complex network of events. Initial studies showed that the hormone itself exerts a controlling feedback effect on its own secretion both *in vivo* and *in vitro*.[21,22] Additionally, thymulin production and secretion is influenced directly or indirectly by the neuroendocrine system. For instance, GH can influence thymulin synthesis and secretion. *In vitro*, human GH can stimulate thymulin release from TEC lines,[23] which are known to possess specific receptors for GH.[24] Animal studies have shown that treatment of aged dogs with bovine GH partially restored their low thymulin serum levels.[25] In old mice, treatment with ovine GH increased their low circulating thymulin levels and enhanced the concanavalin A-dependent proliferative response of their thymocytes as well as interleukin-6 production.[26] In old rats, combined treatment with GH and thyroxine (T$_4$) was also able to partially restore their reduced thymulin levels.[27] In clinical studies, it was reported that in congenitally GH-deficient children who consistently exhibited low plasma thymulin levels GH therapy succeeded in increasing thymic hormone levels to near normal values.[28] Acromegalic middle-aged patients have elevated thymulin serum levels compared to age-matched normal subjects.[23,28] It is likely that these effects of GH are mediated, at least in part, by insulin-like growth factor 1 (IGF-1) as suggested by the fact that the GH-induced enhancement of thymulin production could be prevented by previous treatment with antibodies against IGF-1 or IGF-1 receptor.[23]

There is also evidence for a PRL–thymulin axis. Thus, it is known that TEC possess PRL receptors[29] and that PRL can stimulate thymulin synthesis and secretion both *in vitro* and *in vivo*.[30] Furthermore, administration of PRL to old mice elevated their reduced circulating levels of thymulin.[30]

The thyroid axis also influences thymulin secretion. Thus, T$_4$ has been shown to stimulate thymulin synthesis and secretion in mice.[31] *In vivo* treatment of mice with triiodothyronine enhanced thymulin secretion, whereas treatment of the animals with propylthiouracil, an inhibitor of thyroid hormone synthesis, decreased their circulating thymulin levels.[32] In humans, hyperthyroidism brings about an increase in circulating thymulin levels, whereas hypothyroid patients show depressed levels of this thymic hormone.[33] In *in vitro* studies, it was shown that thyroid hormones stimulate thymulin secretion by a direct action on TEC.[34,35] Interestingly, it has been shown that treatment of aged animals with T$_4$ can reverse their decreased thymulin levels.[31,35]

Although there are no studies documenting a direct effect of gonadotropins or adrenocorticotropic hormone (ACTH) on thymulin secretion, gonadectomy or adrenalectomy in mice is known to induce a transient decrease in serum thymulin levels. This effect is potentiated by the simultaneous removal of the adrenals and gonads.[34] In TEC cultures it was shown that exposure to physiological levels of glucocorticoids or gonadal steroids enhanced thymulin concentration in the cell supernatants.[36,37]

Although there is no rigorous evidence proving the existence of hypothalamic factors able to influence thymulin production by a direct action on TEC, there are two studies that suggest that this may be the case. Treatment of old mice with hypothalamic extracts from young mice resulted in the reappearance of detectable levels of circulating thymulin.[38] Hypothalamic and pituitary extracts from young mice stimulated thymulin release from TEC cultures, but this stimulation declined when the pituitary and hypothalamic extracts were obtained from old mice.[39]

Hypophysiotropic Activity of Thymulin

The multilateral influence that the neuroendocrine system exerts on thymulin secretion suggests that this metallopeptide could, in turn, be part of a feedback loop acting on neuroendocrine structures. This possibility is now supported by a significant body of evidence indicating that thymulin possesses hypophysiotropic activity. Thus, thymulin has been shown to stimulate luteinizing hormone (LH) release from perifused rat pituitaries[40] and ACTH from incubated rat pituitary fragments, the latter being an effect mediated by intracellular cAMP and cGMP accumulation.[41] In an *in vitro* study using pituitary cells obtained from female rats in different days of the estrous cycle, it was observed that thymulin modulates the stimulatory activity of gonadotropin-releasing hormone on LH and follicle-stimulating hormone (FSH) release.[42] Thymulin has been found to stimulate GH, PRL, TSH, and gonadotropin release in dispersed rat pituitary cells at doses from 10^{-8} to 10^{-3} mol/L,[43-45] whereas others have reported that thymulin doses of 10^{-11} mol/L stimulate LH, inhibit PRL release, and have no effect on GH secretion in incubated rat pituitary fragments.[40] The stimulatory effect of thymulin on hormone release in rat pituitary cells declines with the age of the cell donor, which suggests that aging brings about a desensitization of the pituitary gland to thymic signals.[43-45]

There is *in vitro* and *in vivo* evidence suggesting that thymulin plays a role in the regulation of female spontaneous puberty, possibly through effects on pituitary gonadotropin release and ovarian steroidogenesis.[40,42,44-47] Thymulin also modulates gonadotropin-induced testicular steroidogenesis.[48]

Recent immunoneutralization studies have strengthened the hypothesis that thymulin is a physiological mediator of the perinatal influence of the thymus on neuroendocrine maturation. Thus, neonatal immunoneutralization of circulating thymulin in otherwise normal C57BL/6 mice induced significant morphologic alterations in most anterior pituitary endocrine cell populations when the animals reached puberty.[49] Thymulin immunoneutralization from birth to puberty in normal mice also induced serum gonadotropin[50] and serum TSH, PRL, and GH reduction (Goya *et al.*, unpublished results) when the animals reached puberty.

Construction of Synthetic Genes for Thymulin

The prospect of implementing thymic hormone gene therapy appears as an interesting avenue of research aimed at restoring endocrine thymic activity when thymus function is compromised. However, none of the genes coding for the known thymic peptides have been cloned, a situation that hinders the implementation of gene or other molecular therapies for thymic hormones. It was suggested that a possible way to overcome this problem could be to construct "artificial genes" coding for those thymic peptides whose amino acid sequences were short and required no posttranslational processing.[51] This has been recently achieved for thymulin and the corresponding DNA sequence cloned in a recombinant adenoviral (RAd) vector that was subsequently used in a number of experimental gene therapy studies (see below).

In an early study aimed at upscaling thymulin production, a synthetic DNA sequence coding for FTS was inserted into a bacterial expression vector and successfully used to obtain large quantities of purified thymulin retaining full biological activity.[52] More recently, a DNA sequence coding for the biologically active FTS analogue called *metFTS* was constructed and cloned in an adenoviral vector.[53] The design of the DNA sequence for metFTS was optimized for expression in rat systems by choosing, for each amino acid of the native peptide, the codon more frequently used by rat cells (Fig. 1A). A variant of this sequence was used to construct RAd-metFTS, an adenoviral vector that harbors the synthetic gene for metFTS driven by the mouse cytomegalovirus promoter (PmCMV) (Fig. 1B and C). When intramuscularly (i.m.) administered to thymectomized (Tx) mice and rats (whose circulating levels of thymulin are nondetectable), RAd-metFTS induced sustained supraphysiological serum levels of biologically active thymulin that remained high for at least 112 days in mice[53] and for over 320 days in rats. Interestingly, adenovirally mediated expression of the synthetic gene for metFTS in the substantia nigra and hypothalamus of adult Tx rats had a significantly longer duration than adenovirally mediated expression of the gene for green fluorescent protein or *Escherichia coli* β-galactosidase in the same brain regions.[54] This phenomenon could be a result of the anti-inflammatory activity in the brain reported for thymulin and some thymulin analogues.[55,56] Additionally, results from experiments using intracerebroventricular injection of thymulin in rats with experimentally induced brain inflammation

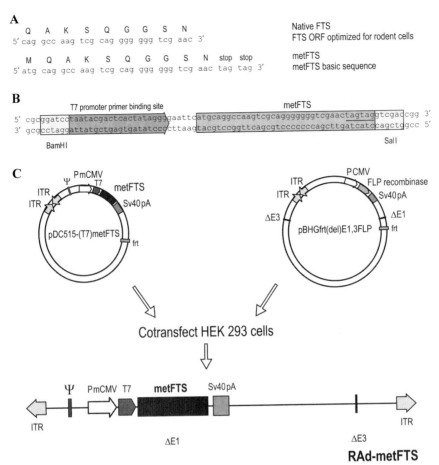

Figure 1. DNA constructs encoding the biologically active serum thymus factor (FTS) analogue (metFTS) and assembly of an adenoviral vector (RAd-metFTS) that harbors the synthetic gene for metFTS. A DNA sequence coding for native FTS was designed for optimal expression in rat cells. By adding an ATG starting codon upstream and two stop codons downstream of this sequence, it was converted into an open reading frame (ORF) for the analogue metFTS (**A**). This metFTS ORF was used to generate a construct to be cloned in the shuttle vector pDC515. The construct included the phage T7 promoter primer-binding site, which was used for sequencing purposes (**B**). The shuttle pDC515-metFTS was generated by inserting the T7-metFTS sequence into the BamHI and SalI sites of the multiple cloning site of the shuttle pDC515. This construct was used to generate RAd-metFTS (**C**). PmCMV, mouse cytomegalovirus promoter; frt, recognition element for the yeast FLP recombinase; ITR, inverted terminal repeats; ΔE1 and ΔE3, deletions in the Ad5 genome; SV40, simian virus 40 polyadenylation signal; ψ, packaging signal. From Ref. 50, used with permission.

suggested that this peptide has a neuroprotective role in the central nervous system and indicate a possible therapeutic use as analgesic and anti-inflammatory drug.[57] The anti-inflammatory activity could prevent the immune system of the vector-injected animals from mounting a destructive response against the transduced cells. The same rationale could explain the long-term persistence of high concentrations of transgenic metFTS in the circulation of RAd-metFTS-injected Tx rodents.[53] Because thymulin has no known toxic effects even at high doses, i.m. injection of RAd-metFTS could generate sustained pharmacologically effective levels of serum and brain thymulin for the amelioration of pathologies involving chronic brain inflammation. This would represent a distinct advantage over alternative anti-inflammatory approaches that use direct brain injection of viral vectors that block the production or actions of pro-inflammatory cytokines.[58]

Gene Therapy for Thymulin

Neonatal Thymulin Gene Therapy Prevents the Disruptive Impact of Athymia on the Reproductive System of Female Mice

A single i.m. injection of RAd-metFTS in newborn nude mice (nude mice have undetectable circulating levels of thymulin) elicited long-term restoration of serum thymulin in these mutants. This treatment was able to prevent the deficits in serum LH and FSH that typically appear in adult female nude mice.[50] Furthermore, neonatal thymulin gene therapy in nude female mice has been found to significantly prevent the ovarian dysgenesis that usually develops in 70-day-old, female, nude mice.[59]

Effect of Neonatal Thymulin Gene Therapy on the Metabolic Dyshomeostasis in Nude Mice

There is evidence that the endocrine thymus may participate in glucose homeostasis. Thus, it has been reported that after 1 month of age, nude BALB/c mice develop spontaneous hyperglycemia and impaired glucose tolerance.[60,61] Furthermore, these animals show peripheral insulin insensitivity with normal pancreatic β-cell reserves and normal lean body mass.[62] Assessment of pancreatic islet-cell populations in hyperglycemic nude mice revealed an increase in the D cell population (somatostatin producing). Also, somatostatin content in pancreatic tissue was higher in the athymic nude mice compared to heterozygous sex- and age-matched counterparts.[63] Adult thymectomy in Wistar rats was reported to in-

crease circulating insulin levels without significant changes in blood glucose.[64] Other studies point to a modulatory activity of thymic factors on lipid metabolism. Thus, a thymic protein factor was reported to reduce serum cholesterol levels in rodents, increase low-density lipoprotein catabolism, and inhibit the activity of hepatic 3-hydroxy-3-methylglutaryl (HMG)-CoA reductase, the rate-limiting enzyme in cholesterol synthesis.[65–67] In adult nude mice it has been reported that the relative percentage of 16:0, 18:1 n9, and 18:1 n7 fatty acids is lower whereas that of 18:0, 20:4 n6, and 22:6 n3 fatty acids is higher in hepatic phospholipids of nu/nu animals compared to nu/+ counterparts. Some of these alterations were completely or partially prevented by neonatal thymulin gene therapy.[68] Neonatal thymulin gene therapy completely prevented the adult-onset hyperglycemia of 70-day-old nude mice (Garcia-Bravo *et al.*, unpublished results).

Concluding Remarks

Thymulin is probably the best characterized of all putative thymic hormones and seems to play a physiological role in thymus–pituitary communication, particularly during perinatal life. Interest in the therapeutic use of thymulin flourished during the 1970s and 1980s when efforts were almost exclusively focused on using thymulin (and other thymic peptides) for the treatment of autoimmune and other immunopathologies as well as cancer.[69,70] Subsequent studies, most of them carried out during the last 15 years, established that thymulin is active on the hypophysis and the brain. This awareness and the recent availability of a synthetic gene for metFTS have opened new avenues for the exploration and eventual exploitation of the therapeutic potential of this metallopeptide.

Acknowledgments

Part of the work from our laboratory reviewed here was supported by National

Institutes of Health Grant #R01AG029798 and Grant #PICT38214 from the National Agency for the Promotion of Science and Technology to RGG and by the Argentine Research Council (CONICET) and the Institut National de la Santé et de la Recherche Médicale (INSERM), France, to M.D. and R.G.G. R.G.G., O.A.B., and C.G.B. are CONICET career researchers. G.M.C. is a career researcher of the Scientific Research Commission of the Province of Buenos Aires (CIC-PBA).

Conflicts of Interest

The authors declare no conflicts of interest.

References

1. Goya, R.G. 1991. The immune-neuroendocrine homeostatic network and ageing. *Gerontology* **37:** 208–213.

2. Solomon, J.B. 1971. Ontogeny of defined immunity in mammals. In *Foetal and Neonatal Immunology. Frontiers of Biology*, Vol. 20. A. Neuberger & E.L. Tatum, Eds.: 234–306. American Elsevier Publishing Co. New York.

3. Jost, A. 1969. The extent of foetal and endocrine autonomy. In *Foetal Autonomy. Ciba Foundation Symposium*. G.E.W. Wolstenholme & M. O'Connor, Eds.: 79–94. Churchill. London.

4. Rebar, R.W., I.C. Morandini, G.F. Erickson, *et al.* 1981. The hormonal basis of reproductive defects in athymic mice. *Endocrinology* **108:** 120–126.

5. Besedovsky, H.O. & E. Sorkin. 1974. Thymus involvement in female sexual maturation. *Nature* **249:** 356–358.

6. Lintern-Moore, S. & E.M. Pantelouris. 1975. Ovarian development in athymic nude mice. I. The size and composition of the follicle population. *Mech. Age. Dev.* **4:** 385–390.

7. Michael, S.D., O. Taguchi & Y. Nishizuka. 1980. Effects of neonatal thymectomy on ovarian development and plasma LH, FSH, GH and PRL in the mouse. *Biol. Reprod.* **22:** 343–350.

8. Nishizuka, Y. & T. Sakakura. 1971. Ovarian dysgenesis induced by neonatal thymectomy in the mouse. *Endocrinology* **89:** 889–893.

9. Pierpaoli, W. & H.O. Besedovsky. 1975. Role of the thymus in programming of neuroendocrine functions. *Clin. Exp. Immunol.* **20:** 323–328.

10. Lintern-Moore, S. & E.M. Pantelouris. 1976. Ovarian development in athymic nude mice. III. The effect of PMSG and oestradiol upon the size and composition of the ovarian follicle population. *Mech. Ageing. Dev.* **5:** 33–38.

11. Goya, R.G., G.M. Cónsole, Y.E. Sosa, *et al.* 2001. Altered functional responses with preserved morphology of gonadotrophic cells in congenitally athymic mice. *Brain Behav. Immun.* **15:** 85–92.

12. Goya, R.G., Y.E. Sosa, G.M. Cónsole, *et al.* 1995. Altered thyrotropic and somatotropic responses to environmental challenges in congenitally athymic mice. *Brain Behav. Immun.* **9:** 79–86.

13. Goya, R.G., Y.E. Sosa, G.M. Cónsole, *et al.* 1996. Altered regulation of serum prolactin in nude mice. *Med. Sci. Res.* **24:** 279–280.

14. Daneva, T., E. Spinedi, R. Hadid, *et al.* 1995. Impaired hypothalamo-pituitary-adrenal axis function in swiss nude athymic mice. *Neuroendocrinology* **62:** 79–86.

15. Savino, W. & M. Dardenne. 2000. Neuroendocrine control of thymus physiology. *Endocrine Rev.* **21:** 412–443.

16. Bach, J.F. 1983. Thymulin (FTS-Zn). *Clin. Immunol. Allergy* **3:** 133–156.

17. Dardenne, M., M. Papiernik, J.F. Bach, *et al.* 1974. Studies on thymus products. III. Epithelial origin of the serum thymic factor. *Immunology* **27:** 299–304.

18. Gastinel, L.N., M. Dardenne, J.M. Pléau, *et al.* 1984. Studies on the zinc-binding site to the serum thymic factor. *Biochim. Biophys. Acta* **797:** 147–155.

19. Dardenne, M., B. Nabarra & P. Lefrancier. 1982. Contribution of zinc and other metals to the biological activity of serum thymic factor (FTS). *Proc. Natl. Acad. Sci. USA* **79:** 5370–5373.

20. Cung, M.T., M. Marraud, P. Lefrancier, *et al.* 1988. NMR study of a lymphocyte differentiating thymic factor. *J. Biol. Chem.* **263:** 5574–5580.

21. Savino, W., M. Dardenne & J.F. Bach. 1983. Thymic hormones containing cells. III. Evidence for a feedback regulation of the secretion of the serum thymic factor (FTS) by thymic epithelial cells. *Clin. Exp. Immunol.* **52:** 7–12.

22. Cohen, S., S. Berrih, M. Dardenne, *et al.* 1986. Feedback regulation of the secretion of a thymic hormone (thymulin) by human thymic epithelial cells in culture. *Thymus* **8:** 109–119.

23. Timsit, J., W. Savino, B. Safieh, *et al.* 1992. GH and IGF-I stimulate hormonal function and proliferation of thymic epithelial cells. *J. Clin. Endocrinol. Metab.* **75:** 183–188.

24. Ban, E., M.C. Gagnerault, H. Jammes, *et al.* 1991. Specific binding sites for growth hormone in cultured mouse thymic epithelial cells. *Life Sci.* **48:** 2141–2148.

25. Goff, B.L., J.A. Roth, L.H. Arp, et al. 1987. Growth hormone treatment stimulates thymulin production in aged dogs. Clin. Exp. Immunol. **68:** 580–587.

26. Goya, R.G., M.C. Gagnerault, M.C. Leite de Moraes, et al. 1992. In vivo effects of growth hormone on thymus function in aging mice. Brain Behav. Immun. **6:** 341–354.

27. Goya, R.G., M.C. Gagnerault, Y.E. Sosa, et al. 1993. Effects of growth hormone and thyroxine on thymulin secretion in aging rats. Neuroendocrinology **58:** 338–343.

28. Mocchegiani, E., P. Paolucci, A. Balsamo, et al. 1990. Influence of growth hormone on thymic endocrine activity in humans. Horm. Res. **33:** 7–14.

29. Dardenne, M., P.A. Kelly, J.F. Bach, et al. 1991. Identification and functional activity of Prl receptors in thymic epithelial cells. Proc. Natl. Acad. Sci. USA **88:** 9700–9704.

30. Dardenne, M., W. Savino, M.C. Gagnerault, et al. 1989. Neuroendocrine control of thymic hormonal production. I. Prolactin stimulates in vivo and in vitro the production of thymulin by human and murine thymic epithelial cells. Endocrinology **125:** 3–12.

31. Fabris, N. & E. Mocchegiani. 1985. Endocrine control of thymic serum factor production in young-adult and old mice. Cell. Immunol. **91:** 325–335.

32. Savino, W., B. Wolf, S. Aratan-Spire, et al. 1984. Thymic hormone containing cells. IV. Fluctuations in the thyroid hormone levels in vivo can modulate the secretion of thymulin by the epithelial cells of young mouse thymus. Clin. Exp. Immunol. **55:** 629–635.

33. Fabris, N., E. Mocchegiani, S. Mariotti, et al. 1986. Thyroid function modulates thymic endocrine activity. J. Clin. Endocrinol. Metab. **62:** 474–478.

34. Villa-Verde, D.M.S., V. Mello-Coelho, D.A. Farias de Oliveira, et al. 1993. Pleiotropic influence of triiodothyronine on thymus physiology. Endocrinology **133:** 867–875.

35. Mocchegiani, E., L. Amadio & N. Fabris. 1990. Neuroendocrine-thymus interactions. I. In vitro modulation of thymic factor secretion by thyroid hormones. J. Endocrinol. Invest. **13:** 139–147.

36. Dardenne, M., W. Savino, D. Duval, et al. 1986. Thymic hormone-containing cells. VII. Adrenals and gonads control the in vivo secretion of thymulin and its plasmatic inhibitor. J. Immunol. **136:** 1303–1308.

37. Savino, W., E. Bartoccioni, F. Homo-Delarche, et al. 1988. Thymic hormone containing cells. IX. Steroids in vitro modulate thymulin secretion by human and murine thymic epithelial cells. J. Steroid Biochem. **30:** 479–484.

38. Folch, H., G. Eller, M. Mena, et al. 1986. Neuroendocrine regulation of thymus hormones: hypothalamic dependence of FTS level. Cell. Immunol. **102:** 211–216.

39. Goya, R.G., M.C. Gagnerault & Y.E. Sosa. 1995. Reduced ability of pituitary extracts from old mice to stimulate thymulin secretion in vitro. Mech. Age. Dev. **83:** 143–154.

40. Zaidi, S.A., M.D. Kendall, B. Gillham, et al. 1988. The release of LH from pituitaries perifused with thymic extracts. Thymus **12:** 253–264.

41. Hadley, A.J., C.M. Rantle & J.C. Buckingham. 1997. Thymulin stimulates corticotrophin release and cyclic nucleotide formation in the rat anterior pituitary gland. Neuroimmunomodulation **4:** 62–69.

42. Hinojosa, L., L. García, R. Domínguez, et al. 2004. Effects of thymulin and GnRH on the release of gonadotropins by in vitro pituitary cells obtained from rats in each day of estrous cycle. Life Sci. **76:** 795–804.

43. Brown, O.A., Y.E. Sosa, F. Bolognani, et al. 1998. Thymulin stimulates prolactin and thyrotropin release in an age-related manner. Mech. Age. Dev. **104:** 249–262.

44. Brown, O.A., Y.E. Sosa, M. Dardenne, et al. 2000. Studies on the gonadotropin-releasing activity of thymulin: changes with age. J. Gerontol. (Biological Sciences) **55:** B170–176.

45. Hinojosa, L., R. Chavira, R. Dominguez, et al. 1999. Effects of thymulin on spontaneous puberty and gonadotrophin-induced ovulation in prepubertal normal and hypothymic mice. J. Endocrinol. **163:** 255–260.

46. García, L., L. Hinojosa, R. Domínguez, et al. 2000. Effects of infantile thymectomy on ovarian functions and gonadotrophin-induced ovulation in prepubertal mice. Role of thymulin. J. Endocrinol. **166:** 381–387.

47. García, L., L. Hinojosa, R. Domínguez, et al. 2005. Effects of injecting thymulin into the anterior or medial hypothalamus or the pituitary on induced ovulation in prepubertal mice. Neuroimmunomodulation **12:** 314–320.

48. Wise, T. 1998. In vitro and in vivo effects of thymulin on rat testicular steroid synthesis. J. Steroid. Biochem. Mol. Biol. **66:** 129–135.

49. Camihort, G., G. Luna, S. Vesenbeckh, et al. 2006. Morphometric assessment of the impact of serum thymulin immunoneutralization on pituitary cell populations in peripubertal mice. Cells Tiss. Organs **184:** 23–30.

50. Goya, R.G., P.C. Reggiani, S.M. Vesenbeckh, et al. 2007. Thymulin gene therapy prevents the reduction in circulating gonadotropins induced by thymulin deficiency in mice. Am. J. Physiol.-Endocrinol. Metab. **293:** E182–E187.

51. Goya, R.G., G.M. Cónsole, C.B. Hereñú, et al. 2002. Thymus and aging: Potential of gene therapy for restoration of endocrine thymic function in thymus-deficient animal models. Gerontology **48:** 325–328.

52. Calenda, A., A. Cordonnier, F. Lederer, *et al.* 1988. Production of biologically active thymulin in Escherichia coli through expression of a chemically synthesized gene. *Biotechnol. Lett.* **10:** 155–160.

53. Reggiani, P.C., C.B. Hereñú, O.J. Rimoldi, *et al.* 2006. Gene therapy for long-term restoration of circulating thymulin in thymectomized mice and rats. *Gene Ther.* **13:** 1214–1221.

54. Morel, G.R., O.A. Brown, P.C. Reggiani, *et al.* 2006. Peripheral and mesencephalic transfer of a synthetic gene for the thymic peptide thymulin. *Brain Res. Bull.* **69:** 647–651.

55. Safieh-Garabedian, B., M. Dardenne, J.-M. Pleau, *et al.* 2002. Potent analgesic and anti-inflammatory actions of a novel thymulin-related peptide in the rat. *Br. J. Pharmacol.* **136:** 947–955.

56. Safieh-Garabedian, B., C.I. Ochoa-Chaar, S. Poole, *et al.* 2003. Thymulin reverses inflammatory hyperalgesia and modulates the increased concentration of proinflammatory cytokines induced by i.c.v. endotoxin injection. *Neuroscience* **121:** 865–873.

57. Dardenne, M., N. Saade & B. Safieh-Garabedian. 2006. Role of thymulin or its analogue as a new analgesic molecule. *Ann. N. Y. Acad. Sci.* **1088:** 153–63.

58. Stone, D., W. Xiong, J.C. Williams, *et al.* 2003. Adenovirus expression of IL-1 and NF-kappaB inhibitors does not inhibit acute adenoviral induced brain inflammation, but delays immune system-mediated elimination of transgene expression. *Mol. Ther.* **8:** 400–411.

59. Reggiani, P.C., C.G. Barbeito, M.A. Flamini, *et al.* 2008. Neonatal thymulin gene therapy prevents the characteristic ovarian atrophy of adult nude mice (Abstract); Presented at the Seventh Meeting of the International Society for Neuroimmunomodulation. Rio de Janeiro, Brazil, 19–23 April.

60. Zeidler, A., C. Tosco, D. Kumar, *et al.* 1982. Spontaneous hyperglycemia and impaired glucose tolerance in athymic nude BALB/c mice. *Diabetes* **31:** 821–825.

61. Zeidler, A., D. Kumar, C. Johnson, *et al.* 1984. Development of a diabetes-like syndrome in an athymic nude Balb/c mouse colony. *Exp. Cell. Biol.* **52:** 145–149.

62. Zeidler, A., N.S. Shargill & T.M. Chan. 1991. Peripheral insulin insensitivity in the hyperglycemic athymic nude mouse: similarity to noninsulin-dependent diabetes mellitus. *Proc. Soc. Exp. Biol. Med.* **196:** 457–460.

63. Zeidler, A., S. Arbuckle, E. Mahan, *et al.* 1989. Assessment of pancreatic islet- cell population in the hyperglycemic athymic nude mouse: immunohistochemical, ultrastructural, and hormonal studies. *Pancreas* **4:** 153–160.

64. Velkov, Z., M. Zafirova, Z. Kemileva, *et al.* 1990. Time course changes in blood glucose and insulin levels of thymectomized rats. *Acta Physiol. Pharmacol. Bulg.* **16:** 64–67.

65. Mondola, P., L. Coscia Porrazzi & C. Falconi. 1979. Cholesterol and triglycerides of a liver after administration of a chromatographic fraction of thymus: variations in tissue and blood. *Horm. Metab. Res.* **11:** 503–505.

66. Mondola, P., M. Santillo, F. Santangelo, *et al.* 1992. Effects of a new calf thymus protein on 3-hydroxy-3-methyl-glutarylCoA reductase activity in rat (rattus bubalus) hepatocyte cells (BRL-3A). *Comp. Biochem. Physiol.* **103B:** 431–434.

67. Mondola, P., M. Santillo, I. Tedesco, *et al.* 1989. Thymus fraction (FIII) effect on cholesterol metabolism: modulation of the low density lipoprotein receptor pathway. *Int. J. Biochem.* **21:** 627–630.

68. García-Bravo, M.M., M.P. Polo, P.C. Reggiani, *et al.* 2006. Partial prevention of hepatic lipid alterations in nude mice by neonatal thymulin gene therapy. *Lipids* **41:** 753–757.

69. Bach, J.F., M. Dardenne & A.L. Goldstein. 1984. Clinical aspects of thymulin (FTS). In *Thymic Hormones and Lymphokines. Basic Chemistry and Clinical Applications.* A.L. Goldstein, Ed.: 593–600. Plenum Press. New York.

70. Sztein, M.B. & A.L. Goldstein. 1986. Thymic hormones—a clinical update. *Springer Sem. Immunopathol.* **9:** 1–18.

Behavior: A Relevant Tool for Brain-immune System Interaction Studies

Frederico Azevedo Costa-Pinto, Daniel Wagner Hamada Cohn, Vanessa Moura Sa-Rocha, Luiz Carlos Sa-Rocha, and Joao Palermo-Neto

Department of Pathology, School of Veterinary Medicine and Animal Science, University of São Paulo, Sao Paulo, Brazil

Neuroimmunomodulation describes the field focused on understanding the mechanisms by which the central nervous system interacts with the immune system, potentially leading to changes in animal behavior. Nonetheless, not many articles dealing with neuroimmunomodulation employ behavior as an analytical endpoint. Even fewer papers deal with social status as a possible modifier of neuroimmune phenomena. In the described sets of experiments, we tackle both, using a paradigm of social dominance and subordination. We first review data on the effects of different ranks within a stable hierarchical relationship. Submissive mice in this condition display more anxiety-like behaviors, have decreased innate immunity, and show a decreased resistance to implantation and development of melanoma metastases in their lungs. This suggests that even in a stable, social, hierarchical rank, submissive animals may be subjected to higher levels of stress, with putative biological relevance to host susceptibility to disease. Second, we review data on how dominant and submissive mice respond differentially to lipopolysaccharide (LPS), employing a motivational perspective to sickness behavior. Dominant animals display decreased number and frequency in several aspects of behavior, particularly agonistic social interaction, that is, directed toward the submissive cage mate. This was not observed in submissive mice that maintained the required behavior expected by its dominant mate. Expression of sickness behavior relies on motivational reorganization of priorities, which are different along different social ranks, leading to diverse outcomes. We suggest that *in vitro* assessment of neuroimmune phenomena can only be understood based on the behavioral context in which they occur.

Key words: neuroimmunomodulation; animal behavior; immunity; social rank; dominant; submissive

Introduction

Reports on mutual influence between the central nervous system and the immune system consist of a vast, albeit somewhat controversial, amount of literature. Over the past decades this area of knowledge has built into a more organized structure, leading to the field referred to as *neuroimmunomodulation* (NIM), *psychoneuroimmunology, immunoneuroendocrinology,* and other synonyms.

A historical mark on the development of NIM must point to the life and work of Hans Selye who compiled observations on a series of physiological, histological, and functional changes in animals submitted to a multitude of diverse "stressful" situations.[1] The so-called general adaptation syndrome anticipated the major role that stress responses would have in modern society. In the words of Robert Sapolsky[2]:

> Stress is not everywhere. Every twinge of dysfunction in our bodies is not a manifestation of

Address for correspondence: Frederico Azevedo Costa-Pinto, Av. Prof. Dr. Orlando Marques de Paiva, 87, São Paulo, SP, Brazil 05508-900. Voice: 551130911373; fax: 551130917829. fpinto@usp.br

Neuroimmunomodulation: Ann. N.Y. Acad. Sci. 1153: 107–119 (2009).
doi: 10.1111/j.1749-6632.2008.03961.x © 2009 New York Academy of Sciences.

stress-related disease. It is true that the real world is full of bad things that we can finesse away by altering our outlook and psychological makeup, but it is also full of awful things that cannot be eliminated by a change in attitude, no matter how heroically, fervently, complexly, ritualistically we may wish. Once we are actually sick with the illness, the fantasy of which keeps us anxiously awake at two in the morning little about our psychological attitude is likely to help. (. . .) But amid this caution, there remains a whole realm of health and disease that is sensitive to the quality of our minds – our thoughts and emotions and behaviors. And sometimes whether we become sick with the diseases that frighten us at two in the morning will reflect this realm of mind. It is here that we must turn from the physicians and their ability to clean up the messes afterward, and recognize our own capacity to prevent some of these problems beforehand in the small steps with which we live our everyday lives.

Ever since Selye's pioneer work, the literature has been flooded by reports ascribing phenomena to neuroimmune interactions in health and disease, both for changes in brain activity and behavior induced by peripheral immune stimuli or reactions[3–26] and for the influence of brain activity and behavior on immunity.[27–52] Overwhelming amounts of data have been gathered from clinical and experimental reports in this regard, constituting unequivocal evidence supporting the biological relevance of NIM interactions in health and disease.

Sickness behavior as a conceptual framework for understanding the biological (theoretical) basis and the mechanistic rationale of the behavior of sick animals is of particular importance here. Prior to the work of Benjamin Hart,[53] other groups had offered evidence that general aspects of sickness represent an important strategy providing physiological means for recovery.[54,55] Nonetheless, usage of the term *sickness behavior* became generally accepted only after work published by Stephen Kent and colleagues.[56]

Sickness behavior in rodents can be modeled by injection of Gram-negative bacteria cell component lipopolysaccharide (LPS), leading to several physiological and behavioral nonspecific changes associated with disease. For its

simplicity and reproducibility, LPS has been widely employed for the study of mechanisms and behavioral patterns displayed in sickness. LPS induces secretion of several cytokines, such as interleukin-1 and tumor necrosis factor, simulating, to a certain extent, parameters of bacterial infection.

Several behavioral paradigms have also been extensively employed in order to assess their influence on immunity. Among them, models dependent on social interaction, such as social confrontation with an aggressive conspecific, intruder–resident models of social stress, or defeat, have all been employed in NIM studies because they not only accurately represent natural life events for experimental subjects, such as rodents, commonly used in biomedical research but also because they may relate to the human condition of social stress and defeat.[40,43,49,57–60] Nonetheless, whether a long-term social condition based on hierarchy leads to stable rank interactions or is perceived by submissive animals as chronic stress appears to rely on the model employed and remains an unresolved area in the field.[34,35,37,61]

We focus on two different approaches from our group on the relevance for assessing behavior in NIM. First, we review data on the importance of social rank, even within a stable hierarchy, on behavior and immunity of mice against tumors.[62] Second, we focus on the strong repercussions of dominance and subordination on the expression of sickness behavior induced by LPS.[63] We believe these experiments strengthen the concept that behavioral analysis is crucial for the comprehension of NIM phenomena because these cannot take place out of the original social context in which they were built.

First Case Study: Effects of Social Rank on Immunity and Resistance to Disease

Several groups working in the field of NIM have focused on the effects of stressful events on host resistance and on possible outcomes of failure in immunity, such as disease. Stress has long been recognized as a major modifier of immunity in which mechanisms, such as increased activity of the hypothalamus–pituitary–adrenal (HPA) axis, with consequent secretion of steroids, and overstimulation of the sympathetic branch of the autonomic nervous system and increased release of cathecolamines play a pivotal role. Social confrontation with aggressive conspecifics may represent a meaningful source of daily stress. In fact, models of social defeat have proven the biological consequences of dealing with a permanent instability of a high-risk/high-stress social environment. On the other hand, what are the consequences of different social ranks in a stable hierarchical rank? In such situations, it is expected that fights and putative confrontations are kept to a minimum because submissive animals have learned to deal and hopefully cope with social subordination. Predicting and anticipating offensive aggressive responses from the standpoint of submissive animals becomes part of their social repertoire employed to preserve stability and reduce chances of conflict. Is it still stressful to submissive animals?[61] In this situation, does maintenance of social status imply, as a trade-off, any biological cost to the submissive animal?

These concerns have been addressed by Sa-Rocha and colleagues.[62] C57BL/6 mice were paired after weaning (21-days old) and kept in dyads until used in the experiments (3-months old). During this period, hierarchical relationships are created and dominance and submission can be detected before the experiment actually takes place. Thus, immediately before group formation, mice were transferred into separate cages and kept apart for 7 min. After reunion, animals were observed for evaluation of fighting and anticipatory aggressive (offensive and defensive) responses based on whether they were dominant or submissive for each individual dyad.[64] This procedure was repeated on the following 2 days to ensure accuracy of rank status representation.

First, the authors focused on behavioral profiling of the mice in order to infer levels of

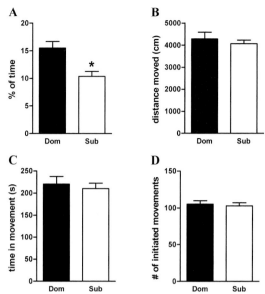

Figure 1. Effects of social rank on behavior in the open field. Submissive animals spent less percentage of session time in the central zone of an open field arena than dominant mice (**A**). This is not determined by decreased motor activity since the distance moved during the test (**B**), the time in movement (**C**), and the number of initiated movements (**D**) do not differ among groups. Data are mean ± SEM; *$P < 0.05$ compared to dominant mice.

anxiety displayed by dominant and submissive animals, employing two, standard, widely accepted models for the assessment of motor activity and anxiety-like responses in rodents, the open field and the elevated plus maze, respectively.[65,66] It should be noted that these experiments were conducted 1 week after determining dominant and submissive animals in order to minimize the influence of that particular stressful encounter on the outcome of this profiling. Figure 1 shows results obtained in the open field arena for dominant and submissive mice. Although the open field is usually employed to evaluate ambulation (or locomotion) as a measure of motor activity,[65] employing a computer-aided system of animal tracking and behavioral recording (Ethovision; Noldus Technology, Wageningen, the Netherlands) enables virtual division of the arena in several zones in which ambulation may also indicate altered levels of anxiety. In this case, time spent exploring the central zone of the arena (farther away from the round walls that surround it) can be associated with lower levels of anxiety-like behavior in rodents because it is an unprotected area. The authors show (Fig. 1A) that submissive animals display a decrease (in about 30%) in preference for this zone, indicating an increased basal (undisturbed) level of anxiety in these animals if compared to dominant mates. Because crossings of the central zone of the apparatus rely on locomotion in general, it should be relevant to stress that no differences in general activity were observed when analyzing total distance moved in the session (Fig. 1B), time spent in movement (Fig. 1C), or percentage of initiated movements (Fig. 1D). It thus seems accurate to describe this behavior as suggestive of increased levels of anxiety.

The authors next confirmed the increased levels of anxiety in mice exposed to the elevated plus maze in which exploration of the open arms correlates with lower levels of anxiety; conversely, preference for the closed arms indicates increased levels of anxiety.[66,67] Figure 2 shows that submissive mice display a significantly reduced preference for the plus maze open arms, represented by fewer entries in these compartments and less time spent exploring them, when compared to their dominant mates. This confirms data from the open field with regard to increased levels of anxiety in submissive mice. Therefore, even in a stable social hierarchy, submissive mice appear subjected to higher levels of daily stressors.

Employing a computer-aided behavioral tracking and analysis system, the authors were able to further characterize the anxiety behavior in submissive mice. Figure 3 depicts data from the same animals described above but includes a more refined analysis of activity in the elevated plus maze. The authors chose to compare only the last third of the open and closed arms (where they all converge farther away from the central platform). The distal third of the open arms is the most unprotected zone of the entire apparatus because it is most dis-

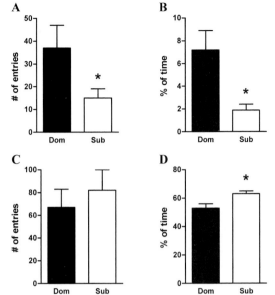

Figure 2. Effects of social rank on behavior in the number of entries and percentage of time spent exploring the open (**A** and **B**, respectively) or closed (**C** and **D**, respectively) arms of the elevated plus maze. Submissive animals display higher levels of anxiety-like behavior as assessed by decreased exploration of the open arms and increased time spent in the closed arms of this apparatus. Data are mean ± SEM; *$P < 0.05$ compared to dominant mice.

tant from the closed arms; on the other hand, the distal third of the closed arms is the most protected area of the arena since three walls converge there. Therefore, the distal third open arms reflects low levels of anxiety, while the distal third closed arms relates to higher levels of anxiety. Accordingly, Figure 3 shows that submissive mice display reduced preference for the unprotected areas than dominant animals; the opposite holds true for the protected zone.

Although participating in a hierarchical arrangement, supposedly more stable submissive animals display a behavioral pattern consistent with higher levels of anxiety compared to dominant mates. Since there is an overwhelming amount of data describing the repercussions of stressors (associated with responses also characterized by anxiety, such as described here), the authors then asked if in this paradigm, i.e., a stable hierarchy of social ranks, there

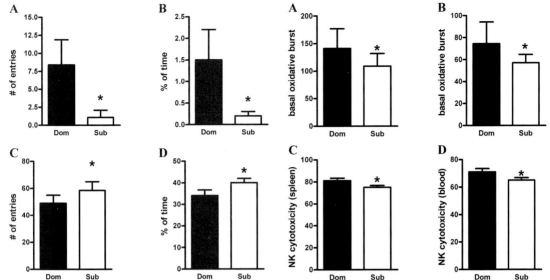

Figure 3. Effects of social rank on exploration of protected or unprotected areas of the elevated plus maze. Number of entries and percentage of time exploring the distal third zone of the open (**A** and **B**, respectively) or closed (**C** and **D**, respectively) arms of the apparatus were compared among dominant and submissive mice. Dominant animals show a higher exploration of the distal third zone of the open arms ("unprotected," panels A and B), while submissive animals enter the distal third zone of the closed arms ("protected," panels C and D) more often and explore it longer than dominant mice. Data are mean ± SEM; *P < 0.05 compared to dominant mice.

Figure 4. Effects of social rank on basal oxidative burst by neutrophils and monocytes and on cytotoxicity performed by natural killer (NK) cells from the spleen or blood. Neutrophils (**A**) and monocytes (**B**) harvested from the blood of submissive mice display a reduced spontaneous oxidative burst. Furthermore, NK cells collected from the spleen (**C**) or blood (**D**) of the same animals show decreased *in vitro* cytotoxicity against B16F10 tumor cells. Data are mean ± SEM; *P < 0.05 compared to dominant mice.

are differences in immunity that could underlie increased susceptibility to disease. They assessed parameters of innate immunity, such as oxidative burst by circulating leukocytes and cytotoxicity of natural killer (NK) cells against a tumor cell line. The relevance of these parameters lies in the fact that they represent not only the first line of responses toward potentially harmful pathogens but also participate in the immune surveillance directed at aberrant cells, such as virus infected or transformed (tumoral).[68]

Figure 4 depicts the basal oxidative burst performed by circulating neutrophils and monocytes as well as an assay of cytotoxicity of NK cells harvested from the blood or from the spleen. Submissive mice have a modest but consistent reduction in oxidative burst (Fig. 4A and

B for neutrophils and monocytes, respectively) and on cytoxicity of NK cells from the spleen (Fig. 4C) or blood (Fig. 4D) targeting the tumor cell line B16F10. Albeit numerically modest, these differences could decrease host resistance to infection or predispose them to the development of tumors.

In order to assess the biological relevance of a putative decrease in innate immunity suggested by the results described above, the authors went further and injected dominant and submissive mice with the same cell line (B16F10) employed *in vitro* for the evaluation of NK cell activity. This is a melanoma line that metastasizes to the lung if injected intravenously to C57BL/6 mice.[69] The authors counted the number of metastases in the lungs of dominant and submissive mice 14 days after inoculation with the tumor cells and found that the average number of metastases per animal

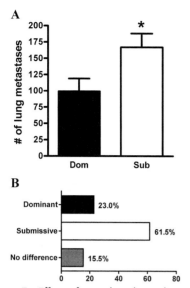

Figure 5. Effect of social rank on the implantation and development of metastases of B16F10 tumor cells. Submissive mice display a higher count of metastases in the lungs than dominant animals; *P < 0.05 compared to dominant mice (**A**). Moreover, assessing each individual pair of mice, the percentage of pairs in which the submissive mouse had a higher count of metastases than its cage mate is 61.5% (**B**), while in only 23% of the pairs did the dominant develop more metastases than its submissive cage mate. No significant differences in the number of metastases between dominant and submissive cage mates were shown in 15.5% of the pairs.

was 50% higher in submissive animals than in their dominant cage mates (Fig. 5A). Furthermore, the percentage of pairs in which the submissive mouse had more metastases than its dominant mate was 61.5%; in only 23% of the pairs did the dominant have more metastases than its submissive mate. This strongly suggests that submissive mice within a stable dyad still have increased susceptibility to develop certain pathological conditions, represented here as the implantation and development of melanoma metastases.

Interestingly, their findings do not seem to rely on altered secretion of corticosterone in submissive mice as their levels did not differ among social ranks. Other mechanisms, such as increased activity of the autonomic nervous system (either sympathetic or parasympa-

thetic branches), could underlie the responses reported here.

Second Case Study: Effects of Social Rank on the Expression of LPS-induced Sickness Behavior

Cohn and colleagues assessed whether dominant and submissive mice kept in a dyad would respond differently to LPS.[15,16,54,63] Male Swiss mice were paired immediately after weaning (21-days old) and shared the same home cage (14 × 30 × 13 cm, transparent, polypropylene cages kept in standard animal housing conditions) in pairs. Animals were paired when still very young, a fact that prevents escalating fights that could lead to serious injury, commonly seen when adults are placed together. Experiments took place when animals were between 65- and 75-days old. Animals were classified either as dominant or submissive within each particular dyad, according to strict criteria described elsewhere: display of attacks, chasing the cage mate, and expressing offensive upright and sideways postures. Conversely, submissive mice exhibited flights and defensive upright and sideways postures.[70]

The main objective of these experiments was to determine if dominant and submissive animals would express sickness behavior, as defined as a set of nonspecific behavioral changes, such as anorexia, lethargy, reduced grooming, and increased sleep, associated with illness.[23,53,56,71] Therefore, after determination of social rank (i.e., which animal of the pair is the dominant and which is the submissive one), each dyad was assigned to either one of the groups: control (none of the animals received LPS), dominant (the dominant mouse in the pair was treated with LPS), or submissive (the submissive animal received LPS). This hypothesis is based on proposals to focus on sickness behavior from a motivational perspective.[72–74] Behaviors displayed by sick animals are not a result of physical debilitation but rather an extremely organized strategy to overcome illness, be it from traumatic injury or infection. From this standpoint, changes in behavior found in sick animals represent a reorganization of priorities that would favor recovery from whatever injury or disease is present. This work tests this hypothesis by comparing dominant and submissive mice in a stable dyad. These animals obviously have different priorities because, in a social environment, some behaviors are expected from submissive animals and not from dominant ones and vice versa. What happens when only one mouse in each dyad gets (pseudo-) sick?

Observation of behavior occurred for 5 consecutive days, 5 min a day, between 14:00 and 15:00 h. It should be mentioned that during the week of observation, animals were kept in the observation chamber (transparent cage with wood shavings, $30 \times 40 \times 15$ cm, with a drinking bottle and a few chow pellets) during the entire day. Animals were removed from the observation chamber for 5 min before joining their cage mates again. This procedure assures the occurrence of social interaction that otherwise would not necessarily occur because animals could be engaged in other activities, such as eating or sleeping.[75] Sessions were taped in the absence of the experimenter (who monitored the behavior from an adjacent room) and were later assessed with the aid of a software package (The Observer; Noldus Technology) specific for behavioral recording and analysis. Behavioral analysis focused on both dominant and submissive animals of each dyad. Ethograms (collections of all behaviors displayed by mice in the observation chamber) were created for all animals and generated logs for dominant and submissive mice of all dyads. The categories employed to describe animal behavior in this study were based on Grant and Mackintosh.[70]

First, the authors focus on the total frequency of behaviors expressed by dominant and submissive animals on the day of treatment [with LPS or with saline (control)]. Total frequency is defined and the sum of all behaviors from any category initiated by an individual mouse, including repetition of the same behav-

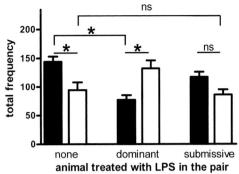

Figure 6. Total frequency of behaviors expressed by dominant (black bars) and submissive (clear bars) mice on observation day 3. The animal within each pair injected with lipopolysaccharide (LPS) on day 3 is indicated below the bars. Administration of saline to both animals in the pair ("none") shows that dominant mice have a naturally higher total frequency of behaviors within each pair when compared to their submissive mates. LPS causes a decrease in total frequency of behaviors in dominant mice compared to untreated submissive cage mates ("dominant"). Conversely, LPS does not lead to decreased total frequency in submissive mice compared to untreated dominant mates ("submissive"). Further comparison of dominant mice from the LPS-treated group ("dominant") to the untreated group ("none") shows that LPS caused a significant decrease in total frequency; a similar comparison for submissive mice does not show the same pattern. Data are mean ± SEM; *$P < 0.05$; "ns" denotes lack of difference.

iors. Figure 6 shows that if none of the animals are treated with LPS, dominant animals initiate more behaviors than submissive mice. Dominant mice receiving LPS express a significantly smaller value of total frequency than their submissive cage mates; they also display decreased total frequency when compared to saline-treated dominant mice. Nonetheless, this reduction in the initiation of all categories of behavior found in LPS-treated dominant mice is not seen when LPS is given only to the submissive mouse. Therefore, this is the first result from their work showing that the expression of sickness behavior differs in dominant and submissive animals within a dyad. Since total frequency includes many types of behavior, which may or may not be directed to the other animal in the cage, the authors then asked if this

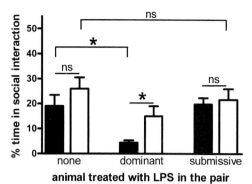

Figure 7. Percentage of session time spent in social interaction by dominant (black bars) or submissive (clear bars) mice on observation day 3. The animal within each pair injected with LPS on day 3 is indicated below the bars. Dominant and submissive mice spend a similar percentage of session time in social interaction when LPS is not used in any animal. LPS administration to dominant mice leads to a decrease in the time spent in social interaction compared to their submissive cage mates or to untreated dominant animals. Conversely, LPS-treated submissive mice spend a similar percentage of session time in social interaction when compared to their dominant cage mates and behave similarly to untreated submissive mice. Data are mean ± SEM; *$P < 0.05$; "ns" denotes lack of difference.

reduction in total frequency is associated with a decrease in social interaction, which is the sum of the duration of any particular behavioral category that involves searching for active contact with the other individual.

Figure 7 shows the percentage of session time spent in social interaction by dominant and submissive individuals. In nontreated pairs, there is no significant difference in time spent in social interaction between dominant and submissive mice. In contrast, when dominant animals receive LPS they spend less time in social interaction than their submissive mates; they also spend less time in social interaction than saline-treated dominant animals. LPS-treated submissive mice do not display this reduction in social interaction shown by dominant animals. The reduction shown in Figure 6 for total frequency of behaviors in LPS-treated dominant mice appears to rely, at least partially, on a decrease in social behavior toward their cage

mates. Conversely, submissive mice maintain their social interaction after treatment with the same amount of LPS that renders dominant animals sick.

It is important to stress that one animal may be engaged in social interaction (e.g., sniffing at the other) while the cage mate expresses a behavior not socially directed, such as eating. Therefore, values for social interaction may differ for each mouse within a particular dyad. Moreover, social interaction includes two types of contacts: investigative (sniffing at the other mouse) or agonistic (attacks, chases, fights, and any offensive or defensive posture). Splitting the analysis into these categories may shed some light on the nature of differential effects of LPS on dominant versus submissive mice. Thus, the authors focus on specific sets of behaviors classified as investigative or agonistic and assess which class is more easily disrupted by LPS treatment. Figure 8 compares the effects of LPS in dominant or submissive mice, splitting the data for social interaction in agonistic (light gray bars) and investigative (dark gray bars) within each experimental group (LPS to submissive or to dominant animal compared to dyads without treatment). When LPS is given to dominant mice, agonistic interactions ceased; in these situation, social behaviors initiated from either the (LPS-treated) dominant or the submissive mouse were investigative.

We might conclude at this point that the decrease in frequency of behaviors found in dominant but not in submissive mice treated with LPS (Fig. 6) is based on reducing social interaction (Fig. 7), particularly ceasing agonistic behaviors between LPS-treated dominant mice and their cage mates (Fig. 8). These results clearly point to a selective change in behavior of dominant mice treated with LPS; they not only initiate behaviors less frequently but show a blunted response in socially driven and focused categories of these behaviors. This is not seen in submissive animals, showing that the expression of sickness-associated behaviors relies on a motivational reorganization and change in

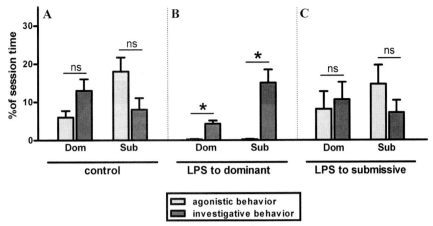

Figure 8. Percentage of session time spent in agonistic (light gray) or investigative (dark gray) social behavior by dominant or submissive mice from different pairs in which LPS was not employed (**A**) or administered to dominant (**B**) or submissive (**C**) mouse within the pair. No statistical differences were found in the percentage of session time spent by dominant or submissive animals when LPS was not used (**A**) or in sessions when the submissive animal had been treated with LPS (**B**). Nonetheless, there is a trend in both situations for dominant mice to concentrate on investigative behavior while submissive mice spend more time in agonistic behavior. Conversely, when LPS is given to dominant mice, agonistic behaviors expressed by these animals practically ceased (**C**). Dominant and submissive animals from pairs in which the dominant mouse had been treated with LPS spend much longer in investigative behaviors than in agonistic behaviors. Data are mean ± SEM; *$P < 0.05$; "ns" denotes lack of difference.

priorities that should differ according to social rank and life experience. Nonetheless, sickness is usually accompanied by a profound decrease in locomotion, evaluated in several apparatuses employed for rodents, such as the open field arena. It could be argued that all effects of LPS on the behavior of dominant mice could simply reflect a reduction in motor activity. Although it was highly unlikely, as submissive animals submitted to a similar treatment with LPS showed completely different results, the authors evaluated locomotion during their observation sessions in order to rule out this possibility. Figure 9 shows results for locomotion, considered the sum of duration of all behaviors in which the animals displayed any movement, represented by the percentage of total session time. Interestingly, LPS-treated dominant mice, regardless of displaying reduced frequency of behaviors (Fig. 6), particularly social behaviors (Fig. 7), toward their mates (agonistic, Fig. 8), do not show any decrease in motor activity following treatment with LPS (on day 3, vertical arrow). The

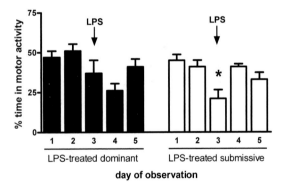

Figure 9. Percentage of time spent in motor activity displayed by animals effectively treated with LPS within each pair. Animals are treated with LPS on day 3 (arrows). LPS causes a decrease in locomotion of submissive (clear bars) but not of dominant (black bars) mice on the day of injection compared to the base line adjusted from the other days of observation. Data are mean ± SEM; *$P < 0.05$.

opposite is reported for submissive mice; although these animals do not display decreased frequency of behaviors after LPS treatment, they do display a reduction of locomotion on day 3 compared to their activity on previous (days 1 and 2) or subsequent (4 and 5) days.

The authors provide compelling evidence that social dominance or submission influences the expression of sickness behavior, pointing to a crucial motivational ground for the behavior of sick animals, induced in that work by LPS.[63] Does the opposite hold true? Is a simulation of disease in a particular animal (especially dominant) in a given dyad capable of modifying, or at least of destabilizing, social hierarchy and dominance? The results are less clear, but preliminary (unpublished) observations from the same group suggest this is the case.

Evidence for LPS-driven Temporary Switch of Social Ranks

When the same authors analyzed dyads that remained paired for much longer than those described above (6–7 months compared to 2–3 months for ordinary dyads), the experiments yielded relevant results concerning the effects of sickness on social ranking. Although the analysis is preliminary, the results are strong and unequivocal: in two out of three dyads of mice housed for over 6 months from weaning, there were clear signs of social destabilization, represented mainly by attacks initiated by the submissive (untreated) directed at the LPS-treated dominant mouse. These attacks happened at night following LPS treatment, in their home cages, leading to serious injuries in dominant mice and unfortunately culminating in death in one case. Obviously, in such an extreme situation, observations were interrupted. Nonetheless, the most interesting results come from a dyad in which destabilization occurred (easily noted by a biting mark on the back of the LPS-treated dominant mouse) but without drastic physical outcomes. When mice from this dyad were observed 24 h after LPS, there was a clear lack of dominance by the (prior) LPS-dominant mouse. The movie file available as supplementary material to this article shows a dispute for a chow pellet that took place during observation on day 4. In several moments the

submissive mouse (indicated by two black pen stripes on his tail) holds the pellet in its possession, obstructing the access to it by the supposedly dominant mouse. This situation would never be expected to occur were social dominance not in question during that 5-min session. Toward the end of the session the dominant mouse regains its rank in the dyad, controlling access to the pellet and preventing the submissive mouse to come near it. This was temporary and could no longer be detected on the following observation day when signs of social instability ceased. This observation, although preliminary, points to a role for health and disease for the maintenance or eventual loss of social dominance in mice submitted to a model of simulated infection.

Concluding Remarks

We stress here the need for better elucidation of the real impact of life events on predisposition to disease and host resistance represented by immunity. Even in a mild stable situation of housing conditions, placement in a particular rank may have drastic consequences in life. Moreover, moving to a more biological standpoint for the comprehension of sickness, such as the one proposed by the "motivational" perspective to behavioral reorganization of priorities, suggests that oversimplification may be even more misleading than not digging deep enough into the cellular and molecular mechanisms that explain the phenomena on which NIM focuses.

Reports, such as those described here, may point to an answer as to why sometimes it is difficult to predict *in vivo* outcomes of NIM studies based on prior *in vitro* data because the latter do not take into account social interaction, rank factors, and life events of the animal in which the response takes place. It is evident that much in the NIM field is owed to *in vitro* studies, particularly recent data generated in knockout and transgenic systems, that clarify obscure bizarre results from the past. Nonetheless, it is also quite obvious to us that artificial paradigms may not be enough to account for the entire complexity of a live organism, even the simplest one, let alone a mammal.

Conflicts of Interest

The authors declare no conflicts of interest.

Supporting Information

Additional Supporting Information may be found in the online version of this article:

MPG file

Please note: Wiley-Blackwell is not responsible for the content or functionality of any supporting materials supplied by the authors. Any queries (other than missing material) should be directed to the corresponding author for the article.

References

1. Selye, H. 1936. A syndrome produced by diverse noxious agents. *Nature* **138:** 32.
2. Sapolsky, R. 2002. *Why Zebras Don't Get Ulcers*. W. H. Freeman and Company. New York.
3. Besedovsky, H. *et al.* 1975. Changes in blood hormone levels during the immune response. *Proc. Soc. Exp. Biol. Med.* **150:** 466–470.
4. Besedovsky, H. & E. Sorkin. 1977. Network of immune-neuroendocrine interactions. *Clin. Exp. Immunol.* **27:** 1–12.
5. Besedovsky, H. *et al.* 1983. The immune response evokes changes in brain noradrenergic neurons. *Science* **221:** 564–566.
6. Blalock, J.E. 1984. The immune system as a sensory organ. *J. Immunol.* **132:** 1067–1070.
7. McCarthy, D.O., M.J. Kluger & A.J. Vander. 1984. The role of fever in appetite suppression after endotoxin administration. *Am. J. Clin. Nutr.* **40:** 310–316.
8. McCarthy, D.O., M.J. Kluger & A.J. Vander. 1985. Suppression of food intake during infections: is interleukin-1 involved? *Am. J. Clin. Nutr.* **42:** 1179–1182.
9. Besedovsky, H. *et al.* 1986. Immunoregulatory feedback between interleukin-1 and glucocorticoid hormones. *Science* **233:** 652–654.
10. Sapolsky, R. *et al.* 1987. Interleukin-1 stimulates the secretion of hypothalamic corticotropin-releasing factor. *Science* **238:** 522–524.
11. Blalock, J.E. 1989. A molecular basis for bidirectional communication between the immune and neuroendocrine systems. *Physiol. Rev.* **69:** 1–32.
12. Ader, R. 1990. Immune-derived modulation of behavior. *Ann. N. Y. Acad. Sci.* **594:** 280–288.
13. Dunn, A.J., M. Antoon & Y. Chapman. 1991. Reduction of exploratory behavior by intraperitoneal injection of interleukin-1 involves brain corticotropin-releasing factor. *Brain Res. Bull.* **26:** 539–542.
14. Felten, D.L. *et al.* 1991. Central neural circuits involved in neural-immune interactions. In *Psychoneuroimmunology*. R. Ader, D.L. Felten & N. Cohen, Eds.: 3–19. Academic Press. San Diego.
15. Bluthe, R.M., R. Dantzer & K.W. Kelley. 1992. Effects of interleukin-1 receptor antagonist on the behavioral effects of lipopolysaccharide in rat. *Brain Res.* **573:** 318–320.
16. Bluthe, R.M. *et al.* 1994. Lipopolysaccharide induces sickness behaviour in rats by a vagal mediated mechanism. *C. R. Acad. Sci. III* **317:** 499–503.
17. Watkins, L.R., S.F. Maier & L.E. Goehler. 1995. Cytokine-to-brain communication: a review & analysis of alternative mechanisms. *Life Sci.* **57:** 1011–1026.
18. Yirmiya, R. 1996. Endotoxin produces a depressive-like episode in rats. *Brain Res.* **711:** 163–174.
19. Fishkin, R.J. & J.T. Winslow. 1997. Endotoxin-induced reduction of social investigation by mice: interaction with amphetamine and anti-inflammatory drugs. *Psychopharmacology (Berl.)* **132:** 335–341.
20. Plata-Salaman, C.R. 1997. Anorexia during acute and chronic disease: relevance of neurotransmitter-peptide-cytokine interactions. *Nutrition* **13:** 159–160.
21. Swiergiel, A.H., G.N. Smagin & A.J. Dunn. 1997. Influenza virus infection of mice induces anorexia: comparison with endotoxin and interleukin-1 and the effects of indomethacin. *Pharmacol. Biochem. Behav.* **57:** 389–396.
22. Goehler, L.E. *et al.* 1999. Interleukin-1beta in immune cells of the abdominal vagus nerve: a link between the immune and nervous systems? *J. Neurosci.* **19:** 2799–2806.
23. Dantzer, R. 2001. Cytokine-induced sickness behavior: where do we stand? *Brain Behav. Immun.* **15:** 7–24.
24. Larson, S.J. & A.J. Dunn. 2001. Behavioral effects of cytokines. *Brain Behav. Immun.* **15:** 371–387.
25. Dunn, A.J. 2002. Mechanisms by which cytokines signal the brain. *Int. Rev. Neurobiol.* **52:** 43–65.
26. Larson, S.J. *et al.* 2002. Effects of interleukin-1beta on food-maintained behavior in the mouse. *Brain Behav. Immun.* **16:** 398–410.

27. Miller, N.E. 1964. Some psychophysiological studies of motivation and of the behavioral effects of illness. *Bull. Br. Psych. Soc.* **17:** 1–20.

28. Ader, R. & N. Cohen. 1975. Behaviorally conditioned immunosuppression. *Psychosom. Med.* **37:** 333–340.

29. Guyre, P.M., J.E. Bodwell & A. Munck. 1981. Glucocorticoid actions on the immune system: inhibition of production of an Fc-receptor augmenting factor. *J. Steroid Biochem.* **15:** 35–39.

30. Visintainer, M.A., J.R. Volpicelli & M.E. Seligman. 1982. Tumor rejection in rats after inescapable or escapable shock. *Science* **216:** 437–439.

31. Guyre, P.M., J.E. Bodwell & A. Munck. 1984. Glucocorticoid actions on lymphoid tissue and the immune system: physiologic and therapeutic implications. *Prog. Clin. Biol. Res.* **142:** 181–194.

32. Locke, S.E. *et al.* 1984. Life change stress, psychiatric symptoms, and natural killer cell activity. *Psychosom. Med.* **46:** 441–453.

33. Felten, D.L. *et al.* 1985. Noradrenergic and peptidergic innervation of lymphoid tissue. *J. Immunol.* **135:** 755s-765s.

34. Fauman, M.A. 1987. The relation of dominant and submissive behavior to the humoral immune response in BALB/c mice. *Biol. Psychiatry* **22:** 776–779.

35. Hardy, C.A. *et al.* 1990. Altered T-lymphocyte response following aggressive encounters in mice. *Physiol. Behav.* **47:** 1245–1251.

36. Irwin, M. *et al.* 1990. Sympathetic nervous system mediates central corticotropin-releasing factor induced suppression of natural killer cytotoxicity. *J. Pharmacol. Exp. Ther.* **255:** 101–107.

37. Lyte, M., S.G. Nelson & B. Baissa. 1990. Examination of the neuroendocrine basis for the social conflict-induced enhancement of immunity in mice. *Physiol. Behav.* **48:** 685–691.

38. File, S.E. 1991. Interactions of anxiolitic and antidepressant drugs with hormones of the hypothalamic–pituitary–adrenal axis. In *Psychopharmacology of Anxiolytics and Antidepressants.* P. Simon, P. Soubrie & P. Wildlocher, Eds.: 29–55. Pergamon. New York.

39. Felten, D.L. 1993. Direct innervation of lymphoid organs: substrate for neurotransmitter signaling of cells of the immune system. *Neuropsychobiology* **28:** 110–112.

40. Azpiroz, A. *et al.* 1994. Fighting experience and natural killer cell activity in male laboratory mice. *Aggressive Behav.* **20:** 67–72.

41. Madden, K.S., V.M. Sanders & D.L. Felten. 1995. Catecholamine influences and sympathetic neural modulation of immune responsiveness. *Annu. Rev. Pharmacol. Toxicol.* **35:** 417–448.

42. Song, C., B. Earley & B.E. Leonard. 1995. Behavioral, neurochemical, and immunological responses to CRF administration. Is CRF a mediator of stress? *Ann. N. Y. Acad. Sci.* **771:** 55–72.

43. Barnard, C.J. & J.M. Behnke. 1996. Social status and resistance to disease in house mice (Mus musculus): status-related modulation of hormonal responses in relation to immunity costs in different social and physical environments. *Ethology* **102:** 63–84.

44. Sobrian, S.K. *et al.* 1997. Gestational exposure to loud noise alters the development and postnatal responsiveness of humoral and cellular components of the immune system in offspring. *Environ. Res.* **73:** 227–241.

45. Shakhar, G. & S. Ben-Eliyahu. 1998. In vivo beta-adrenergic stimulation suppresses natural killer activity and compromises resistance to tumor metastasis in rats. *J. Immunol.* **160:** 3251–3258.

46. Elenkov, I.J. *et al.* 2000. The sympathetic nerve—an integrative interface between two supersystems: the brain and the immune system. *Pharmacol. Rev.* **52:** 595–638.

47. Bartolomucci, A. *et al.* 2001. Social status in mice: behavioral, endocrine and immune changes are context dependent. *Physiol. Behav.* **73:** 401–410.

48. Zorrilla, E.P. *et al.* 2001. The relationship of depression and stressors to immunological assays: a meta-analytic review. *Brain Behav. Immun.* **15:** 199–226.

49. Cacho, R. *et al.* 2003. Endocrine and lymphoproliferative response changes produced by social stress in mice. *Physiol. Behav.* **78:** 505–512.

50. Devoino, L., E. Alperina & T. Pavina. 2003. Immunological consequences of the reversal of social status in C57BL/6J mice. *Brain Behav. Immun.* **17:** 28–34.

51. Palermo-Neto, J., C. de Oliveira Massoco & W. Robespierre deSouza. 2003. Effects of physical and psychological stressors on behavior, macrophage activity, and Ehrlich tumor growth. *Brain Behav. Immun.* **17:** 43–54.

52. Morgulis, M.S. *et al.* 2004. Cohabitation with a sick cage mate: consequences on behavior and on ehrlich tumor growth. *Neuroimmunomodulation* **11:** 49–57.

53. Hart, B.L. 1988. Biological basis of the behavior of sick animals. *Neurosci. Biobehav. Rev.* **12:** 123–137.

54. Kluger, M.J. 1991. Fever: role of pyrogens and cryogens. *Physiol. Rev.* **71:** 93–127.

55. Murray, M.J. & A.B. Murray. 1979. Anorexia of infection as a mechanism of host defense. *Am. J. Clin. Nutr.* **32:** 593–596.

56. Kent, S. *et al.* 1992. Sickness behavior as a new target for drug development. *Trends Pharmacol. Sci.* **13:** 24–28.

57. Barnard, C.J. & J.M. Behnke. 2001. From psychoneuroimmunology to ecological immunology: life history

strategies and immunity trade-offs. In *Psychoneuroimmunology*. R. Ader, D.L. Felten & N. Cohen, Eds.: 35–47. Academic Press. New York.

58. de Groot, J. *et al.* (1999. A single social defeat transiently suppresses the anti-viral immune response in mice. *J. Neuroimmunol.* **95:** 143–151.
59. Ginsburg, B. & W.C. Allec. 1942. Some effects of conditioning on social dominance and subordination in inbred strains of mice. *Physiol. Zool.* **15:** 485–506.
60. Kundryavsteva, N.N. 1991. A sensory contact model for the study of agressive and submissive behavior in male mice. *Aggressive Behav.* **17:** 285–291.
61. Vekovishcheva, O.Y., I.A. Sukhotina & E.E. Zvartau. 2000. Co-housing in a stable hierarchical group is not aversive for dominant and subordinate individuals. *Neurosci. Behav. Physiol.* **30:** 195–200.
62. Sa-Rocha, V.M., L.C. Sa-Rocha & J. Palermo-Neto. 2006. Variations in behavior, innate immunity and host resistance to B16F10 melanoma growth in mice that present social stable hierarchical ranks. *Physiol. Behav.* **88:** 108–115.
63. Cohn, D.W. & L.C. de Sa-Rocha. 2006. Differential effects of lipopolysaccharide in the social behavior of dominant and submissive mice. *Physiol. Behav.* **87:** 932–937.
64. Moyer, E.K. 1976. *The Psychobiology of Aggression.* Harper and Row, Publisher. New York.
65. Kelley, A.E. 1993. Locomotor activity and exploration. In *Methods in Behavioral Pharmacology.* F. Van Haaren, Ed.: 499–518. Elsevier Science. New York.
66. Pellow, S. *et al.* 1985. Validation of open:closed arm entries in an elevated plus-maze as a measure of anxiety in the rat. *J. Neurosci. Methods* **14:** 149–167.
67. Lister, R.G. 1987. The use of a plus-maze to measure anxiety in the mouse. *Psychopharmacology (Berl.)* **92:** 180–185.
68. Smyth, M.J., D.I. Godfrey & J.A. Trapani. 2001. A fresh look at tumor immunosurveillance and immunotherapy. *Nat. Immunol.* **2:** 293–299.
69. Brown, L.M., D.R. Welch & S.R. Rannels. 2002. B16F10 melanoma cell colonization of mouse lung is enhanced by partial pneumonectomy. *Clin. Exp. Metastasis* **19:** 369–376.
70. Grant, E.C. & J.H. Mackintosh. 1963. A comparison of the social postures of some common laboratory rodents. *Behavior* **21:** 247–259.
71. Hart, B.L. 1990. Behavioral adaptations to pathogens and parasites: five strategies. *Neurosci. Biobehav. Rev.* **14:** 273–294.
72. Aubert, A. 1999. Sickness and behaviour in animals: a motivational perspective. *Neurosci. Biobehav. Rev.* **23:** 1029–1036.
73. Aubert, A. *et al.* 1997. Differential effects of lipopolysaccharide on pup retrieving and nest building in lactating mice. *Brain Behav. Immun.* **11:** 107–118.
74. Aubert, A., K.W. Kelley & R. Dantzer. 1997. Differential effect of lipopolysaccharide on food hoarding behavior and food consumption in rats. *Brain Behav. Immun.* **11:** 229–238.
75. Sieber, B., H.R. Frischknecht & P.G. Waser. 1981. Behavioral effects of hashish in mice. IV. Social dominance, food dominance, and sexual behavior within a group of males. *Psychopharmacology (Berl.)* **73:** 142–146.

Immunology, Signal Transduction, and Behavior in Hypothalamic–Pituitary–Adrenal Axis-related Genetic Mouse Models

Susana Silberstein,[a] **Annette M. Vogl,**[b] **Juán José Bonfiglio,**[a] **Wolfgang Wurst,**[b,c] **Florian Holsboer,**[b] **Eduardo Arzt,**[a] **Jan M. Deussing,**[b] **and Damián Refojo**[b]

[a]*Laboratorio de Fisiología y Biología Molecular, Departamento de Fisiología y Biología Molecular y Celular, Facultad de Ciencias Exactas y Naturales, Universidad de Buenos Aires, and IFYBINE: Instituto de Fisiología, Biología Molecular y Neurociencias–Consejo Nacional de Investigaciones Científicas y Técnicas, Buenos Aires, Argentina*

[b]*Max-Planck Institute of Psychiatry, Munich, Germany*

[c]*Institute of Developmental Genetics, Helmholtz Zentrum München, German Research Center for Environmental Health, Munich, Germany*

A classical view of the neuroendocrine–immune network assumes bidirectional interactions where pro-inflammatory cytokines influence hypothalamic–pituitary–adrenal (HPA) axis-derived hormones that subsequently affect cytokines in a permanently servo-controlled circle. Nevertheless, this picture has been continuously evolving over the last years as a result of the discovery of redundant expression and extended functions of many of the molecules implicated. Thus, cytokines are not only expressed in cells of the immune system but also in the central nervous system, and many hormones present at hypothalamic–pituitary level are also functionally expressed in the brain as well as in other peripheral organs, including immune cells. Because of this intermingled network of molecules redundantly expressed, the elucidation of the unique roles of HPA axis-related molecules at every level of complexity is one of the major challenges in the field. Genetic engineering in the mouse offers the most convincing method for dissecting *in vivo* the specific roles of distinct molecules acting in complex networks. Thus, various immunological, behavioral, and signal transduction studies performed with different HPA axis-related mutant mouse lines to delineate the roles of β-endorphin, the type 1 receptor of corticotropin-releasing hormone (CRHR1), and its ligand CRH will be discussed here.

Key words: HPA axis; mouse models; β-endorphin; CRH; CRF; ERK; MAPK; stress; behavior; forced swim test; stress-coping behavior

Introduction

In a classical view, the hypothalamic–pituitary–adrenal (HPA) axis is constituted by

Address for correspondence: Dr. Damian Refojo or Dr. Jan Deussing, Max-Planck Institute of Psychiatry, Kraepelinstrasse 2-10, 80804 Munich, Germany. Voice: +49 (0)89 30622-240; fax: +49 (0)89 30622-610. refojo@mpipsykl.mpg.de; Voice: +49 (0)89 30622-639; fax: +49 (0)89 30622-610. deussing@mpipsykl.mpg.de

Dr. Eduardo Arzt, Laboratorio de Fisiologia y Biologia Molecular, FCEN, Universidad de Buenos Aires; Ciudad Universitaria, 1428 Buenos Aires, Argentina. Voice: +54-11-4576-3368/86; fax: +54-11-4576-3321. earzt@fbmc.fcen.uba.ar

the parvocellular corticotropin-releasing hormone (CRH)-positive neurons of the hypothalamic paraventricular nucleus (PVN), the corticotrophs, and the adrenal cortex.[1] But in a wider sense, the HPA axis belongs to a more complex and intermingled system built by many different tissues and organs of the body as well as a great number of nuclei in the nervous system. Whereas the HPA axis exhibits *per se* a clear axial conformation, many of the molecules that constitute this axis, for instance CRH, adrenocorticotropic hormone

Neuroimmunomodulation: Ann. N.Y. Acad. Sci. 1153: 120–130 (2009).
doi: 10.1111/j.1749-6632.2008.03967.x © 2009 New York Academy of Sciences.

(ACTH), β-endorphin, glucocorticoids (GCs), and all their receptors, are widely expressed throughout the brain and in a myriad of cells, tissues, and organs of the periphery.[2,3] All these molecules maintain a close anatomical and functional cross-communication establishing an intricate working network where every molecular member has additive, synergistic, and complementary but also overlapping and compensatory functions over other members of the network.[3,4] In this context, the elucidation of the molecular and physiological roles of individual genes in specific locations has been and continues to be one of the major challenges in neuroimmunomodulation. The use of genetic engineering tools to achieve the disruption or overexpression of a gene of interest in a conditionally controlled manner, offers the most valuable tool to dissect *in vivo* the role of single molecules acting in complex circuitries.[5,6]

In the present revision we will focus on three molecules of the HPA axis: β-endorphin, CRH, and its type 1 receptor (CRHR1). β-endorphin is expressed in the brain stem and diencephalon of the central nervous system (CNS), in pituitary corticotrophs, and also in peripheral immunocytes. Different endocrine and immunological aspects of β-endorphin with special focus on studies performed in β-endorphin-mutant mice will be analyzed. CRH and its receptor CRHR1 exert key roles in triggering and controlling the stress response[7–10] as well as in the development of chronic stress-related disorders, such as anxiety and depression.[2,11] To elucidate the mechanism of action of these molecules in the brain, a set of experiments performed with different mutant mouse models will be discussed.

In Vivo Dissection of β-Endorphin Roles in Neuroimmunomodulation

Proopiomelanocortin (POMC)-derived peptides are expressed not only in the hypothalamic arcuate nucleus and anterior-intermediate pituitary cells but also in immunocompetent cells.[12,13] In particular, β-endorphin is synthesized and released by splenocytes, peripheral blood lymphocytes, and monocytes,[14,15] a process enhanced by mitogens and T cell activation.[16]

There are substantial data underpinning the effects of β-endorphin and opioids on the immune system, but a general agreement about the net effect has not yet been reached.[17,18]

β-endorphin enhances lipopolysaccharide (LPS)-induced interleukin (IL)-1 production by macrophages[19,20] and stimulates the basal expression of the IL-1 receptor antagonist.[21] Nevertheless, opposite effects of β-endorphin have also been reported in primary cell cultures, macrophage cell lines, and peripheral blood mononuclear cells.[22,23] A similar situation is present in the case of lymphocytes where both stimulatory[24–26] and inhibitory[27,28] roles of β-endorphin on lymphocyte proliferation have been reported.

Taking all this into consideration, divergent or even opposite effects of β-endorphin have been observed at different levels of the immune response. Gene targeting to create null mutations is a powerful tool to dissect complex phenotypes. In order to clarify the *in vivo* function of β-endorphin on the immune function, we studied the cell proliferation response of lymphocytes and the secretion of pro-inflammatory cytokines in mice lacking β-*endorphin*.[29]

Splenocytes obtained from wild-type (WT) mice and mice lacking β-*endorphin* were stimulated with different mitogens: LPS, pokeweed, and concanavalin A (Con A). Basal proliferative rates did not differ between genotypes. However, the mitogen-induced proliferation was significantly higher in β-*endorphin*-deficient mice. Accordingly, Con A-treated lymphocytes derived from β-*endorphin*-null mice showed higher levels of IL-2 than that of control animals.[30] Next, the production of inflammatory cytokines was evaluated in splenic macrophage cultures. Both tumor necrosis factor and IL-6 production in response to LPS was significantly increased in macrophage cultures from mice lacking β-*endorphin* compared to WT mice. Similarly, after LPS administration *in vivo*, IL-6 plasma levels rose in both genotypes but were significantly higher in β-*endorphin* knockout (KO) mice. These results strongly suggest that local endogenous β-*endorphin* would exert local anti-inflammatory and antiproliferative actions.

To address the endocrine aspect under β-endorphin-deficient conditions, we evaluated the HPA axis response to LPS *in vivo*. Basal plasma ACTH and corticosterone levels showed no differences between genotypes, as previously reported.[29] However, the stimulated responses of both plasma ACTH and corticosterone levels to systemic LPS, were significantly attenuated in mice lacking β-*endorphin* compared to WT mice.[30] Interestingly, the blunted ACTH and corticosterone responses of β-endorphin-deficient mice to LPS, represent a stress-specific differential response because basal and stimulated corticosterone levels in response to restraint- and ether-induced stress were normal in these mutant mice.[29]

A global analysis of the immunological and endocrine parameters studied, emphasizes the concept that β-endorphin exerts anti-inflammatory and immunosuppressive actions both directly at immunological levels and indirectly by means of the potentiation of the HPA axis activation after immunological challenge and its concomitant increase in circulating GCs.

Beyond Receptor: Elucidating the Brain Specificity of CRHR1-mediated MAPK Activation

CRH is a 41-amino acid peptide that exerts a key role in the adjustment of neuroendocrine and behavioral adaptations to stress.[1,2,7,8,10] By means of the activation of ACTH release, the hypothalamic CRH neurons drive both basal and stress-induced HPA activation. Besides the hypothalamus, CRH is widely distributed throughout the CNS,[31] where it acts as a neuroregulator in extrahypothalamic circuits to develop and integrate a complex response to

stress, controlling numerous behaviors, such as anxiety, arousal, locomotor activity, sexual behavior, sleep, and memory formation.[2,7–10] As will be highlighted below, alterations in this system may influence the development of affective disorders and other stress-related clinical conditions.[2,11,32–34]

CRH exerts its actions by means of two subtypes of CRH receptors (CRHR1 and CRHR2) that display different localization throughout the brain.[35,36] CRH is a high-affinity ligand for CRHR1 and binds poorly to the CRHR2 for which other ligands, such as urocortin (Ucn), have stronger affinity.[32,33,37] *CRHR1* KO mice exhibit reduced anxiety-related behavior and an impaired basal and stress-induced HPA axis response.[38,39]

CRHRs are G protein-coupled seven transmembrane receptors linked to a number of intracellular signaling pathways.[37,40] In the corticotroph cell line, AtT20, one of the most used cellular models for studying CRH-dependent signaling, CRH activates, via cAMP–protein kinase A (PKA)-dependent cascades, the transcription factor cAMP response element binding as well as the orphan receptor Nur77, which finally drive the transcription of the *POMC* gene.[37,40,41] Using this cell line we demonstrated that CRH activates extracellular signal-regulated kinase (ERK)1/2 via a PKA–calcium/calmodulin-dependent protein kinase 2 alpha (CamKIIa)-dependent pathway to induce the full activation of the transcription factor Nur77.[42] Likewise, in Chinese hamster ovary cells stably expressing CRHR1, both Ucn I and CRH phosphorylate ERK1/2, a process mediated by PKA.[43] Nevertheless, the CRHR1-dependent activation of ERK–mitogen-activated protein kinase (MAPK) is not an obligate step in every cell system because, for instance, in human embryonic kidney 293 cells stably transfected with the type 1 receptor, CRH was ineffective in triggering ERK activation.[44] Similarly, in hippocampal or cerebellar primary cultures CRH does not trigger ERK activation[45] whereas in neuronal cell lines or hippocampal and cerebellar

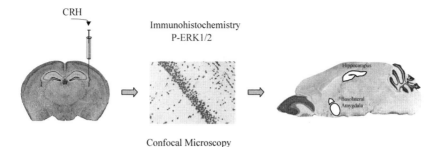

Figure 1. General strategy for the detection of corticotropin-releasing hormone (CRH)-induced extracellular signal-regulated kinase (ERK) activation in the brain *in vivo*. CRH was injected intracerebroventricularly (i.c.v.) into brains of *CRHR1$^{loxP/loxP}$-Camk2a-cre* and *CRHR1$^{loxP/loxP}$-Camk2a* control mice. Brains were removed and phospho (P)-ERK activation was evaluated by immunohistochemistry of P-ERK1/2. The analysis, performed by confocal microscopy, revealed a limbic-specific CRH-receptor1 (CRHR1)-dependent increase of P-ERK1/2 in the CA1 and CA3 region of the hippocampus as well as in the basolateral amygdala.

organotypic cultures it does.[46,47] These results clearly indicate that the cellular context crucially determines the final outcome of CRH-dependent signaling, further underlining the importance of studying CRHR1-downstream pathways under physiological conditions *in vivo*.

ERK1 and ERK2 are widely expressed in the brain although they show some differences in their expression patterns. While both kinases are strongly expressed in the basolateral complex (BLA) of the amygdala, only ERK2 is present at high levels in the pyramidal cell layer of the hippocampus.[48] Acute restraint stress increases ERK2 phosphorylation in hippocampus and prefrontal cortex,[49,50] and pharmacological manipulations of the ERK pathway affect different parameters in anxiety and stress-coping behavior tests.[49,51–53]

To elucidate the link between CRH, CRHRs (in particular CRHR1), and ERK signaling, we conducted functional *in vivo* experiments in WT mice and in mice carrying a *CRHR1* deletion in the anterior forebrain, including limbic structures.[54]

In the first set of experiments, CRH was injected intracerebroventricularly (i.c.v.) in undisturbed freely moving mice. After 10 and 30 min the central activation of ERK was evaluated by immunohistochemistry and confocal microscopy, using phospho-specific (anti-

P-ERK1/2) antibodies (Fig. 1). The acute administration of CRH induced a limbic-specific ERK activation pattern restricted to the hippocampus and amygdala.[54] In the hippocampal formation, only the pyramidal cells of the layer CA1 and CA3 were activated, whereas the dentate gyrus, a structure that contains both CRHR1/R2, remained virtually absent of activation, underlining the specificity of the activation pattern. A low basal phosphorylation level present both in the cortex and in the PVN was not altered by the CRH injection. In the amygdala, only the BLA became activated by the peptide, while all the other amygdaloid nuclei remained unchanged. The fact that CRH injection triggers such a specific activation pattern even though ERK1/2 kinases and CRHRs are widely expressed throughout the brain[35,36,48] suggests that a molecular and functional link between the CRHRs and downstream MAPKs may be present only on these structures.

In order to further confirm specificity and to determine the CRHR subtype involved in the CRH-induced activation of P-ERK1/2, we carried out i.c.v. CRH or vehicle injections in *CRHR1$^{loxP/loxP}$-Camk2a-cre* and *CRHR1$^{loxP/loxP}$*-control mice.[55] In the *CRHR1$^{loxP/loxP}$*-control line, exons 8–13 of the *CRHR1* gene are flanked by loxP recombination sites. By breeding with a *Camk2a-cre* line that expresses the Cre recombinase in forebrain structures, it was possible to delete *CRHR1* only in anterior limbic structures. This conditional approach offers the advantage of conserving the pituitary expression of CRHR1, thus leaving the HPA axis unaffected. This is a crucial feature for analyzing ERK activation because MAPKs are known targets of corticosteroids, and a virtual hypocorticosterone state could obscure the interpretation of the results. Consequently, the same injection protocol was conducted in the *CRHR1*-mutant animals.

Immunohistochemical analysis showed that CRH-induced activation of ERK at both CA1/CA3 and BLA were strongly reduced in *CRHR1^{loxP/loxP}-Camk2a-cre* mice, providing evidence for a critical role of CRHR1 in the CRH signaling process.

Thus, CRH preferentially activates ERK in limbic structures closely related with learning and memory, environmental information processing, and behavioral aspects of stress but not in other structures, such as the hypothalamus, or the central amygdala involved in autonomic and neuroendocrine adaptation to stress. These results suggest that ERK kinases could also be linked to the effects of CRH in chronic stress-related disorders. Nevertheless, limbic P-ERK2 is decreased in chronic stress models in rodents,[50,56] and suicide victims exhibit decreased levels of ERK in the prefrontal cortex and hippocampus.[57] The effects of the ERK pathway on several anxiety and depression-related behavioral parameters have been analyzed, but a clear picture of its role remains elusive. Experiments with pharmacological inhibitors have shown opposite results in different tests used to evaluate anxiety, such as fear conditioning, fear startle response, and elevated plus maze.[49,58,59] Immobility in the forced swim test (FST)—a paradigm used to measure efficiency of antidepressant drugs—is a parameter that indicates behavioral despair. The peripheral administration of mitogen-activated protein/extracellular signal-regulated kinase (MEK) inhibitors has been reported to decrease,[51] increase,[52] and not

to affect[53] immobility in rodents. The causes of these discrepancies remain unclear, but recent experiments demonstrate that the temporal dimension may be fundamental in understanding the fine-tuned role of ERK1/2 in mood disorders. Whereas acute injections of an MEK inhibitor strongly reduced immobility and latency escapes in learned helplessness models, subacute administration has the opposite effect.[52] Thus ERK kinases could not only have different roles on different brain structures but these effects could also change over time. In this context, the role of MAPKs under chronic CRH exposition is still unclear, and new investigations are being conducted to elucidate it.

Conditional Region-specific Overexpression of CRH in the Brain: Modeling Stress-coping Behavior

Dysregulation of the CRH system and accompanying chronically elevated CRH levels play a role in human stress-related and affective disorders, including anxiety disorders and major depression.[2,11,32–34] However, after years of enormous research effort, a complete picture of the etiology and mechanisms underlying mood disorders remains unknown. This failure has been explained by the fact that the lack of known pathophysiological mechanisms gives rise to two negative consequences: (1) the absence of new molecular targets for drug discovery and (2) the impossibility of replicating genetic causes of the diseases in animal models.[60]

The HPA axis in general and the central CRH/CRHR system in particular arguably offer one of the strongest basis for understanding the mechanistic processes involved in mood disorders.[11,32,33,40] Elevated CRH levels in cerebrospinal fluid and a blunted ACTH release in response to exogenous CRH are observed in depressed patients.[61,62] CRH expression in the hypothalamic PVN is increased,[63] while CRH binding in the prefrontal cortex of depressed patients who committed suicide is diminished.[64] In addition, an acute increase in central CRH concentrations results in depression-like symptomatology in laboratory animals.[65]

The problem of the lack of *bona fide* animal models for mood disorders is due to the fact that all existing animal models rely on the exposure of healthy animals to different stress paradigms. However, these models have not led to the discovery of compounds with truly new mechanisms of action. At this point, as was stated by others previously,[60,66] a circular paradox emerges: good animal models are required to better understand depression, but development of such models requires a better understanding of the etiology of the disorder. Thus, genetically engineered mice might circumvent this problem, thereby providing new models to more precisely dissect genetic influences on behavior in basic psychiatric research.[5,6,60]

Taking all this into consideration, genetic manipulations of the central CRH system would certainly offer a reliable *in vivo* system to model specific mood disorder-related endophenotypes and at the same time to investigate the pathophysiological role of the CRH system in chronic stress-related disorders.

Two CRH overexpressing (OE) transgenic mouse lines have been established in the past, expressing CRH either under the control of the broadly active methallothionein (*MTI–CRH–OE*[67] or the CNS-restricted Thy-1.2 promoter (*Thy–CRH–OE*).[68] In both cases CRH overexpression resulted in elevated GC levels and Cushing-like symptoms. GCs are known to influence anxiety-related behavior.[2,69] Therefore, the behavioral phenotype of these animals may result from CRH overexpression itself or, alternatively, from increased GC levels. To solve this unclear outcome we developed a mouse model, which permits conditional CRH overexpression in the absence of marked neuroendocrine disturbances. Transgenic mouse lines conditionally overexpressing CRH were generated by combining the knock-in of the murine *CRH* cDNA into the *ROSA26 (R26)* locus with

the versatile Cre/loxP system (Fig. 2).[70] This conditional mouse model enables us to overexpress CRH in a spatio-temporally regulated fashion.

CNS-restricted CRH overexpression, achieved by breeding with Nestin-Cre mice (*CRH–COE^Nes*), did not alter the basal status of the HPA axis. Corticosterone and ACTH plasma levels determined either in the morning or afternoon remained unchanged, showing no effects of the CRH overexpression on HPA axis circadian rhythmicity. Nevertheless, CRH overexpression driven by the *Nestin* promoter resulted in a stress-induced, gender-specific, HPA axis hyperactivity (present in male but not female mice), displayed by elevated plasma ACTH and corticosterone levels after restraint stress. The *Nestin* promoter is expressed in the hypothalamus, including the PVN, and consequently an increased expression of CRH would be expected to result in high corticosterone levels in mice. However, adaptive mechanisms occur at hypothalamic level, resulting in significantly downregulated basal levels of endogenous CRH, keeping the total CRH constant. This could explain the normal concentrations of HPA axis hormones.

One of the main features of depression is the increased stress-reactivity status.[71] The evaluation of immobility in the Porsolt FST used after drug administration is highly predictive for clinically effective monoamine-targeting antidepressants. However, under nonpharmacological conditions, the FST also involves a strong component of stress-coping behavior, arousal, and alertness; all behavioral parameters dependent on catecholaminergic neurotransmisson as well.

Thus, *CRH-COE^Nes* mice showed an increased, active, stress-coping behavior in the FST and tail suspension test.[70] The reduction in immobility, resulting from mimicking the behavioral consequences of stress-mediated activation of the endogenous CRH system by exogenous CRH overexpression, is indicative of an enhanced responsiveness of these mice to a stressful stimulus.

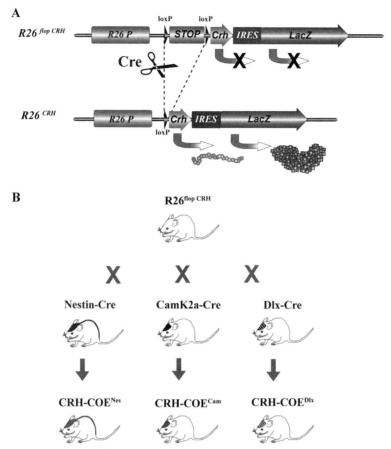

Figure 2. Generation of conditional CRH overexpressing mouse lines. (**A**) A *CRH-IRES–LacZ* construct was knocked into the ubiquitously active *ROSA26 locus*. To prevent expression of CRH and LacZ in the absence of Cre recombinase, a transcriptional stop cassette flanked by two loxP sites was inserted between the *ROSA26 promoter* (R26 P) and the *CRH-IRES-LacZ* construct. By using homologous recombination in embryonic stem cells, the *R26flopCRH* mouse line was generated. (**B**) To achieve overexpression of CRH in the whole central nervous system (CNS), this floxed mouse line (*R26flopCRH*) was bred to a *Nestin-Cre* transgenic line. After Cre-mediated excision of the stop cassette, CRH and LacZ are overexpressed in the whole CNS of the new line generated (*CRH-COENes*). Breeding the *R26flopCRH* to the *Camk2a-Cre* mouse line resulted in a new line (*CRH-COECam*) specifically overexpressing CRH in principal neurons of the forebrain. To restrict CRH overexpression to GABAergic interneurons, the *R26flopCRH* mouse was bred to *Dlx-Cre* mice. IRES, internal ribosome entry site.

Restricting CRH overexpression to principal neurons in forebrain structures (by breeding with a *Camk2a-Cre* line) and GABAergic interneurons (by breeding with the *Dlx5/6-Cre* mice) (Fig. 2) failed to affect the stress-coping behavior in the FST, suggesting that more caudal brain regions may be responsible for the observed behavioral phenotype.

Accordingly, the forced swimming-induced neuronal activation in the locus coeruleus (measured by means of c-fos and Zif268 *in situ* hybridization) was strongly enhanced in *CRH-COENes* mice. Moreover, the pharmacological blockade of catecholamine synthesis by alpha-methyl-p-tyrosine but not of serotonin synthesis by p-chlorophenylalanine, reversed the FST phenotype in these animals, further suggesting a noradrenaline involvement in the decreased immobility observed in *CRH-COENes* mice.[70] Nevertheless, in the *Thy-CRH-OE* mouse line this phenotype could not be replicated.[68] Although these discrepancies might be due to the presence of different levels of circulating corticosteroids (normal in *CRH-COE[Nes]* but elevated in *Thy-CRH-OE* mice), this is most probably not the case because the other CRH-OE line with high corticosterone levels (*MTI-CRH-OE*) also displays less immobility in the FST.[72] Thus, other influences related to differences in compensatory mechanisms triggered by different promoters, behavioral test conditions, and background of strains could explain these differences. Interestingly, both *Thy-CRH-OE* and *CRH-COE[Nes]* mice showed no differences in anxiety-like behavior in the elevated plus maze and dark–light box tests (Lu and Deussing, Unpublished results).[68,70] In contrast, acute injection of CRH induces anxiety-like behaviors and *CRHR1* KO mice exhibit decreased anxiety in respective behavioral tests.[39,55,73] The explanation for such a discrepancy remains elusive, but a plausible explanation might be related to the concentration of and the time that CRH is active in the synapses. Hence the permanent presence of bioactive CRH in the brain might trigger compensatory mechanisms that counterregulate the chronic anxious response. This opens up the question of whether the link between CRH hyperfunction and anxiety disorders requires a concentration window where either too little or too much CRH keeps the resilience and avoids the appearance of anxiety, whereas sustained intermediate to high levels of CRH switch on the anxiogenic circuits. This question will definitively be addressed in the near future by means of new mouse models carrying inducible promoters where the expression of the Cre recombinase could be tightly controlled by tamoxifen or doxycycline.

In conclusion, we have generated a flexible animal model for CRH overproduction, which will help to determine the contribution of CRH-sensitive pathways involved in the transition from physiological to pathological stress response, a crucial event in the development of affective disorders. In addition, *CRH-COE[Nes]* mice represent a robust genetic model for testing new candidate drugs for treatment of chronic stress-related disorders, such as CRHR1 antagonists.

General Conclusions

β-endorphin, CRH, and CRHR1 are three clear examples of molecules expressed in different regions of the brain and in different cells and organs of the periphery. The full comprehension of their roles in every localization is essential for understanding the functioning of the networks to which they belong. Until now, conditional gene targeting permitted the development of mutant mice with a tight control of spatial expression. In the near future this spatial control must be improved with the arrival of new Cre lines driven by HPA-related promoters that will allow the targeting of specific cell populations. Finally the field will need to improve the temporal aspect of genetic control with the introduction of inducible lines.

Acknowledgments

This work was supported by grants from the Max Planck Society, Germany; the University of Buenos Aires (UBA), the Consejo Nacional de Investigaciones Científicas y Técnicas (CONICET), and Agencia Nacional de Promoción Científica y Tecnológica (ANPCYT), Argentina. D.R. is supported by the European Molecular Biology Organization. J.D. is supported by the Fonds der Chemischen Industrie.

Conflicts of Interest

The authors declare no conflicts of interest.

References

1. Smith, S.M. & W.W. Vale. 2006. The role of the hypothalamic-pituitary-adrenal axis in neuroendocrine responses to stress. *Dialogues Clin. Neurosci.* **8:** 383–395.

2. de Kloet, E.R., M. Joels & F. Holsboer. 2005. Stress and the brain: from adaptation to disease. *Nat. Rev. Neurosci.* **6:** 463–475.

3. Hillhouse, E.W. & D.K. Grammatopoulos. 2006. The molecular mechanisms underlying the regulation of the biological activity of corticotropin-releasing hormone receptors: implications for physiology and pathophysiology. *Endocr. Rev.* **27:** 260–286.

4. Besedovsky, H.O. & R.A. del Rey. 1996. Immune-neuro-endocrine interactions: facts and hypotheses. *Endocr. Rev.* **17:** 64–102.

5. Branda, C.S. & S.M. Dymecki. 2004. Talking about a revolution: the impact of site-specific recombinases on genetic analyses in mice. *Dev. Cell* **6:** 7–28.

6. Deussing, J.M. & W. Wurst. 2005. Dissecting the genetic effect of the CRH system on anxiety and stress-related behaviour. *C.R. Biol.* **328:** 199–212.

7. Bale, T.L. & W.W. Vale. 2004. CRF and CRF receptors: role in stress responsivity and other behaviors. *Annu. Rev. Pharmacol. Toxicol.* **44:** 525–557.

8. Herman, J.P., H. Figueiredo, N.K. Mueller, *et al.* 2003. Central mechanisms of stress integration: hierarchical circuitry controlling hypothalamo-pituitary-adrenocortical responsiveness. *Front Neuroendocrinol.* **24:** 151–180.

9. Korosi, A. & T.Z. Baram. 2008. The central corticotropin releasing factor system during development and adulthood. *Eur. J. Pharmacol.* **583:** 204–214.

10. Smagin, G.N., S.C. Heinrichs & A.J. Dunn. 2001. The role of CRH in behavioral responses to stress. *Peptides* **22:** 713–724.

11. Arborelius, L., M.J. Owens, P.M. Plotsky, *et al.* 1999. The role of corticotropin-releasing factor in depression and anxiety disorders. *J. Endocrinol.* **160:** 1–12.

12. Buzzetti, R., L. McLoughlin, P.M. Lavender, *et al.* 1989. Expression of pro-opiomelanocortin gene and quantification of adrenocorticotropic hormone-like immunoreactivity in human normal peripheral mononuclear cells and lymphoid and myeloid malignancies. *J. Clin. Invest.* **83:** 733–737.

13. Lyons, P.D. & J.E. Blalock. 1997. Pro-opiomelanocortin gene expression and protein processing in rat mononuclear leukocytes. *J. Neuroimmunol.* **78:** 47–56.

14. Cabot, P.J., L. Carter, C. Gaiddon, *et al.* 1997. Immune cell-derived beta-endorphin. Production, release, and control of inflammatory pain in rats. *J. Clin. Invest.* **100:** 142–148.

15. Smith, E.M. & J.E. Blalock. 1981. Human lymphocyte production of corticotropin and endorphin-like substances: association with leukocyte interferon. *Proc. Natl. Acad. Sci. USA* **78:** 7530–7534.

16. Kavelaars, A., R.E. Ballieux & C.J. Heijnen. 1989. The role of IL-1 in the corticotropin-releasing factor and arginine-vasopressin-induced secretion of immunoreactive beta-endorphin by human peripheral blood mononuclear cells. *J. Immunol.* **142:** 2338–2342.

17. Blalock, J.E. 1998. Beta-endorphin in immune cells. *Immunol. Today* **19:** 191–192.

18. Panerai, A.E. & P. Sacerdote. 1997. Beta-endorphin in the immune system: a role at last? *Immunol. Today* **18:** 317–319.

19. Apte, R.N., S.K. Durum & J.J. Oppenheim. 1990. Opioids modulate interleukin-1 production and secretion by bone-marrow macrophages. *Immunol. Lett.* **24:** 141–148.

20. Hosoi, J., H. Ozawa & R.D. Granstein. 1999. beta-Endorphin binding and regulation of cytokine expression in Langerhans cells. *Ann. N. Y. Acad. Sci.* **885:** 405–413.

21. Kovalovsky, D., M.P. Pereda, G.K. Stalla, *et al.* 1999. Differential regulation of interleukin-1 receptor antagonist by proopiomelanocortin peptides adrenocorticotropic hormone and beta-endorphin. *Neuroimmunomodulation* **6:** 367–372.

22. Belkowski, S.M., C. Alicea, T.K. Eisenstein, *et al.* 1995. Inhibition of interleukin-1 and tumor necrosis factor-alpha synthesis following treatment of macrophages with the kappa opioid agonist U50, 488H. *J. Pharmacol. Exp. Ther.* **273:** 1491–1496.

23. Chao, C.C., T.W. Molitor, K. Close, *et al.* 1993. Morphine inhibits the release of tumor necrosis factor in human peripheral blood mononuclear cell cultures. *Int. J. Immunopharmacol.* **15:** 447–453.

24. Fontana, L., A. Fattorossi, R. D'Amelio, *et al.* 1987. Modulation of human concanavalin A-induced lymphocyte proliferative response by physiological concentrations of beta-endorphin. *Immunopharmacology* **13:** 111–115.

25. Gilmore, W. & L.P. Weiner. 1989. The opioid specificity of beta-endorphin enhancement of murine lymphocyte proliferation. *Immunopharmacology* **17:** 19–30.

26. Van den Bergh, P., J. Rozing & L. Nagelkerken. 1991. Two opposing modes of action of beta-endorphin on lymphocyte function. *Immunology* **72:** 537–543.

27. Puppo, F., G. Corsini, P. Mangini, *et al.* 1985. Influence of beta-endorphin on phytohemagglutinin-induced lymphocyte proliferation and on the expression of mononuclear cell surface antigens in vitro. *Immunopharmacology* **10:** 119–125.

28. Panerai, A.E., B. Manfredi, F. Granucci, *et al.* 1995. The beta-endorphin inhibition of mitogen-induced splenocytes proliferation is mediated by central and peripheral paracrine/autocrine effects of the opioid. *J. Neuroimmunol.* **58:** 71–76.

29. Rubinstein, M., J.S. Mogil, M. Japon, *et al.* 1996. Absence of opioid stress-induced analgesia in mice lacking beta-endorphin by site-directed mutagenesis. *Proc. Natl. Acad. Sci. USA* **93:** 3995–4000.

30. Refojo, D., D. Kovalovsky, J.I. Young, *et al*. 2002. Increased splenocyte proliferative response and cytokine production in beta-endorphin-deficient mice. *J. Neuroimmunol.* **131:** 126–134.

31. Swanson, L.W., P.E. Sawchenko, J. Rivier, *et al*. 1983. Organization of ovine corticotropin-releasing factor immunoreactive cells and fibers in the rat brain: an immunohistochemical study. *Neuroendocrinology* **36:** 165–186.

32. Grigoriadis, D.E. 2005. The corticotropin-releasing factor receptor: a novel target for the treatment of depression and anxiety-related disorders. *Expert. Opin. Ther. Targets* **9:** 651–684.

33. Holsboer, F. & M. Ising. 2008. Central CRH system in depression and anxiety—evidence from clinical studies with CRH1 receptor antagonists. *Eur. J. Pharmacol.* **583:** 350–357.

34. Todorovic, C., O. Jahn, H. Tezval, *et al*. 2005. The role of CRF receptors in anxiety and depression: implications of the novel CRF1 agonist cortagine. *Neurosci. Biobehav. Rev.* **29:** 1323–1333.

35. Bittencourt, J.C. & P.E. Sawchenko. 2000. Do centrally administered neuropeptides access cognate receptors?: an analysis in the central corticotropin-releasing factor system. *J. Neurosci.* **20:** 1142–1156.

36. Van Pett, K., V. Viau, J.C. Bittencourt, *et al*. 2000. Distribution of mRNAs encoding CRF receptors in brain and pituitary of rat and mouse. *J. Comp. Neurol.* **428:** 191–212.

37. Hauger, R.L., V. Risbrough, O. Brauns, *et al*. 2006. Corticotropin releasing factor (CRF) receptor signaling in the central nervous system: new molecular targets. *CNS Neurol. Disord. Drug Targets* **5:** 453–479.

38. Timpl, P., R. Spanagel, I. Sillaber, *et al*. 1998. Impaired stress response and reduced anxiety in mice lacking a functional corticotropin-releasing hormone receptor 1. *Nat. Genet.* **19:** 162–166.

39. Smith, G.W., J.M. Aubry, F. Dellu, *et al*. 1998. Corticotropin releasing factor receptor 1-deficient mice display decreased anxiety, impaired stress response, and aberrant neuroendocrine development. *Neuron* **20:** 1093–1102.

40. Arzt, E. & F. Holsboer. 2006. CRF signaling: molecular specificity for drug targeting in the CNS. *Trends Pharmacol. Sci.* **27:** 531–538.

41. Philips, A., S. Lesage, R. Gingras, *et al*. 1997. Novel dimeric Nur77 signaling mechanism in endocrine and lymphoid cells. *Mol. Cell Biol.* **17:** 5946–5951.

42. Kovalovsky, D., D. Refojo, A.C. Liberman, *et al*. 2002. Activation and induction of NUR77/NURR1 in corticotrophs by CRH/cAMP: involvement of calcium, protein kinase A, and MAPK pathways. *Mol. Endocrinol.* **16:** 1638–1651.

43. Brar, B.K., A. Chen, M.H. Perrin, *et al*. 2004. Specificity and regulation of extracellularly regulated kinase1/2 phosphorylation through corticotropin-releasing factor (CRF) receptors 1 and 2beta by the CRF/urocortin family of peptides. *Endocrinology* **145:** 1718–1729.

44. Grammatopoulos, D.K., H.S. Randeva, M.A. Levine, *et al*. 2000. Urocortin, but not corticotropin-releasing hormone (CRH), activates the mitogen-activated protein kinase signal transduction pathway in human pregnant myometrium: an effect mediated via R1alpha and R2beta CRH receptor subtypes and stimulation of Gq-proteins. *Mol. Endocrinol.* **14:** 2076–2091.

45. Bayatti, N., J. Zschocke & C. Behl. 2003. Brain region-specific neuroprotective action and signaling of corticotropin-releasing hormone in primary neurons. *Endocrinology* **144:** 4051–4060.

46. Elliott-Hunt, C.R., J. Kazlauskaite, G.J. Wilde, *et al*. 2002. Potential signalling pathways underlying corticotrophin-releasing hormone-mediated neuroprotection from excitotoxicity in rat hippocampus. *J. Neurochem.* **80:** 416–425.

47. Swinny, J.D., F. Metzger, J. IJkema-Paassen, *et al*. 2004. Corticotropin-releasing factor and urocortin differentially modulate rat Purkinje cell dendritic outgrowth and differentiation in vitro. *Eur. J. Neurosci.* **19:** 1749–1758.

48. Di Benedetto B., C. Hitz, S.M. Holter, *et al*. 2007. Differential mRNA distribution of components of the ERK/MAPK signalling cascade in the adult mouse brain. *J. Comp. Neurol.* **500:** 542–556.

49. Ailing, F., L. Fan, S. Li, *et al*. 2008. Role of extracellular signal-regulated kinase signal transduction pathway in anxiety. *J. Psychiatr. Res.* **43:** 55–63.

50. Meller, E., C. Shen, T.A. Nikolao, *et al*. 2003. Region-specific effects of acute and repeated restraint stress on the phosphorylation of mitogen-activated protein kinases. *Brain Res.* **979:** 57–64.

51. Einat, H., P. Yuan, T.D. Gould, *et al*. 2003. The role of the extracellular signal-regulated kinase signaling pathway in mood modulation. *J. Neurosci.* **23:** 7311–7316.

52. Duman, C.H., L. Schlesinger, M. Kodama, *et al*. 2007. A role for MAP kinase signaling in behavioral models of depression and antidepressant treatment. *Biol. Psychiatry* **61:** 661–670.

53. Tronson, N.C., C. Schrick, A. Fischer, *et al*. 2008. Regulatory mechanisms of fear extinction and depression-like behavior. *Neuropsychopharmacology* **33:** 1570–1583.

54. Refojo, D., C. Echenique, M.B. Muller, *et al*. 2005. Corticotropin-releasing hormone activates ERK1/2 MAPK in specific brain areas. *Proc. Natl. Acad. Sci. USA* **102:** 6183–6188.

55. Muller, M.B., S. Zimmermann, I. Sillaber, *et al.* 2003. Limbic corticotropin-releasing hormone receptor 1 mediates anxiety-related behavior and hormonal adaptation to stress. *Nat. Neurosci.* **6:** 1100–1107.

56. Qi, X., W. Lin, J. Li, *et al.* 2006. The depressive-like behaviors are correlated with decreased phosphorylation of mitogen-activated protein kinases in rat brain following chronic forced swim stress. *Behav. Brain Res.* **175:** 233–240.

57. Dwivedi, Y., H.S. Rizavi, R.C. Roberts, *et al.* 2001. Reduced activation and expression of ERK1/2 MAP kinase in the post-mortem brain of depressed suicide subjects. *J. Neurochem.* **77:** 916–928.

58. Di Benedetto B., M. Kallnik, D.M. Weisenhorn, *et al.* 2008. Activation of ERK/MAPK in the Lateral Amygdala of the Mouse is Required for Acquisition of a Fear-Potentiated Startle response. *Neuropsychopharmacology* In press.

59. Fischer, A., M. Radulovic, C. Schrick, *et al.* 2007. Hippocampal Mek/Erk signaling mediates extinction of contextual freezing behavior. *Neurobiol. Learn. Mem.* **87:** 149–158.

60. Berton, O. & E.J. Nestler. 2006. New approaches to antidepressant drug discovery: beyond monoamines. *Nat. Rev. Neurosci.* **7:** 137–151.

61. Nemeroff, C.B., E. Widerlov, G. Bissette, *et al.* 1984. Elevated concentrations of CSF corticotropin-releasing factor-like immunoreactivity in depressed patients. *Science* **226:** 1342–1344.

62. Holsboer, F., U. von Bardeleben, A. Gerken, *et al.* 1984. Blunted corticotropin and normal cortisol response to human corticotropin-releasing factor in depression. *N. Engl. J. Med.* **311:** 1127.

63. Raadsheer, F.C., W.J. Hoogendijk, F.C. Stam, *et al.* 1994. Increased numbers of corticotropin-releasing hormone expressing neurons in the hypothalamic paraventricular nucleus of depressed patients. *Neuroendocrinology* **60:** 436–444.

64. Nemeroff, C.B., M.J. Owens, G. Bissette, *et al.* 1988. Reduced corticotropin releasing factor binding sites in the frontal cortex of suicide victims. *Arch. Gen. Psychiatry* **45:** 577–579.

65. Dunn, A.J. & C.W. Berridge. 1990. Physiological and behavioral responses to corticotropin-releasing factor administration: is CRF a mediator of anxiety or stress responses? *Brain Res. Brain Res. Rev.* **15:** 71–100.

66. Tamminga, C.A., C.B. Nemeroff, R.D. Blakely, *et al.* 2002. Developing novel treatments for mood disorders: accelerating discovery. *Biol. Psychiatry* **52:** 589–609.

67. Stenzel-Poore, M.P., V.A. Cameron, J. Vaughan, *et al.* 1992. Development of Cushing's syndrome in corticotropin-releasing factor transgenic mice. *Endocrinology* **130:** 3378–3386.

68. Groenink, L., T. Pattij, J.R. De, *et al.* 2003. 5-HT1A receptor knockout mice and mice overexpressing corticotropin-releasing hormone in models of anxiety. *Eur. J. Pharmacol.* **463:** 185–197.

69. Tronche, F., C. Kellendonk, O. Kretz, *et al.* 1999. Disruption of the glucocorticoid receptor gene in the nervous system results in reduced anxiety. *Nat. Genet.* **23:** 99–103.

70. Lu, A., M.A. Steiner, N. Whittle, *et al.* 2008. Conditional mouse mutants highlight mechanisms of corticotropin-releasing hormone effects on stress-coping behavior. *Mol. Psychiatry* **13:** 1028–1042.

71. Hasler, G., W.C. Drevets, H.K. Manji, *et al.* 2004. Discovering endophenotypes for major depression. *Neuropsychopharmacology* **29:** 1765–1781.

72. van Gaalen, M.M., J.H. Reul, A. Gesing, *et al.* 2002. Mice overexpressing CRH show reduced responsiveness in plasma corticosterone after a5-HT1A receptor challenge. *Genes Brain Behav.* **1:** 174–177.

73. Steckler, T. & F. Holsboer. 1999. Corticotropin-releasing hormone receptor subtypes and emotion. *Biol. Psychiatry* **46:** 1480–1508.

Behavior and Stress Reactivity in Mouse Strains with Mitochondrial DNA Variations

Ulrike Gimsa,[a] Ellen Kanitz,[a] Winfried Otten,[a] and Saleh M. Ibrahim[b]

[a]Research Unit Behavioural Physiology, Research Institute for the Biology of Farm Animals, Dummerstorf, Germany

[b]Section of Immunogenetics, University of Rostock, Rostock, Germany

We studied the behavior and neuroendocrine regulation under social disruption stress of C57BL/6J mice in which mitochondria were substituted by mitochondria from AKR/J or FVB/N strains. C57BL/6J-mt$^{FVB/N}$ mice were significantly more anxious in the elevated plus-maze test than C57BL/6J-mt$^{AKR/J}$ and C57BL/6J mice at base line. In addition, they showed a reduced corticosterone response and an activation of serotonergic and dopaminergic neurotransmitter systems after repeated challenge, i.e., social defeat and elevated plus-maze test. Our findings suggest that mitochondrial variations could affect anxiety-like behavior as well as corticosterone and neurotransmitter response to psychological stress.

Key words: conplastic mouse strain; mitochondrial substitution; HPA reactivity; psychosocial stress; depression; corticosterone; serotonin; dopamine; noradrenaline; elevated plus maze; mtDNA; ATP8

Introduction

In humans, a growing body of evidence suggests that mitochondrial dysfunctions are involved in psychiatric disorders, such as schizophrenia, bipolar disease, and major depression.[1] In mice, a reduced expression of the *Bcl-2* gene in mitochondria, which is linked with mitochondrial dysfunction, has been shown to induce increased anxiety-like behavior.[2] Monoaminergic neurotransmitter systems have been in the focus of neurobiological studies of anxiety disorders and depression.[3–5] Monoamine oxidase inhibitors, which are among the most potent anxiolytics and antidepressants, have been shown to improve mitochondrial efficiency.[6]

Psychological stress has been shown to be associated with higher oxidative stress[7] and a reduced availability of antioxidants[8] in humans. On the other hand, psychological stress increased anxiety-like behavior in rats while at the same time reducing the supply of antioxidant enzymes. Pretreatment with antioxidants, such as α-tocopherol and N-acetylcysteine, attenuated the behavioral stress response.[9]

To examine differences that can only be caused by particular mitochondrial genes, we used mitochondrial substitution strains, also called conplastic strains. Mitochondria of C57BL/6J mice were substituted by mitochondria of AKR/J or FVB/N mice. The mitochondrial DNA (mtDNA) of AKR/J mice differs from the mtDNA of C57BL/6J mice in the number of adenine repeats in the tRNA of arginine being nine compared to eight in C57BL/6J. Mitochondria of FVB/N mice also have these nine adenine repeats but in addition they have a G7778T mutation in the ATPase subunit-8. This mutation leads to an increased production of reactive oxygen species (ROS) in C57BL/6J-mt$^{FVB/N}$ (manuscript submitted). Here, we tested whether these differences affect behavior,

Address for correspondence: Ulrike Gimsa, Research Unit Behavioural Physiology, Research Institute for the Biology of Farm Animals, Wilhelm-Stahl-Allee 2, D-18196 Dummerstorf, Germany. Voice: +49-38208-68803; fax: +49-38208-68802. gimsa@fbn-dummerstorf.de

Neuroimmunomodulation: Ann. N.Y. Acad. Sci. 1153: 131–138 (2009).
doi: 10.1111/j.1749-6632.2008.03960.x © 2009 New York Academy of Sciences.

activity of the hypothalamo–pituitary–adrenal (HPA) axis, and dopaminergic, serotonergic, and noradrenergic neurotransmitter systems at base line and in response to psychosocial stress. We examined the effects of social disruption stress (SDR) leading to social defeat in a group of subdominant young male mice after repeated encounters with an aggressive dominant intruder.

Materials and Methods

Conplastic Mouse Strains

The inbred strains C57BL/6J, AKR/J, FVB/N and NZB/B1n were obtained from the Jackson Laboratory (Bar Harbor, MA). To generate conplastic strains, we crossed AKR/J and FVB/N donor strain female mice with male C57BL/6J mice and then backcrossed the female offspring to male C57BL/6J mice. Such backcrosses were performed for 10 subsequent generations. The offspring of the 10th generation was regarded as the conplastic strains C57BL/6J-mt$^{AKR/J}$ or C57BL/6J-mt$^{FVB/N}$ that carried the nuclear genome from C57BL/6J and the mitochondrial genome from the donor strain. Animals were housed at the animal facility at the University of Rostock, Germany, and all procedures were pre-approved by the local Animal Care Committee.

Social Disruption Stress

Six-week-old male mice of the strains C57BL/6J, C57BL/6J-mt$^{AKR/J}$, or C57BL/6J-mt$^{FVB/N}$ were either received from Harlan–Winkelmann (Borchen, Germany) at 3 weeks of age (C57BL/6J) or reared as siblings (C57BL/6J-mt$^{AKR/J}$ or C57BL/6J-mt$^{FVB/N}$) in our facility. Cages of three mice were randomly assigned as either control or SDR groups. Control mice remained undisturbed in their home cage. Stressed mice experienced two SDR events over the course of 2 days: stress was induced by introducing an aggressive intruder,

i.e., a retired old breeder male (NZB/B1n mice, >1 year of age) into the home cage for 6 h (7 AM to 1 PM) and again from 6:30 AM to 9:30 AM the following day. Behavior was observed to ensure that the intruder attacked the residents and that the residents showed submissive postures. All of the attacked mice received small back or tail bite wounds. None of the group-housed control mice were injured. After the second SDR cycle, mice were either killed by cervical dislocation or tested on an elevated plus maze for 10 min and killed immediately afterward.

Sample Collection

After cervical dislocation mice were rapidly decapitated and their trunk blood was collected. Brains were isolated, snap frozen in liquid nitrogen, and stored at $-80°$C until neurotransmitter analysis. Blood was allowed to clot for 2 h and was centrifuged at 2000 g for 10 min. Sera were stored frozen at $-20°$C until corticosterone analysis.

Behavioral Test

The elevated plus-maze tests the conflict between the tendency to explore a novel environment and the aversive properties of brightly lit, open, and elevated areas. The elevated plus maze consists of four arms of 30-cm length and 5-cm width each. Two opposing arms are enclosed in opaque 15-cm high side and end walls. The elevation of the structure was 60 cm. We tested anxiety based on the parameters: (i) percentage of entries into open arms; (ii) percentage of time spent in open arms; and (iii) distance in open arms. The conflict between approaching or avoiding risk, i.e., to enter the "dangerous" open arms was tested by (i) time in central position; (ii) returns into closed arms; and (iii) time in closed arms. Locomotor activity was determined as (i) total entries into open and closed arms; (ii) entries into closed arms; and (iii) distance in closed arms. In addition, risk assessment behavior in order to gather information in the form of head dipping from the center platform toward the open arms was registered.

Approximately half of the mice were tested on the elevated plus maze for their anxiety and locomotor activity. Mice were put into the central position of the maze and left undisturbed for 10 min. Their behavior was recorded by video camera and later analyzed by a blinded observer. Control and SDR-stressed mice were tested alternately to minimize influences of time progression after SDR stress and time of day.

Corticosterone Analysis

Serum corticosterone concentrations were measured in duplicate using a commercially available double antibody rat corticosterone ^{125}I-RIA kit (DRG Diagnostics, Marburg, Germany) according to the manufacturer's instructions. Cross-reactivities of the antibody used to any potentially competing plasma steroids were lower than 0.5%. The test sensitivity was 7.2 ng/mL, and intra-assay and interassay coefficents of variation were 6.9% and 8.1%, respectively.

Neurotransmitter Analyses

Whole brain concentrations of noradrenaline (NA), its metabolite 3-methoxy-4-hydroxyphenylglycol (MHPG), dopamine (DA), its metabolites 3,4-dihydroxyphenylacetic acid (DOPAC) and homovanillic acid (HVA), 5-hydroxytryptamine (5-HT), and its metabolite 5-hydroxyindole-3-acetic acid (5-HIAA) were determined in duplicate by high-performance liquid chromatography (HPLC) with electrochemical detection. Brains were weighed and homogenized on ice for 5 min with a hand homogenizer in 4 mL of 0.2 mol/L perchloric acid followed by centrifugation at 45,000 *g* for 10 min at 4°C. The procedure was repeated after collection of the supernatants. Pooled supernatants of the repeated extractions were again centrifuged at 45,000 *g* for 10 min at 4°C. Samples (20 μL) were then injected directly into the HPLC system equipped with a 125-mm × 4-mm reversed-phase column packed with Prontosil C18 AQ (Bischoff Analysentechnik, Leonberg, Germany). As the mobile phase, 58 mmol/L sodium hydrogen phosphate buffer containing 1.2 mmol/L octansulfonic acid, 0.3 mmol/L EDTA, 0.2 mmol/L potassium chloride, and 6% methanol at pH 3.8 was used at a flow rate of 1.2 mL/min. Electrochemical detection was achieved by an ISAAC cell with a glassy carbon working electrode set at a potential of 600 mV (Axel Semrau, Sprockhövel, Germany). Dihydroxybenzylamine was used as an internal standard for quantification, and tissue contents of the above neurotransmitters and their metabolites were expressed as nanograms per gram of wet tissue weight. As an index of NA, DA, and 5-HT turnover, the MHPG/NA, DOPAC/DA, HVA/DA, and 5-HIAA/5-HT ratios were calculated.

Statistical Analysis

We compared data of mouse strains with the nonparametric Mann–Whitney test. In all statistical tests, $P < 0.05$ was considered to be statistically significant. We used GraphPad InStat^{TM} software (GraphPad Software Inc., La Jolla, CA).

Results

To examine the stress reactivity by means of behavioral and endocrine changes as an effect of the ATP8 mutation, we exposed male mice of the mitochondrial substitution strain C57BL/6J-mt$^{FVB/N}$ and its control strains C57BL/6J and C57BL/6J-mt$^{AKR/J}$ to two cycles of SDR exerted by an aggressive intruder. As one measure of their stress reactivity was anxiety, we tested the mice in the elevated plus maze. Interestingly, C57BL/6J-mt$^{FVB/N}$ were significantly more anxious than C57BL/6J-mt$^{AKR/J}$ and C57BL/6J mice at base line, i.e., without SDR stress (Fig. 1A).

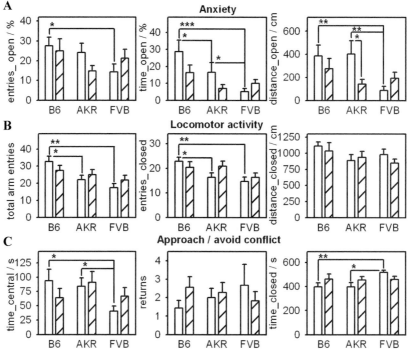

Figure 1. Elevated plus-maze behavior of C57BL/6J (B6), C57BL/6J-mt$^{AKR/J}$ (AKR), and C57BL/6J-mt$^{FVB/N}$ (FVB) mice without (plain bars) and with (hatched bars) prior exposure to social disruption stress (SDR). (**A**) Anxiety was tested as percentage of entries into open arms, percentage of time spent in open arms, and distance mice walked in open arms. (**B**) Locomotor activity was recorded as total entries into open and closed arms, the number of times mice entered closed arms, and the distance mice walked in closed arms. (**C**) The conflict between the tendency to explore and avoidance of risk ("approach/avoid conflict") was assessed as the time spent in the central position, the number of returns into the closed arms, and the time spent in closed arms. Data represent means and SEM of 9–12 mice per strain and treatment. Asterisks indicate significant differences (*$P < 0.05$; **$P < 0.01$; ***$P < 0.001$; Mann–Whitney test).

They entered the open arms less often than C57BL/6J mice, spent less time in the open arms of the maze, and walked shorter distances in open arms than C57BL/6J-mt$^{AKR/J}$ and C57BL/6J mice. Total arm entries and entries into closed arms were reduced in C57BL/6J-mt$^{AKR/J}$ and C57BL/6J-mt$^{FVB/N}$ compared to C57BL/6J mice, whereas distances the mice walked in closed arms were equal (Fig. 1B). Entries into open arms and even entries into closed arms might be reduced by anxiety because in order to enter, the mice have to leave the "safe" environment of the closed arms. By contrast, distances the mice walk in closed arms are rather independent of anxiety. Therefore, we believe that the general locomotor activity of

C57BL/6J-mt$^{AKR/J}$ and C57BL/6J-mt$^{FVB/N}$ does not differ from that of C57BL/6J mice and is not affected by SDR stress. C57BL/6J-mt$^{FVB/N}$ mice were also more cautious than the other strains. They entered the central position less often (data not shown) and spent less time there and more time in the closed arms (Fig. 1C). Along that line, control C57BL/6J-mt$^{FVB/N}$ mice showed more head dipping from the center platform toward the open arms than C57BL/6J mice (30.0 ± 2.4 versus 20.4 ± 2.1; $P = 0.019$). SDR stress before behavioral testing did not change plus-maze behavior of C57BL/6J-mt$^{FVB/N}$ mice while it decreased the distance C57BL/6J-mt$^{AKR/J}$ mice walked in open arms. C57BL/6J mice did not develop

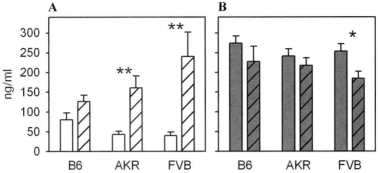

Figure 2. Serum corticosterone concentrations of C57BL/6J (B6), C57BL/6J-mt$^{AKR/J}$ (AKR), and C57BL/6J-mt$^{FVB/N}$ (FVB) mice without (plain bars) and with (hatched bars) prior exposure to SDR stress. (**A**) Animals without behavioral testing. (**B**) Animals that were tested on the elevated plus maze. Data represent means and SEM of 9–13 mice per strain and treatment. Asterisks indicate significant differences (*P < 0.05; **P < 0.01; Mann–Whitney test).

anxiety from SDR stress. Defecation and urination did not show any differences between strains.

To test their stress level we determined serum corticosterone concentrations either immediately after SDR or after SDR stress, followed by an elevated plus-maze test (Fig. 2). Corticosterone levels were significantly increased by SDR in C57BL/6J-mt$^{AKR/J}$ and C57BL/6J-mt$^{FVB/N}$ mice but not in C57BL/6J mice (Fig. 2A). The plus maze itself, however, constituted an even stronger stressor as it significantly increased corticosterone levels of control mice of all strains (P < 0.001) and SDR-stressed C57BL/6J mice (P < 0.01). Interestingly, of mice that underwent behavioral testing, SDR-stressed C57BL/6J-mt$^{FVB/N}$ mice had lower levels of serum corticosterone than their controls (Fig. 2B).

Concentrations of brain neurotransmitters and their metabolites were differentially affected by SDR stress and the stress exerted by the behavioral test in the three mouse strains. SDR stress alone had only minor effects. In C57BL/6J mice, 5-HIAA levels and the HVA/DA ratio increased as a result of SDR stress from 480 ± 26 to 609 ± 43 ng/g brain (P = 0.034) and from 0.185 ± 0.015 to 0.235 ± 0.016 (P = 0.044), respectively. C57BL/6J-mt$^{AKR/J}$ mice showed a higher HVA/DA ratio in stressed versus control mice,

with 0.244 ± 0.013 versus 0.179 ± 0.018 (P = 0.027). SDR stress did not change base line neurotransmitter levels in C57BL/6J-mt$^{FVB/N}$ mice (data not shown).

The elevated plus-maze test was clearly a challenge for C57BL/6J-mt$^{AKR/J}$ and C57BL/6J-mt$^{FVB/N}$ mice. In control C57BL/6J-mt$^{AKR/J}$ mice, behavioral testing increased 5-HT, DOPAC, and HVA levels from 794 ± 38 to 911 ± 41 ng/g brain (P = 0.041), from 109 ± 4 to 130 ± 6 ng/g brain (P = 0.016), and from 220 ± 13 to 280 ± 18 ng/g brain (P = 0.026), respectively. In control C57BL/6J-mt$^{FVB/N}$ mice, behavioral testing increased HVA levels from 238 ± 17 to 296 ± 23 ng/g brain (P = 0.031) and the DOPAC/DA ratio from 0.080 ± 0.005 to 0.098 ± 0.005 (P = 0.025). Further, it decreased NA levels from 668 ± 38 to 570 ± 44 ng/g brain (P = 0.038).

In SDR-stressed C57BL/6J and C57BL/6J-mt$^{AKR/J}$ mice, the additional challenge of behavioral testing did not change neurotransmitter levels. By contrast, behavioral testing increased HVA levels in SDR-stressed C57BL/6J-mt$^{FVB/N}$ mice from 272 ± 12 to 326 ± 18 ng/g brain (P = 0.032). Further, the combination of SDR stress and behavioral testing decreased 5-HT levels in C57BL/6J-mt$^{AKR/J}$ mice and markedly increased the 5-HIAA concentration and the 5-HIAA/5-HT

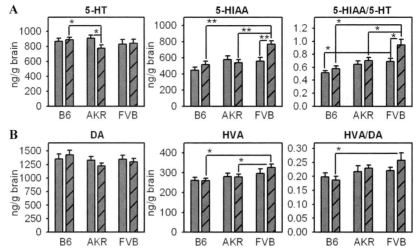

Figure 3. Genetic and stress influences on brain neurotransmitters and their turnover in C57BL/6J (B6), C57BL/6J-mt$^{AKR/J}$ (AKR), and C57BL/6J-mt$^{FVB/N}$ (FVB) mice after behavioral testing without (plain bars) and with (hatched bars) prior exposure to SDR stress. **(A)** Effects on the serotonergic system characterized by 5-hydroxytryptamine (5-HT), 5-hydroxyindole-3-acetic acid (5-HIAA), and the 5-HIAA/5-HT ratio. **(B)** Effects on the dopaminergic system characterized by dopamine (DA), homovanillic acid (HVA), and the HVA/DA ratio. Data represent means and SEM of 8–13 mice per strain and treatment. Asterisks indicate significant differences (*$P < 0.05$; **$P < 0.01$; Mann–Whitney test).

ratio in C57BL/6J-mt$^{FVB/N}$ mice. The values in C57BL/6J-mt$^{FVB/N}$ mice were significantly higher than in the other strains (Fig. 3A). An enhanced response of C57BL/6J-mt$^{FVB/N}$ mice to the combined challenge of SDR stress and behavioral testing was also observed in HVA levels compared to C57BL/6J and C57BL/6J-mt$^{AKR/J}$ mice and in the HVA/DA ratio compared to C57BL/6J mice (Fig. 3B).

Discussion

Mitochondria are considered "cellular power plants" as their main function is ATP production. Our study indicates that they may also influence behavior and neuroendocrine regulation. In this study, we found that mitochondrial genes influence anxiety-like behavior, HPA reactivity, and brain neurotransmitter systems at base line and in response to psychological stress. In particular, a DNA polymorphism in the ATPase subunit-8 gene that leads

to an increased production of ROS (manuscript submitted) exerts profound effects.

The behavioral pattern of C57BL/6J-mt$^{FVB/N}$ mice, which carry the ATPase mutation, differs from the other strains at base line, i.e., without SDR stress. C57BL/6J-mt$^{FVB/N}$ mice are more anxious than the other strains. C57BL/6J-mt$^{AKR/J}$ mice became more anxious from exposure to SDR stress than C57BL/6J mice. The anxiety measures of C57BL/6J-mt$^{AKR/J}$ mice after SDR stress resemble those of C57BL/6J-mt$^{FVB/N}$ mice with and without SDR stress.

The elevated plus-maze test clearly exposes mice to a challenging situation in a novel environment and must be considered a psychologically stressful event itself. Thus, mice that were exposed to SDR stress experienced a second stressful event when tested on the elevated plus maze. Accordingly, we characterized the three mouse strains in four groups each: mice with and without SDR stress that were either tested or not tested on the elevated plus maze. SDR stress induced a strong

HPA response in C57BL/6J-mt$^{FVB/N}$ and C57BL/6J-mt$^{AKR/J}$ mice but not in C57BL/6J mice. While base line corticosterone levels of control mice of all strains were equal, it is interesting to observe that a repeated exposure to a stressful event, i.e., the elevated plus maze, shortly after SDR apparently reduced HPA reactivity in C57BL/6J-mt$^{FVB/N}$ mice. It is likely that this is related to enhanced feedback inhibition of the HPA axis activity in the repeatedly stressed mice.[10,11] C57BL/6J-mt$^{AKR/J}$ mice show a stronger reaction to SDR stress than C57BL/6J mice both in behavior and corticosterone production.

SDR stress, but even more pronounced the psychological stress from elevated plus-maze testing, activated dopaminergic and serotonergic neurotransmitter systems of the brain differentially in the three mouse strains. As we did not determine which region of the brain is responsible for the observed neurotransmitter concentrations, changes in brain neurotransmitter levels are difficult to interpret. However, C57BL/6J-mt$^{FVB/N}$ mice show the strongest neurotransmitter responses to repeated psychological stress compared to the other strains. In mood disorders, serotonergic, dopaminergic, and noradrenergic neurotransmission play a prominent role.[12] A reduction of 5-HT, DA, and NA levels has been associated with depression.[13] Accordingly, our mouse strain exhibiting an anxious phenotype is characterized by a reduction of NA levels and increased serotonergic and dopaminergic turnover.

The mechanisms of the observed differences between C57BL/6J-mt$^{FVB/N}$ mice and their control strains are unclear. It could be speculated that ROS, which are amply produced by cells of these mice, might indirectly affect behavior via nuclear factor-kappa beta (NF-κβ), which gets activated by ROS.[14,15] NF-κβ itself has been shown to be involved in anxious behavior.[16] The bases for the differences in corticosterone and neurotransmitter levels remain to be elucidated. NF-κβ is involved in the regulation of glucocorticoid receptor (GR) expression, and transcriptional activity[17] and GR are responsible for feedback inhibition of corticosterone production.[18] We therefore assume a link between ROS and HPA axis reactivity.

In summary, we established a mouse model for studying the role of single nucleotide exchanges in mtDNA in the response to psychological stress. Our study shows that genetic differences in a single molecule are able to alter stress reactivity. C57BL/6J-mt$^{FVB/N}$ mice have a mutation in their mitochondrial ATPase subunit-8 gene. In humans, an A8537G mutation in ATPase subunit-6 and -8 genes were found in patients with a family history of bipolar disorder with manic and depressive episodes for which maternal transmission was suspected.[19] C57BL/6J-mt$^{FVB/N}$ mice show a strikingly higher anxiety and stress reactivity, particularly to recurring stress. Thus, this conplastic mouse strain might be a useful animal model for studying anxiety as an aspect of bipolar disorder.

Acknowledgments

The authors wish to thank Ilona Klamfuss and Claudia Voigt for animal care and technical assistance and Jan Gimsa for helpful comments on the manuscript. This study has been supported by the Hertie foundation (1.01.1/07/001).

Conflicts of Interest

The authors declare no conflicts of interest.

References

1. Shao, L., M.V. Martin, S.J. Watson, *et al.* 2008. Mitochondrial involvement in psychiatric disorders. *Ann. Med.* **40:** 281–295.
2. Einat, H., P. Yuan & H.K. Manji. 2005. Increased anxiety-like behaviors and mitochondrial dysfunction in mice with targeted mutation of the Bcl-2 gene: further support for the involvement of mitochondrial function in anxiety disorders. *Behav. Brain Res.* **165:** 172–180.

3. Esposito, E. 2006. Serotonin-dopamine interaction as a focus of novel antidepressant drugs. *Curr. Drug Targets* **7:** 177–185.

4. Alex, K.D. & E.A. Pehek. 2007. Pharmacologic mechanisms of serotonergic regulation of dopamine neurotransmission. *Pharmacol. Ther.* **113:** 296–320.

5. Konradi, C., M. Eaton, M.L. MacDonald, *et al*. 2004. Molecular evidence for mitochondrial dysfunction in bipolar disorder. *Arch. Gen. Psychiatry* **61:** 300–308.

6. Marcocci, L., U. De Marchi, M. Salvi, *et al*. 2002. Tyramine and monoamine oxidase inhibitors as modulators of the mitochondrial membrane permeability transition. *J. Membr. Biol.* **188:** 23–31.

7. Epel, E.S., E.H. Blackburn, J. Lin, *et al*. 2004. Accelerated telomere shortening in response to life stress. *Proc. Natl. Acad. Sci. USA* **101:** 17312–17315.

8. Eskiocak, S., A.S. Gozen, S.B. Yapar, *et al*. 2005. Glutathione and free sulphydryl content of seminal plasma in healthy medical students during and after exam stress. *Hum. Reprod.* **20:** 2595–2600.

9. Chakraborti, A., K. Gulati, B.D. Banerjee & A. Ray. 2007. Possible involvement of free radicals in the differential neurobehavioral responses to stress in male and female rats. *Behav. Brain Res.* **179:** 321–325.

10. Gadek-Michalska, A. & J. Bugajski. 2003. Repeated handling, restraint, or chronic crowding impair the hypothalamic-pituitary-adrenocortical response to acute restraint stress. *J. Physiol. Pharmacol.* **54:** 449–459.

11. Anisman, H., M.D. Zaharia, M.J. Meaney & Z. Merali. 1998. Do early-life events permanently alter behavioral and hormonal responses to stressors? *Int. J. Dev. Neurosci.* **16:** 149–164.

12. Morilak, D.A. & A. Frazer. 2004. Antidepressants and brain monoaminergic systems: a dimensional approach to understanding their behavioural effects in depression and anxiety disorders. *Int. J. Neuropsychopharmacol.* **7:** 193–218.

13. Ruhe, H.G., N.S. Mason & A.H. Schene. 2007. Mood is indirectly related to serotonin, norepinephrine and dopamine levels in humans: a meta-analysis of monoamine depletion studies. *Mol. Psychiatry* **12:** 331–359.

14. Cadenas, S. & A.M. Cadenas. 2002. Fighting the stranger-antioxidant protection against endotoxin toxicity. *Toxicology* **180:** 45–63.

15. Haddad, J.J. 2002. Antioxidant and prooxidant mechanisms in the regulation of redox(y)-sensitive transcription factors. *Cell Signal.* **14:** 879–897.

16. Kassed, C.A. & M. Herkenham. 2004. NF-kappaB p50-deficient mice show reduced anxiety-like behaviors in tests of exploratory drive and anxiety. *Behav. Brain Res.* **154:** 577–584.

17. Webster, J.C., R.H. Oakley, C.M. Jewell & J.A. Cidlowski. 2001. Proinflammatory cytokines regulate human glucocorticoid receptor gene expression and lead to the accumulation of the dominant negative beta isoform: a mechanism for the generation of glucocorticoid resistance. *Proc. Natl. Acad. Sci. USA* **98:** 6865–6870.

18. De Kloet, E.R., E. Vreugdenhil, M.S. Oitzl & M. Joels. 1998. Brain corticosteroid receptor balance in health and disease. *Endocr. Rev.* **19:** 269–301.

19. Kato, T., H. Kunugi, S. Nanko & N. Kato. 2001. Mitochondrial DNA polymorphisms in bipolar disorder. *J. Affect. Disord.* **62:** 151–164.

The Role of Stress Factors during Aging of the Immune System

Moisés E. Bauer,[a] **Cristina M. Moriguchi Jeckel,**[b] **and Clarice Luz**[c]

[a]*Faculdade de Biociências and Instituto de Pesquisas Biomédicas and* [b]*Faculdade de Farmácia, Pontifícia Universidade Católica do Rio Grande do Sul, Porto Alegre, Brazil*

[c]*LabVitrus, Porto Alegre, Brazil*

This manuscript reviews current evidence suggesting that aging of the immune system (immunosenescence) may be closely related to chronic stress and stress factors. Healthy aging has been associated with emotional distress in parallel to increased cortisol to dehydroepiandrosterone (DHEA) ratio. The impaired DHEA secretion together with the increase of cortisol results in an enhanced exposure of lymphoid cells to deleterious glucocorticoid actions. The lack of appropriated growth hormone signaling during immunosenescence is also discussed. It follows that altered neuroendocrine functions could be underlying several immunosenescence features. Indeed, changes in both innate and adaptive immune responses during aging are also similarly reported during chronic glucocorticoid exposure. In addition, chronically stressed elderly subjects may be particularly at risk of stress-related pathology because of further alterations in both neuroendocrine and immune systems. The accelerated senescent features induced by chronic stress include higher oxidative stress, reduced telomere length, chronic glucocorticoid exposure, thymic involution, changes in cellular trafficking, reduced cell-mediated immunity, steroid resistance, and chronic low-grade inflammation. These senescent features are related to increased morbidity and mortality among chronically stressed elderly people. Overall, these data suggest that chronic stress leads to premature aging of key allostatic systems involved in the adaptation of the organisms to environmental changes. Stress management and psychosocial support may thus promote a better quality of life for elderly people and at the same time reduce hospitalization costs.

Key words: aging; immunosenescence; glucocorticoids; lymphocytes

Introduction

Aging is a continuous and slow process that compromises the normal functioning of various organs and systems in both qualitative and quantitative terms. Aging has been associated with several dynamic immunological alterations that are collectively called immunosenescence. The popular knowledge of immunosenescence is the decline of immune functions. The updated view is a remodeling of major immunological components involving multiple reorganization and developmentally regulated changes.[1] Immunosenescence could be the result of the adaptation of the body to the continuous challenge of bacterial and viral infections. These remodeling features can be demonstrated by significant decrements in adaptive immunity in parallel with overall maintenance or increased innate immune functions during aging. The remodeling immune system is particularly observed in centenarians,

Address for correspondence: Dr. Moisés E. Bauer, Instituto de Pesquisas Biomédicas, Pontifícia Universidade Católica do Rio Grande do Sul (PU-CRS), Av. Ipiranga 6690, 2° andar, P.O. Box 1429, Porto Alegre, RS 90.610-000, Brazil. mebauer@pucrs.br

Neuroimmunomodulation: Ann. N.Y. Acad. Sci. 1153: 139–152 (2009).
doi: 10.1111/j.1749-6632.2008.03966.x © 2009 New York Academy of Sciences.

who present many intact adaptive or innate immune functions and are thus good examples of successful aging.

The clinical consequences of immunosenescence may include increased susceptibility to infectious diseases, neoplasias, and autoimmune disease.[2] This altered morbidity is not evenly distributed and should be influenced by other immune-modulating factors, including the genetic background and chronic stress exposure.[3] Indeed, several immunosenescence-related changes resemble those observed following chronic stress[4] or glucocorticoid (GC) treatment.[5] The present paper summarizes recent findings suggesting that stress factors may accelerate immunosenescence.

Changes in Adaptive Immunity

One of the major features of human immunosenescence is thymic involution, characterized by a progressive age-related reduction in size of the thymus and replacement of lymphoid by fat tissue and associated with the loss of thymic epithelial cells and impairment in thymopoiesis.[6] This thymic involution has been proposed to be a result of changes in the thymic microenvironment that result in its failure to support thymopoiesis.[7] The decline in the output of newly developed T cells results in a diminished number of circulating naive T cells (CD45RA+) and impaired cell-mediated immunity. In contrast, one of the major characteristics of immunosenescence is the accumulation of expanded clones of memory (CD45RO+) and effector T cells as a consequence of the continuous life-long exposure to a variety of antigens.[8] In particular, this phenomenon is faster and more marked in CD8+ T cells.[9,10] The end result is a filling of the immunological space with memory and effector cells.[11]

In addition, a decrease of CD28+ T cells in parallel with a progressive accumulation of CD28− T cells with aging has been observed.[10,12] These cells display several aspects of senescence, such as oligoclonal expansion, shortened telomeres, limited proliferative potential or replicative senescence, production of tumor necrosis factor (TNF)-α and interleukin (IL)-6, and resistance to apoptosis.[12–16] When diseased subjects are excluded, immunosenescence involves impaired humoral responses to new antigens, lower cytotoxicity, and blunted T cell proliferation. The latter is one of the most documented age-related changes observed during aging.[17,18] The effector phases adaptive immune responses are largely mediated by cytokines. Different subpopulations of CD4+ T cells synthesize specific cytokines and have been designated Th1 [interferon (IFN)-γ, IL-2, lymphotoxin α] or Th2 (IL-4, IL-10) cells. Both human and mouse models have demonstrated that aging is associated with a Th1 to Th2 shift in cytokine production.[19,20] This altered cytokine profile could be further involved with reduced T cell functions, including lymphocyte proliferation and development of different T cell subsets.

Immunologists have recently characterized a new T cell subset (CD4+C25+ FoxP3+) with an important regulatory role in suppressing excessive or misguided immune responses that can be harmful to the host. These lymphocytes are called regulatory T (Treg) cells and are responsible for turning off immune responses against self antigens in autoimmune disease, allergy, or commensal microbes in certain inflammatory diseases.[21,22] It is interesting that aging, GC, or chronic stress can increase peripheral Treg cell numbers.[23]

Also, there are some qualitative changes associated with remodeling adaptive immune responses. In particular, the T cell receptor (TCR) repertoire seems to be shortened during aging. Data on the variable segment β (Vβ) families of the TCR show a progressive shrinkage of the TCR repertoire in the CD4+ and CD8+ subsets and a concomitant marked clonal expansion of single Vβ families. This repertoire has been shaped by the selective action of specific T cell clones able to modulate the immune response to endogenous and exogenous antigens.[24,25]

Changes in Innate Immunity

The innate immunity constitutes the first line of defense against a broad range of infectious agents. The nonspecific identification of antigens requires binding to pathogen-associated molecular patterns via pattern recognition receptors [e.g., toll-like receptors (TLR)] expressed on various leukocytes, including macrophages, neutrophils, dendritic cells (DC), and natural killer (NK) cells. The mononuclear phagocyte lineage plays a pivotal role in innate immunity. Aged phagocytes, such as macrophages and neutrophils, showed an impaired respiratory burst and reactive nitrogen intermediate production with a decreased ability to destroy pathogens.[26,27]

The antigen-presenting cell function of DC is generally well retained in elderly people[28] but their numbers (and their precursors) are reduced with age.[29] Monocyte-derived DC from elderly individuals were not impaired in their ability to induce T cell responses[30] or proliferation of T cell lines.[31] Recently, a study measuring the induction of the costimulatory ligands CD80 and CD86 on monocytes found that TLR-mediated induction was compromised in elderly individuals and, importantly, that this correlated with decreased response to the influenza vaccination.[32]

NK cells are a population of heterogeneous lymphocytes that provide a critical role of the innate immune response against a broad variety of infections and tumors. Most studies report increased NK cell numbers in contrast to impaired cytotoxic function during aging.[33,34] This impaired function has been associated with reduced intracellular stores of cytotoxic molecules, such as perforin.[35] Moreover, the impaired NK cell cytotoxicity represents a high risk factor for the appearance of infections in advanced age.[36] An NK cell count in the lowest quartile was associated with a threefold increase in mortality of all causes in the subsequent 2 years.[37]

Chronic low-grade inflammation has repeatedly been observed during aging, as suggested by increased serum pro-inflammatory cytokines (TNF-α, IL-1, IL-6), acute phase proteins [C-reactive protein (CRP)], and soluble IL-2 receptors (sIL-2Rs).[38] It was postulated that inflammatory responses appear to be the prevalent triggering mechanism driving tissue damage associated with different age-related diseases, and the term *inflammaging* has been coined to explain the underlining inflammatory changes common to most age-associated diseases.[39] Inflammaging appears to be a universal phenomenon that accompanies the aging process and which is related to frailty, morbidity, and mortality in the elderly. Indeed, chronic inflammation is considered to be involved in the pathogenesis of major age-related diseases, including Alzheimer's disease, atherosclerosis, diabetes, major depression, sarcopenia, and cancer. In addition, low-grade increases in levels of circulating TNF-α, IL-6, sIL-2R, and CRP and low levels of albumin and cholesterol, which also act as inflammatory markers, are strong predictors of all-cause mortality risk in several longitudinal studies of elderly cohorts. However, low-grade inflammation could be observed in strictly healthy elderly individuals,[40] suggesting that inflammaging could be better associated with pathological aging or with common morbidities frequently observed during aging, including hypertension.

Major Endocrine Changes

In addition to immunosenescence, the endocrine system also undergoes important changes during aging (endocrinosenescence). A decline in growth hormone (GH), sex hormones, and dehydroepiandrosterone (DHEA) with aging has been demonstrated.[41] DHEA is the major secretory product of the human adrenal and is synthesized from cholesterol stores. The hormone is uniquely sulfated (DHEAS) before entering the plasma, and this prohormone is converted to DHEA and its metabolites in various peripheral tissues.[42] Following secretion, total DHEA in the circulation consists mainly of DHEAS—the serum concentration of free DHEA is less than

1%. Serum DHEA levels decrease by the second decade of life, reaching about 5% of the original level in elderly people.[43] It has been suggested that DHEAS/DHEA may antagonize many physiological changes of endogenous GCs, including enhancing immunomodulatory properties.[3]

There is also evidence suggesting that aging is associated with significant activation of the hypothalamic–pituitary–adrenal (HPA) axis in increased production of cortisol in humans.[40,44] The HPA axis is pivotal for the homeostasis of the immune system and its dysregulation has been associated with several immune-mediated diseases. For instance, HPA axis overactivation, as occurs during chronic stress, can affect susceptibility to or severity of infectious disease through the immunosuppressive effect of the GCs.[45,46] In contrast, blunted HPA axis responses are associated with enhanced susceptibility to autoimmune inflammatory disease.[47] It is noteworthy to mention that elderly subjects are particularly at risk for both infectious and chronic inflammatory diseases. Furthermore, chronic inflammatory diseases may be associated with premature aging of the immune system and present several similarities of immunosenescence, including shortening of cellular telomeres, decreased TCR specificities, loss of naive T cells, and increased production of pro-inflammatory cytokines.[48] Dysregulation of the HPA axis may contribute to—but it is not solely responsible for—immunosenescence. Chronically stressed elderly subjects may be at risk of stress-related pathology because of further alterations in GC immunoregulation (immune signaling).

Interplay between Cytokines and Hormones during Aging

Recent work suggests that cytokines and hormones could be considered as possible links between endocrinosenescence and immunosenescence.[49] Indeed, it has long been known that pro-inflammatory cytokines can readily activate the HPA axis during infection in animals[50] or after administration in humans.[51] Other studies have linked the age-related decline in DHEA production to increased serum levels of IL-6.[52,53] In addition, increased plasma TNF-α levels were correlated to major depression in the elderly.[54] However, we do not know exactly to what extent these changes may be related to altered psychological and HPA axis functions in elderly people.

We have investigated whether the psychoneuroendocrine status of healthy elderly individuals was associated with changes in lipopolysaccharide-induced monocyte production of pro-inflammatory cytokines (TNF-α and IL-6) and sIL-2Rα production by T cells *in vitro*.[40] Cells of healthy elderly individuals produced equivalent pro-inflammatory cytokines and sIL-2Rα when compared to cells of young adults. These data are in disagreement with previous work showing that human aging was associated with increased serum[53] or monocyte pro-inflammatory cytokines.[55,56] However, these data should be interpreted with caution because cellular sources other than monocytes can produce cytokines and thus increase serum levels. Considering that our cohort of elderly subjects was significantly distressed, we hypothesize this could have normalized the cytokines investigated in this study as a result of anti-inflammatory GC actions. On the other hand, there is also some evidence of increased pro-inflammatory cytokines during major depression.[54,57,58] Therefore, it becomes difficult to dissociate the cytokine changes observed in elderly subjects with those induced by psychological stimuli.

Healthy Aging Is Associated with Significant Distress

Psychological distress may be an important risk factor for immunosenescence. Human aging has been associated with several psychological and behavioral changes, including difficulty in concentrating, progressive cognitive impairments, and sleep disturbances.[59,60] Although individually identified, these alterations may be associated with major depression. Indeed, depression is highly prevalent in several age-related chronic degenerative diseases, including cardiovascular diseases, Parkinson's disease, Alzheimer's dementia, cancer, and rheumatoid arthritis.[61] In addition, both aging[55] and major depression[57,58] have been associated with increased levels of pro-inflammatory cytokines and could thus contribute to further immunological diseases in frail elderly individuals.

We have recently demonstrated that healthy aging was associated with significant psychological distress. In particular, it was found that strictly healthy (SENIEUR) elderly individuals were significantly more stressed, anxious, and depressed than young adults.[40,62] The literature regarding age-related psychological changes is controversial, and other researchers did not find these changes.[63] This could be a result of methodological issues because specific clinical interviews are required to assess depression in elderly people.

In parallel with psychological distress, we have also observed that SENIEUR elderly individuals have significantly higher (approximately 45%) salivary cortisol production throughout the day compared to young adults.[40] Cortisol peaked in the morning and presented a nadir at night, with a regular circadian pattern for both groups. These data further suggest that healthy aging is associated with significant activation of the HPA axis.[44,64–66] Increased cortisol levels are also seen in demented patients,[67] major depression,[68] or during chronic stress.[69,70]

In addition, it was observed that healthy elderly individuals had lower DHEA levels (a reduction of 54%) throughout the day compared to young adults.[71] Furthermore, elderly individuals also displayed a flat circadian pattern for DHEA secretion. The morphological correlates of the age-related changes of DHEAS/DHEA secretion are progressive atrophy of the zona reticularis of adrenal glands.[72] The lack of appropriate DHEA levels could be another detrimental factor during immunosenescence because this hormone has immune-enhancing properties (as further discussed in this chapter).

Higher cortisol levels in parallel with lower DHEA levels will consequently lead to higher C/D ratios throughout the day. The assessment of molar concentrations constitutes another way to evaluate the adrenal function in the organism.[49,72,73] The measurement of isolated hormonal samples may be an oversimplification, and the C/D ratio may contribute to the effective determination of functional hypercortisolemia. The impaired DHEA secretion, together with the increase of cortisol, results in enhanced exposure of various bodily systems (including brain and immune system) to the cytotoxic and modulatory effects of GCs and thus more allostatic load. Some brain cells (hypocampus) and lymphocytes are specially targeted by the cortisol because they express higher densities of mineralo-receptors and GC receptors.[4] The peripheral tissues of elderly people may thus be more vulnerable to the GC actions in a milieu of low-protective DHEA levels. The antagonist action of DHEA to cortisol in the brain suggests that measurement of cortisol alone may provide an incomplete estimate of hypercortisolemia.

In our previous study, psychological distress was positively related to salivary cortisol levels and negatively correlated to DHEA levels during aging.[40] Therefore, it becomes difficult to dissociate these neuroendocrine changes observed in elderly individuals with those produced by psychological stimuli. It should also be pointed out that endocrinosenescence includes a substantial decline in several hormones, including GH, testosterone, progesterone, and aldosterone—all of which with reported immunomodulatory properties. Thus endocrinosenescence may be considered as an important risk factor for immunosenescence.

Similarities between Aging, Stress, and Glucocorticoid Treatment

All leukocytes exhibit receptors for the neuroendocrine products of the HPA and sympathetic-adrenal medullary axes. It seems reasonable to speculate that increased cortisol and lower DHEA may thus contribute to immunological changes observed during aging. This section provides evidence that the age-related immunological changes are not exclusively observed during aging. In fact, they are also similarly found during chronic GC exposure, as observed during psychological stress or GC treatments *in vitro* or *in vivo*.

Most, if not all, immunological changes are similarly observed during aging or chronic GC exposure. Changes in cellular trafficking are the major changes produced during chronic GC exposure. Trafficking or redistribution of peripheral immune cells in the body is of pivotal importance for effective cell-mediated immune responses. Stress-related increase in GC[74] or GC treatment[5] also atrophy the thymus and, to a lesser extent, other lymphoid tissues, triggering apoptotic death in immature T and B cell precursors and mature T cells.[75] Therefore, thymic involution is not an exclusive phenomenon of aging. In addition, both naive or memory T cell subsets decline during chronic stress or treatment with GC.[4,76,77] Interestingly, GC or chronic stress can also increase peripheral Treg cell numbers.[78,79] In spite of the several similarities among age- and stress-related immunological alterations, only a few studies have addressed the role of stress factors on human immunosenescence. Overall, these results indicate that there are complex psychoneuroendocrine interactions involved with the regulation of the peripheral pool of lymphocytes. In particular, both psychological stress and GCs may synergize during aging to produce alterations in T cell trafficking.

Changes in cell-mediated immunity are also similarly described in aging, chronic stress, or GC exposure. For instance, blunted T cell proliferation is one of the most documented age-related changes observed during aging.[17,18] Yet, these changes are not exclusive of aging, and stress or GC treatment are also associated with decrements of T cell proliferation.[75,76] Indeed, we have observed that healthy SENIEUR

elderly individuals were significantly more distressed, had activated HPA axis, and had significant lower (a reduction of 53.6%) T cell proliferation compared to young adults.[71] Interestingly, the HPA axis may be implicated with this change because salivary cortisol levels were found negatively correlated to T cell proliferation. Similarly to aging, psychological stress[76,80] or GC treatment[81,82] is also associated with a Th1 to Th2 shift in cytokine production.

Role of DHEA during Immunosenescence

The lack of appropriate DHEAS levels during aging could be another detrimental factor for immunosenescence. This androgen and its metabolites have reported immune-enhancing properties in contrast to the immunosuppressive action of GCs. Indeed, this hormone may be considered a natural antagonist of GCs, and the impaired DHEA secretion, together with the increase of cortisol, results in enhanced exposure of lymphoid cells to deleterious GC actions. Therefore, previous studies have evaluated the immunomodulatory DHEA(S) effects *in vitro* as well as DHEA(S) properties during *in vivo* supplementation. The immunomodulatory *in vitro* effects include increased mitogen-stimulated IL-2 production,[83,84] increased rodent or human lymphocyte proliferation,[85] stimulated monocyte-mediated cytotoxicity,[86] diminished TNF-α or IL-6 production,[53,87] and enhanced NK cell activity.[88]

DHEA(S) replacement therapy has yielded significant beneficial effects for healthy elderly individuals, including increased well-being, memory performance, bone mineral density, and altered immune function.[89] It has been shown that DHEA supplementation significantly increased NK cell counts and activity and decreased IL-6 production and T cell proliferation in elderly subjects.[90] These data highlight the potential use of DHEA as an anti-aging hormone and suggest that DHEA supplementation would attenuate chronic low-grade inflammation and age-related frailty by inhibiting production of pro-inflammatory cytokines.

Because of its enhanced immunomodulatory properties, several studies investigated the potential of DHEA(S) as adjuvants in vaccine preparations. Initial studies reported increased adjuvant effects on the immunization of aged mice with recombinant hepatitis B surface antigen[91] or influenza.[92] These studies reported increased antibody titers to vaccines or even effective protection against challenge with the influenza infection.[92] More recently we studied the adjuvant effects of DHEAS during immunization to *Mycobaterium tuberculosis* in mice.[93] Only young mice co-immunized with *M. tuberculosis* heat shock protein 70 (HSP70) and DHEAS showed an early increase in specific IgG levels compared to old mice. However, splenocytes of both young and old mice that received DHEAS showed increased IFN-γ production following priming *in vitro* with HSP70. These data further highlight the importance of DHEAS as a hormonal adjuvant as a result of the role of this cytokine in the cellular response against mycobacteria. However, these animal data are in contrast to previous studies reporting DHEA(S) with minor[94] or no adjuvant effects[95–97] during immunization to influenza or tetanus in human elderly populations. Therefore, extrapolation from studies on murine models to humans should be regarded with caution—especially because of lower circulating DHEA(S) levels in rodents.

Role of Growth Hormone during Aging

Previous studies have demonstrated that serum GH levels are significantly reduced during aging[98] (somatosenescence). The lack of peripheral GH-immune signaling may be detrimental for immunosenescence. In particular, in GH-deficient rodents, there is significant immune dysfunction, which is reversed after GH replacement.[99] In addition, treatment with recombinant human GH or insulin-like growth factor (IGF)-1 enhances immune function in monkeys.[100] The GH, directly or through GH induction of IGF-1, has been implicated in lymphocyte development and function. It has been shown to maintain competence of macrophages, T cells, and B cells, and stimulate antibody production and NK-cell activity.[101]

However, GH is not exclusively produced by pituitary gland, and human immune cells are also capable of secreting several neuropeptides, including GH.[102,103] The role of lymphocyte-derived hormones in immune responses is not well understood, although they might have a role in modulating cell function within the microenvironment of lymphoid organs. The immunoreactive GH has shown several immuno-enhancing proprieties and may be important in modulating both humoral and cellular immune function.[102,104]

In a recent study we investigated whether somatosenescence could be correlated with respective reduced immunoreactive GH levels. We also analyzed the role of psychological distress of healthy SENIEUR elderly subjects on GH levels.[71] We found that elderly individuals had significantly lower (a reduction of 77%) serum GH levels compared to young adults. In contrast, no changes in GH production by activated monocytes or lymphocytes were observed between elderly and young adult subjects.[71] Interestingly, psychological distress (stress, anxiety, and depression) was found negatively correlated to serum GH levels only. No differences in serum GH levels were observed between groups when controlling for psychological variables. Chronic psychological stress may produce severe effects on the production of GH by lymphoid cells. Indeed, a significantly reduced expression (a reduction of 60%) of GH mRNA has been observed in peripheral lymphocytes in stressed elderly individuals (caregivers of patients with Alzheimer's disease) compared to controls.[105] These data suggest that age-related psychological distress may be implicated with impaired GH production and that immunoreactive GH is probably dissociated from pituitary GH levels.

Ghrelin, an endogenous ligand of the GH secretagogue receptor, has recently been demonstrated to inhibit the expression and production of pro-inflammatory cytokines (TNF-α, IL-1β, and IL-6).[106] This effect was mediated via binding on ghrelin receptors expressed on peripheral T cells and monocytes. There is some evidence for increased stomach ghrelin production in the aged rat.[107] Increased peripheral ghrelin levels may thus attenuate cytokine levels during aging. It remains to be investigated, however, whether psychological stress is capable of producing significant effects on stomach or immunoreactive ghrelin levels.

Chronic Stress and Aging Are Associated with Resistance to Glucocorticoids

The functional effect of a stress hormone will depend on the sensitivity of the target tissue for that particular hormone. It has been shown that GC sensitivity changes dramatically during ontogeny. Kavelaars and colleagues have shown that cord blood T cells of human newborns appear to be extremely sensitive to inhibition of the proliferative response.[108] At 1 year of age, the adult response pattern has been acquired. It is interesting that the increased sensitivity of the immune system to GC inhibition occurs at a period in life when the endogenous levels of GC are low.[109]

Recent evidence suggests that aging, chronic stress, or chronic GC levels are associated with significant resistance to GC effects. We have assessed the effects of GC in suppressing T cell proliferation *in vitro* and so examined whether aging was associated with alterations in neuroendocrine immunoregulation.[71] It was found that strictly healthy elderly subjects had a reduced (a reduction of 19%) *in vitro* lymphocyte sensitivity to dexamethasone when compared to young adults. This phenomenon has previously been described during chronic stress,[70,110] major depression,[77,111,112] or in clinical situations where GCs are administered, including

treatment of autoimmune diseases, organ transplantation, and allergies. It has also been shown that aging is associated with changes in GC sensitivity of pro-inflammatory cytokine (TNF-α and IL-6) production following psychosocial stress testing.[113] These data suggest that psychological factors may be implicated in regulating peripheral GC sensitivity during healthy aging. The acquired resistance to GC may have an important physiological significance of protecting cells from the dangerous effects of prolonged GC-related immunosuppression. Additionally, altered steroid immunoregulation may have important therapeutic implications in clinical situations where GCs are administered, including treatment of autoimmune diseases, organ transplantation, and allergies.

The Impact of Chronic Stress on Strictly Healthy Aging—Damaging and Protecting Effects

The caregiving to demented patients is a recognized model to study the impact of chronic stress in elderly populations.[45,70,114] Care of the chronically ill is a demanding task that is associated with increased stress, depression, and poorer immune function.[115] Furthermore, providing care for a relative with dementia typically falls on the partners who are themselves elderly and often ill prepared for the physical and emotional demands placed upon them.

The daily stress experienced by the caregivers of Alzheimer's disease patients may accelerate many age-related changes, particularly on neuroendocrine and immune systems. We have previously demonstrated that caregivers of demented patients had a blunted T cell proliferation in association with increased cortisol levels compared to nonstressed elderly adults.[70] Furthermore, lymphocytes of elderly caregivers were more resistant to GC treatment *in vitro* compared to elderly non-caregivers. When stressed elderly individuals are compared to healthy elderly and young adults, these immunological changes are found in similar

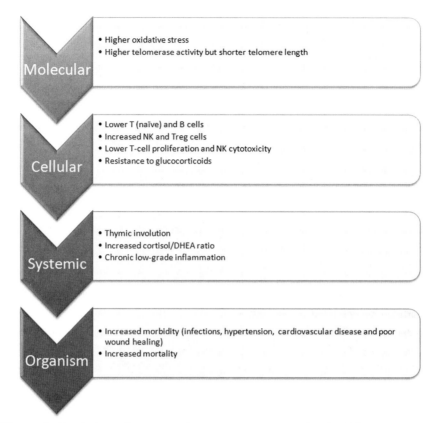

Figure 1. Psychological stress accelerates aging at various levels. Abbreviations: DHEA, dehydroepiandrosterone; NK, natural killer. (In color in *Annals* online.)

magnitude to increased cortisol levels.[3] These data suggest that chronic stress and cortisol would thus accelerate human senescence. Indeed, it has recently been observed that psychological stress (both perceived stress and chronicity of stress) was significantly associated with higher oxidative stress, lower telomerase activity, and shorter telomere length, which are known determinants of cell senescence and longevity.[116] Therefore, chronic stress may accelerate key allostatic systems and senescent features can be described at various levels (Fig. 1).

Several studies have implicated caregiving as a risk factor for the health of elderly populations. Compared with non-caregivers, subjects who provide care to a spouse with a stroke or dementia report more infectious illness episodes,[114] they have poorer immune responses to influenza virus[45,46] and pneumococ-

cal pneumonia vaccines,[117] they present a slow wound healing,[118] they are at greater risk for developing mild hypertension,[119] and they may be at greater risk for coronary heart disease.[120] In addition, a prospective longitudinal study found that the relative risk for mortality among caregivers was significantly higher (63%) than non-caregiving controls.[121] A recent study indicates that a pro-inflammatory cytokine (IL-6) may be involved with this increased morbidity in caregiving populations.[122]

Recent data produced by our laboratory have suggested that the maintenance of health status during aging may protect elderly people from chronic stress exposure. We have recruited strictly healthy (SENIEUR) elderly caregivers from a large population of primary caregivers of demented patients ($n = 342$). Only 12% of caregivers were considered "strictly healthy" according to this stringent protocol, and this may further confirm that chronic stress exposure is associated with increased morbidity in elderly populations. Therefore, we investigated whether a stringent health status would protect caregivers from chronic stress exposure and compared psychoneuroendocrine and immunological changes to nonstressed controls. Although the SENIEUR elderly caregivers were significantly distressed, their salivary cortisol levels remained unchanged compared to nonstressed controls (C. M. Moriguchi Jeckel *et al.*, submitted for publication). This could be of beneficial value for the caregiver and may indicate that a stringent health status in elderly individuals can buffer the impact of chronic stress on neuroendocrine responses. Therefore, healthy caregivers would be protected from the deleterious effects of cortisol excess in the organism. The peripheral lymphoid cells could be spared from the increased and deleterious cortisol signaling normally observed during chronic stress exposure. Indeed, it was observed that healthy caregivers had increased T cell proliferation when compared to nonstressed healthy controls. Taken together, these results suggest that a strictly healthy (SENIEUR) aging may buffer or attenuate many deleterious neuroendocrine and immunological effects associated with chronic stress exposure.

Conclusions and Outlook

The studies reviewed here support the notion that immunological changes observed during healthy aging may be closely related to both psychological distress and stress hormones. Of note, changes in cellular trafficking as well as cell-mediated immunity observed during aging are similarly found following stress or chronic GC exposure. These changes are mainly produced via engagement of specific intracellular adrenal receptors expressed on peripheral lymphocytes. The impaired DHEAS secretion, together with increased cortisol levels, would result in an enhanced exposure of various bodily systems (including brain and immune system) to the cytotoxic/immunomodulatory effects of GCs.

Human aging is associated with changes in allostatic systems (endocrine and immune) that play major roles in the adaptation of organisms to outside forces that are threatening the homeostasis of the internal milieu. In particular, healthy aging is associated with significant psychological distress and activation of the HPA axis (increased cortisol and reduced DHEA). Over weeks, months, or years, exposure to increased secretion of stress hormones would result in allostatic load ("wear and tear") and its pathophysiologic consequences.[123] Given the findings that even discrete HPA axis activation may impair cognitive function[124] and induce sleep disturbances,[125] conditions frequently associated in the elderly, psychological or pharmacological strategies attenuating or preventing increased HPA function during aging might be of considerable benefit for the elderly population.

Chronic stressed elderly subjects may be particularly at risk of stress-related pathology because of further increases in tissue exposure to cortisol. Elderly individuals who experience chronic stress exhibit poorer immune functions, and thus increased disease vulnerability, than nonstressed controls. Overall, these data suggest that chronic stress leads to premature aging of key allostatic systems involved in the adaptation of the organisms to environmental changes. Stress management and psychosocial support may thus promote a better quality of life for the elderly individual as well as reducing hospitalization costs.

Conflicts of Interest

The authors declare no conflicts of interest.

References

1. Franceschi, C. *et al.* 1996. Successful imunosenescence and the remodelling of immune responses with ageing. *Nephrol. Dial. Transplant.* **11:** 18–25.

2. Castle, S.C. 2000. Clinical relevance of age-related immune dysfunction. *Clin. Infec. Dis.* **31:** 578–585.

3. Bauer, M.E. 2005. Stress, glucocorticoids and ageing of the immune system. *Stress* **8:** 69–83.

4. McEwen, B. *et al.* 1997. The role of adrenocorticosteroids as modulators of immune function in health and disease: neural, endocrine and immune interactions. *Brain Res. Rev.* **23:** 79–133.

5. Fauci, A. 1975. Mechanisms of corticosteroid action on lymphocyte subpopulations. *Immunology* **28:** 669–679.

6. Aspinall, R. & D. Andrew. 2000. Thymic atrophy in the mouse is a soluble problem of the thymic environment. *Vaccine* **18:** 1629–1637.

7. Henson, S.M., J. Pido-Lopez & R. Aspinall. 2004. Reversal of thymic atrophy. *Exp. Gerontol.* **39:** 673–678.

8. Hannet, I. *et al.* 1992. Developmental and maturational changes in human blood lymphocyte subpopulations. *Immunol. Today* **13:** 215, 218.

9. Franceschi, C. *et al.* 1995. The immunology of exceptional individuals: the lesson of centenarians. *Immunol. Today* **16:** 12–16.

10. Fagnoni, F.F. *et al.* 1996. Expansion of cytotoxic CD8 +CD28- T cells in healthy ageing people, including centenarians. *Immunology* **88:** 501–507.

11. Franceschi, C., M. Bonaf & S. Valensini. 2000. Human immunosenescence: the prevailing of innate immunity, the failing of clonotypic immunity, and the filling of immunological space. *Vaccine* **18:** 1717–1720.

12. Effros, R. 1997. Loss of CD28 expression on T lymphocytes: a marker of replicative senescence. *Dev. Comp. Immunol.* **21:** 471–478.

13. Zhang, X. *et al.* 2002. Aging leads to disturbed homeostasis of memory phenotype CD8(+) cells. *J. Exp. Med.* **195:** 283–293.

14. Batliwalla, F. *et al.* 1996. Oligoclonality of CD8+ T cells in health and disease: aging, infection, or immune regulation? *Hum. Immunol.* **48:** 68–76.

15. Effros, R.B. *et al.* 2005. The role of CD8+ T-cell replicative senescence in human aging. *Immunol. Rev.* **205:** 147–157.

16. Brzezinska, A. *et al.* 2004. Proliferation and apoptosis of human CD8(+)CD28(+) and CD8(+)CD28(-) lymphocytes during aging. *Exp. Gerontol.* **39:** 539–544.

17. Liu, J. *et al.* 1997. The monitoring biomarker for immune function os lymphocytes in the elderly. *Mech. Ageing Dev.* **94:** 177–182.

18. Murasko, D., P. Weiner & D. Kaye. 1987. Decline in mitogen induced proliferation of lymphocytes with increasing age. *Clin. Exp. Immunol.* **70:** 440–448.

19. Ginaldi, L. *et al.* 2001. Immunosenescence and infectious diseases. *Microbes Infection.* **3:** 851–857.

20. Globerson, A. & R. Effros. 2000. Ageing of lymphocytes and lymphocytes in the aged. *Immunol. Today* **21:** 515–521.

21. Fontenot, J.D., M.A. Gavin & A.Y. Rudensky. 2003. Foxp3 programs the development and function of CD4+CD25+ regulatory T cells. *Nat. Immunol.* **4:** 330–336.

22. Sakaguchi, S. 2000. Regulatory T cells: key controllers of immunologic self-tolerance. *Cell* **101:** 455–458.

23. Trzonkowski, P. *et al.* 2006. CD4+CD25+ T regulatory cells inhibit cytotoxic activity of CTL and NK cells in humans-impact of immunosenescence. *Clin. Immunol.* **119:** 307–316.

24. Wack, A. *et al.* 1998. Age-related modifications of the human alphabeta T cell repertoire due to different clonal expansions in the CD4+ and CD8+ subsets. *Int. Immunol.* **10:** 1281–1288.

25. Kohler, S. *et al.* 2005. Post-thymic in vivo proliferation of naive CD4+ T cells constrains the TCR repertoire in healthy human adults. *Eur. J. Immunol.* **35:** 1987–1994.

26. Plackett, T.P. *et al.* 2004. Aging and innate immune cells. *J. Leukoc. Biol.* **76:** 291–299.

27. Di Lorenzo, G. *et al.* 1999. Granulocyte and natural killer activity in the elderly. *Mech. Ageing Dev.* **108:** 25–38.

28. Agrawal, A. *et al.* 2007. Altered innate immune functioning of dendritic cells in elderly humans: a role of phosphoinositide 3-kinase-signaling pathway. *J. Immunol.* **178:** 6912–6922.

29. Della Bella, S. *et al.* (2007. Peripheral blood dendritic cells and monocytes are differently regulated in the elderly. *Clin. Immunol.* **122:** 220–228.

30. Grewe, M. 2001. Chronological ageing and photoageing of dendritic cells. *Clin. Exp. Dermatol.* **26:** 608–612.

31. Steger, M.M., C. Maczek & B. Grubeck-Loebenstein. 1997. Peripheral blood dendritic cells reinduce proliferation in in vitro aged T cell populations. *Mech. Ageing Dev.* **93:** 125–130.

32. van Duin, D. *et al.* 2007. Prevaccine determination of the expression of costimulatory B7 molecules in activated monocytes predicts influenza vaccine responses in young and older adults. *J. Infect. Dis.* **195:** 1590–1597.

33. Ginaldi, L. *et al.* 1999. Immunological changes in the elderly. *Aging Clin. Exp. Res.* **11:** 281–286.

34. Krishnaraj, R. 1997. Senescence and cytokines modulate the NK cell expression. *Mech. Ageing Dev.* **96:** 89–101.

35. Rukavina, D. *et al.* 1998. Age-related decline of perforin expression in human cytotoxic T lymphocytes and natural killer cells. *Blood* **92:** 2410–2420.

36. Mocchegiani, E. & M. Malavolta. 2004. NK and NKT cell functions in immunosenescence. *Aging Cell.* **3:** 177–184.

37. Pawelec, G. 1999. Immunosenescence: impact in the young as well as the old? *Mech. Ageing Dev.* **108:** 1–7.

38. Licastro, F. *et al.* 2005. Innate immunity and inflammation in ageing: a key for understanding age-related diseases. *Immun. Ageing.* **2:** 8.

39. Franceschi, C. *et al.* 2000. Inflamm-aging. An evolutionary perspective on immunosenescence. *Ann. N. Y. Acad. Sci.* **908:** 244–254.

40. Luz, C. *et al.* 2003. Impact of psychological and endocrine factors on cytokine production of healthy elderly people. *Mech. Ageing Dev.* **124:** 887–895.

41. Roshan, S., S. Nader & P. Orlander. 1999. Ageing and hormones. *Eur. J. Clin. Invest.* **29:** 210–213.

42. Canning, M.O. *et al.* 2000. Opposing effects of dehydroepiandrosterone and dexamethasone on the generation of monocyte-derived dendritic cells. *Eur. J. Endocrinol.* **143:** 687–695.

43. Migeon, C. *et al.* 1957. Dehydroepiandrosterone and androsterone levels in human plasma: effects of age, sex, day to day diurnal variations. *J. Clin. Endocrinol. Metab.* **17:** 1051.

44. Heuser, I. *et al.* 1998. Increased diurnal plasma concentrations of dehydroepiandrosterone in depressed patients. *J. Clin. Endocrinol. Metab.* **83:** 3130–3133.

45. Vedhara, K. *et al.* 1999. Chronic stress in elderly carers of dementia patients and antibody response to influenza vaccination. *Lancet* **353:** 627–631.

46. Kiecolt-Glaser, J.K. *et al.* 1996. Chronic stress alters the immune response to influenza virus vaccine in older adults. *Proc. Natl. Acad. Sci. USA* **93:** 3043–3047.

47. Sternberg, E. 2002. Neuroendocrine regulation of autoimmune/inflammatory disease. *J. Endocrinol.* **169:** 429–435.

48. Straub, R., J. Schölmerich & M. Cutolo. 2003. The multiple facets of premature aging in rheumatoid arthritis. *Arthritis Rheumatism* **48:** 2713–2721.

49. Straub, R. *et al.* 2000. Cytokines and hormones as possible links between endocrinosenescence and immunosenescence. *J. Neuroimmunol.* **109:** 10–15.

50. Besedovsky, H. *et al.* 1977. Hypothalamic changes during the immune response. *Eur. J. Immunol.* **7:** 323–325.

51. Mastorakos, G., G.P. Chrousos & J. Weber. 1993. Recombinant IL-6 activates the hypothalamic-pituitary-adrenal axis in humans. *J. Clin. Endocrinol. Metab.* **77:** 1690–1694.

52. Daynes, R. *et al.* 1993. Altered regulation of IL-6 production with normal aging—possible linkage to the age-associated decline in dehydroepiandros-

terone and its sulfated derivative. *J. Immunol.* **150:** 5219–5230.

53. Straub, R.H. *et al.* 1998. Serum dehydroepiandrosterone (DHEA) and DHEA sulfate are negatively correlated with serum interleukin-6 (IL-6), and DHEA inhibits IL-6 secretion from mononuclear cells in man in vitro: possible link between endocrinosenescence and immunosenescence. *J. Clin. Endocrinol. Metab.* **83:** 2012–2017.

54. Vetta, F. *et al.* 2001. Tumor necrosis factor-alpha and mood disorders in the elderly. *Arch. Gerontol. Geriat.* Suppl. **7:** 442.

55. Gabriel, P., I. Cakman & L. Rink. 2002. Overproduction of monokines by leukocytes after stimulation with lipopolysaccharide in the elderly. *Exp. Gerontol.* **37:** 235–247.

56. Fagiolo, U. *et al.* 1993. Increased cytokine production in mononuclear cells of healthy elderly people. *Eur. J. Immunol.* **23:** 2375–2378.

57. Schiepers, O.J., M.C. Wichers & M. Maes. 2005. Cytokines and major depression. *Prog. Neuropsychopharmacol. Biol. Psychiatry* **29:** 201–217.

58. Trzonkowski, P. *et al.* 2004. Immune consequences of the spontaneous pro-inflammatory status in depressed elderly patients. *Brain. Behav. Immun.* **18:** 135–148.

59. Piani, A. *et al.* 2004. Sleep disturbances in elderly: a subjective evaluation over 65. *Arch. Gerontol. Geriatr.* Suppl. 325–331.

60. Howieson, D.B. *et al.* 2003. Natural history of cognitive decline in the old old. *Neurology* **60:** 1489–1494.

61. Reynolds, C.F. 3rd *et al.* 1998. Effects of age at onset of first lifetime episode of recurrent major depression on treatment response and illness course in elderly patients. *Am. J. Psychiatry* **155:** 795–799.

62. Collaziol, D. *et al.* 2004. Psychoneuroendocrine correlates of lymphocyte subsets during healthy ageing. *Mech. Ageing Dev.* **125:** 219–227.

63. Nolen-Hoeksema, S. & C. Ahrens. 2002. Age differences and similarities in the correlates of depressive symptoms. *Psychol. Aging* **17:** 116–124.

64. Deuschle, M. *et al.* 1997. With aging in humans the activity of the hypothalamus-pituitary-adrenal system increases and its amplitude flattens. *Life Sci.* **61:** 2239–2246.

65. Ferrari, E. *et al.* 2000. Pineal and pituitary-adrenocortical function in physiological aging and in senile dementia. *Exp. Gerontol.* **35:** 1239–1250.

66. Van Cauter, E., R. Leproult & D.J. Kupfer. 1996. Effects of gender and age on the levels and circadian rhythmicity of plasma cortisol. *J. Clin. Endocrinol. Metab.* **81:** 2468–2473.

67. Maeda, K. *et al.* 1991. Elevated urinary free cortisol in patients with dementia. *Neurobiol. Aging* **12:** 161–163.

68. Gold, P., F. Goodwin & G. Chrousos. 1988. Clinical and biochemical manifestations of depression I. *N. Engl. J. Med.* **319:** 348–413.

69. Kirschbaum, C. *et al.* 1995. Persistent high cortisol responses to repeated psychological stress in a subpopulation of healthy men. *Psychol. Med.* **57:** 468–474.

70. Bauer, M.E. *et al.* 2000. Chronic stress in caregivers of dementia patients is associated with reduced lymphocyte sensitivity to glucocorticoids. *J. Neuroimmunol.* **103:** 84–92.

71. Luz, C. *et al.* 2006. Healthy aging is associated with unaltered production of immunoreactive growth hormone but impaired neuroimmunomodulation. *Neuroimmunomodulation* **13:** 90–99.

72. Ferrari, E. *et al.* 2001. Age-related changes of the hypothalamic-pituitary-adrenal axis: pathophysiological correlates. *Eur. J. Endocrinol.* **144:** 319–329.

73. Butcher, S.K. & J.M. Lord. 2004. Stress responses and innate immunity: aging as a contributory factor. *Aging Cell.* **3:** 151–160.

74. Selye, H. 1936. A syndrome produced by diverse nocuous agents. *Nature* **138:** 32.

75. Sapolsky, R.M., L.M. Romero & A.U. Munck. 2000. How do glucocorticoids influence stress responses? Integrating permissive, suppressive, stimulatory, and preparative actions. *Endocr. Rev.* **21:** 55–89.

76. Biondi, M. 2001. Effects of stress on immune functions: an overview. In *Psychoneuroimmunonology*, Vol. 2. R. Ader, D. Felten & N. Cohen, Eds.: 189–226. Academic Press. San Diego.

77. Bauer, M.E. *et al.* 2002. Dexamethasone-induced effects on lymphocyte distribution and expression of adhesion molecules in treatment resistant major depression. *Psychiat. Res.* **113:** 1–15.

78. Hoglund, C.O. *et al.* 2006. Changes in immune regulation in response to examination stress in atopic and healthy individuals. *Clin. Exp. Allergy* **36:** 982–992.

79. Navarro, J. *et al.* 2006. Circulating dendritic cells subsets and regulatory T-cells at multiple sclerosis relapse: differential short-term changes on corticosteroids therapy. *J. Neuroimmunol.* **176:** 153–161.

80. Glaser, R. *et al.* 2001. Evidence for a shift in the Th-1 to Th-2 cytokine response associated with chronic stress and aging. *J. Gerontol. Med. Sci.* **56A:** M477–M482.

81. Galon, J. *et al.* 2002. Gene profiling reveals unknown enhancing and suppressive actions of glucocorticoids on immune cells. *FASEB J.* **16:** 61–71.

82. Ramirez, F. *et al.* 1996. Glucocorticoids promote a Th2 cytokine response by CD4+ T cells in vitro. *J. Immunol.* **156:** 2406–2412.

83. Daynes, R., D. Dudley & B. Araneo. 1990. Regulation of murine lymphokine production in vivo. II. Dehydroepiandrosterone is a natural enhancer of interleukin-2 synthesis by helper T cells. *Eur. J. Immunol.* **20:** 793–802.

84. Suzuki, T. *et al.* 1991. Dehydroepiandrosterone enhances IL2 production and cytotoxic effector function of human T cells. *Clin. Immunol. Immunopathol.* **61:** 202–211.

85. Padgett, D.A. & R. Loria. 1994. In vitro potentiation of lymphocyte activation by dehydroepiandrosterone, androstenediol, and androstenetriol. *J. Immunol.* **153:** 1544–1552.

86. McLachlan, J.A., C.D. Serkin & O. Bakouche. 1996. Dehydroepiandrosterone modulation of lipopolysaccharide-stimulated monocyte cytotoxicity. *J. Immunol.* **156:** 328–335.

87. Di Santo, E., M. Sironi & T. Mennini. 1996. A glucocorticoid receptor independent mechanism for neurosteroid inhibition of tumor necrosis factor production. *Eur. J. Pharmacol.* **299:** 179–186.

88. Solerte, S.B. *et al.* 1999. Dehydroepiandrosterone sulfate enhances natural killer cell cytotoxicity in humans via locally generated immunoreactive insulin-like growth factor I. *J. Clin. Endocrinol. Metab.* **84:** 3260–3267.

89. Buvat, J. 2003. Androgen therapy with dehydroepiandrosterone. *World J. Urol.* **21:** 346–355.

90. Casson, P.R. *et al.* 1993. Oral dehydroepiandrosterone in physiologic doses modulates immune function in postmenopausal women. *Am. J. Obstet. Gynecol.* **169:** 1536–1539.

91. Araneo, B., M. Woods & R. Daynes. 1993. Reversal of the immunosenescent phenotype by dehydroepiandrosterone: hormone treatment provides an adjuvant effect on the immunization of aged mice with recombinant hepatitis B surface antigen. *J. Infect. Dis.* **167:** 830–840.

92. Danenberg, H. *et al.* 1995. Dehydroepiandrosterone (DHEA) treatment reverses the impaired immune response of old mice to influenza vaccination and protects from influenza infection. *Vaccine* **13:** 1445–1448.

93. Ribeiro, F. *et al.* 2007. Dehydroepiandrosterone sulphate enhances IgG and interferon-gamma production during immunization to tuberculosis in young but not aged mice. *Biogerontology* **8:** 209–220.

94. Degelau, J., D. Guay & H. Hallgren. 1997. The effect of DHEAS on influenza vaccination in aging adults. *J. Amer. Geriatr. Soc.* **45:** 747–751.

95. Evans, T.G. *et al.* 1996. The use of oral dehydroepiandrosterone sulfate as an adjuvant in tetanus

and influenza vaccination of the elderly. *Vaccine* **14:** 1531–1537.

96. Ben-Yehuda, A. *et al*. 1998. The influence of sequential annual vaccination and DHEA administration on the efficacy of the immune response to influenza vaccine in the elderly. *Mech. Ageing Dev.* **102:** 299–306.

97. Danenberg, H.D. *et al*. 1997. Dehydroepiandrosterone treatment is not beneficial to the immune response to influenza in elderly subjects. *J. Clin. Endocrinol. Metab.* **82:** 2911–2914.

98. Corpas, S., M. Harman & M.R. Blackmann. 1993. Human growth hormone and human aging. *Endocr. Rev.* **14:** 20–39.

99. Kelley, K.W. 1990. The role of growth hormone in modulation of the immune response. *Ann. N. Y. Acad. Sci.* **594:** 95–103.

100. LeRoith, D. *et al*. 1996. The effects of growth hormone and insulin-like growth factor I on the immune system of aged female monkeys. *Endocrinology* **137:** 1071–1079.

101. Welniak, L.A., R. Sun & W.J. Murphy. 2002. The role of growth hormone in T-cell development and reconstitution. *J. Leukoc. Biol.* **71:** 381–387.

102. Weigent, D.A. *et al*. 1988. Production of immunoreactive growth hormone by mononuclear leukocytes. *Faseb J.* **2:** 2812–2818.

103. Hattori, N. *et al*. 1994. Spontaneous growth hormone (GH) secretion by unstimulated human lymphocytes and the effects of GH-releasing hormone and somatostatin. *J. Clin. Endocrinol. Metab.* **79:** 1678–1680.

104. Malarkey, W.B. *et al*. 2002. Human lymphocyte growth hormone stimulates interferon gamma production and is inhibited by cortisol and norepinephrine. *J. Neuroimmunol.* **123:** 180–187.

105. Wu, H. *et al*. 1999. Chronic stress associated with spousal caregiving of patients with Alzheimer's dementia is associated with downregulation of B-lymphocyte GH mRNA. *J. Gerontol. A Biol. Sci. Med. Sci.* **54:** M212–215.

106. Dixit, V.D. *et al*. 2004. Ghrelin inhibits leptin- and activation-induced proinflammatory cytokine expression by human monocytes and T cells. *J. Clin. Invest.* **114:** 57–66.

107. Englander, E.W., G.A. Gomez & G.H. Greeley, Jr. 2004. Alterations in stomach ghrelin production and in ghrelin-induced growth hormone secretion in the aged rat. *Mech. Ageing Dev.* **125:** 871–875.

108. Kavelaars, A. *et al*. 1996. Ontogeny of the response of human peripheral blood T cells to glucocorticoids. *Brain Behav. Immun.* **10:** 288–297.

109. Sippell, W.G. *et al*. 1978. Longitudinal studies of plasma aldosterone, corticosterone, deoxycorticosterone, progesterone, 17-hydroxyprogesterone, cortisol, and cortisone determined simultaneously in mother and child at birth and during the early neonatal period. I. Spontaneous delivery. *J. Clin. Endocrinol. Metab.* **46:** 971–985.

110. Rohleder, N. *et al*. 2002. Age and sex steroid-related changes in glucocorticoid sensitivity of proinflammatory cytokine production after psychosocial stress. *J. Neuroimmunol.* **126:** 69–77.

111. Miller, G.E. *et al*. 2005. Clinical depression and regulation of the inflammatory response during acute stress. *Psychosom. Med.* **67:** 679–687.

112. Bauer, M.E. *et al*. 2003. Altered glucocorticoid immunoregulation in treatment resistant depression. *Psychoneuroendocrinology* **28:** 49–65.

113. Kirschbaum, C., K.M. Pirke & D.H. Hellhammer. 1993. The 'Trier Social Stress Test'—a tool for investigating psychobiological stress responses in a laboratory setting. *Neuropsychobiology* **28:** 76–81.

114. Kiecolt-Glaser, J. *et al*. 1991. Spousal caregivers of dementia victims: longitudinal changes in immunity and health. *Psychosom. Med.* **53:** 345–362.

115. Redinbaugh, E., R. McCallum & J. Kiecolt-Glaser. 1995. Recurrent syndromal depression in caregivers. *Psychol. Aging* 358–368.

116. Epel, E.S. *et al*. 2004. Accelerated telomere shortening in response to life stress. *Proc. Natl. Acad. Sci. USA* **101:** 17312–17315.

117. Glaser, R. *et al*. 2000. Chronic stress modulates the immune response to a pneumococcal pneumonia vaccine. *Psychosom. Med.* **62:** 804–807.

118. Kiecolt-Glaser, J. *et al*. 1995. Slowing of wound healing by psychological stress. *Lancet* **346:** 1194–1196.

119. Shaw, W.S. *et al*. 1999. Accelerated risk of hypertensive blood pressure recordings among Alzheimer caregivers. *J. Psychosom. Res.* **46:** 215–227.

120. Vitaliano, P.P. *et al*. 2002. A path model of chronic stress, the metabolic syndrome, and coronary heart disease. *Psychosom. Med.* **64:** 418–435.

121. Schulz, R. & S.R. Beach. 1999. Caregiving as a risk factor for mortality: the Caregiver Health Effects Study. *Jama* **282:** 2215–2219.

122. Kiecolt-Glaser, J.K. *et al*. 2003. Chronic stress and age-related increases in the proinflammatory cytokine IL-6. *Proc. Natl. Acad. Sci. USA* **100:** 9090–9095.

123. McEwen, B. 1998. Protective and damaging effects of stress mediators. *N. Engl. J. Med.* **338:** 171–179.

124. Lupien, S. *et al*. 1994. Basal cortisol levels and cognitive deficits in human aging. *J. Neurosci.* **14:** 2893–2903.

125. Starkman, M., D. Schteingart & M. Schork. 1981. Depressed mood and other psychiatric manifestations of Cushing's syndrome: relationship to hormone levels. *Psychosom. Med.* **43:** 3–18.

Modulation of the Immune System by Ouabain

Sandra Rodrigues-Mascarenhas,[a]
Andreia Da Silva de Oliveira,[b] **Nívea Dias Amoedo,**[b]
Ottilia R. Affonso-Mitidieri,[b] **Franklin D. Rumjanek,**[b]
and Vivian M. Rumjanek[b]

[a]*Laboratório de Tecnologia Farmacêutica, Departamento de Fisiologia e Patologia,
Universidade Federal da Paraíba, João Pessoa, Brazil*

[b]*Instituto de Bioquímica Médica, Universidade Federal do Rio de Janeiro,
Rio de Janeiro, Brazil*

Ouabain, a known inhibitor of the Na,K-ATPase, has been shown to regulate a number of lymphocyte functions *in vitro* and *in vivo*. Lymphocyte proliferation, apoptosis, cytokine production, and monocyte function are all affected by ouabain. The ouabain-binding site occurs at the α subunit of the enzyme. The α subunit plays a critical role in the transport process, and four different α-subunit isoforms have been described with different sensitivities to ouabain. Analysis by RT-PCR indicates that α1, α2, and α3 isoforms are all present in murine lymphoid cells obtained from thymus, lymph nodes, and spleen. In these cells ouabain exerts an effect at concentrations that do not induce plasma membrane depolarization, suggesting a mechanism independent of the classical inhibition of the pump. In other systems, the Na,K-ATPase acts as a signal transducer in addition to being an ion pump, and ouabain is capable of inducing the activation of various signal transduction cascades. Neither resting nor concanavalin A (Con A)-activated thymocytes had their levels of phosphorylated-extracellular signal-regulated kinase (P-ERK) modified by ouabain. However, ouabain decreased p38 phosphorylation induced by Con A in these cells. The pathway induced by ouabain in lymphoid cells is still unclear but might vary with the type and state of activation of the cell.

Key words: ouabain; lymphocytes; immune system; Na,K-ATPase alpha subunit isoforms; p38; MAPK; plasma membrane depolarization

Introduction

Ouabain is a cardiotonic glycoside originally isolated from plants, such as *Acocanthera ouabaio* and *Strophantus gratus*. This glycoside has been widely used in therapy for congestive heart failure. For many years the existence of an endogenous equivalent of digitalis has been suggested and searched for,[1] and it is now known that an endogenous mammalian analogue of ouabain can be isolated from human plasma and plasma from different species.[2,3] The adrenal seems to be a source of circulating ouabain, as the secretion of endogenous ouabain from this organ has been identified both *in vivo* and *in vitro*.[4-9] Adrenocorticotropic hormone (ACTH)[7,9-12] and angiotensin II[13,14] were shown to stimulate the adrenal secretion of endogenous ouabain. However, the adrenal cortex is not the only source of endogenous ouabain as this steroid has been identified in the brain, mainly in the hypothalamus and pituitary.[3,15-18]

Address for correspondence: Vivian M. Rumjanek, Laboratório de Imunologia Tumoral, Instituto de Bioquímica Médica, Centro de Ciências da Saúde – Bloco H02 – Sala 003, Universidade Federal do Rio de Janeiro, 21941-590 – Rio de Janeiro – RJ – Brazil. Fax: +055 021 2270 1635. vivian@bioqmed.ufrj.br

Neuroimmunomodulation: Ann. N.Y. Acad. Sci. 1153: 153–163 (2009).
doi: 10.1111/j.1749-6632.2008.03969.x © 2009 New York Academy of Sciences.

Ouabain has been proposed to act as a neuroregulator,[19–26] and we now extend its role as an immunomodulator.[27]

Ouabain and the Immune System

The first evidence of ouabain action on lymphoid cells involved inhibition of lymphocyte proliferation induced by the mitogen phytohemagglutinin.[28] It has now been reported that ouabain inhibits proliferation induced by a variety of stimuli, including not only mitogens[29–31] but phorbol ester,[32,33] anti-CD3,[34] calcium ionophore,[35] and interleukin (IL)-2.[36] It is also clear that, despite the absence of proliferation, these cells start by being responsive to the stimulus as they show an increase in c-Myc[31] and CD69.[37] These results are in accordance with those of Brodie *et al.*[33] indicating that ouabain did not interfere with early activation events. Activated lymphocytes do not progress through the cell cycle as they fail to express CD25 and/or to secrete IL-2.[33,37–40] Thymocytes exposed to ouabain and concanavalin A (Con A) show decreased levels of nuclear factor of activated T cells transcription complex (NFATc),[41] which is in accordance with the fact that, under normal circumstances, the mitogen Con A activates NFAT synthesis and nuclear entry, which is essential for the production of the cytokine IL-2.[42]

Despite inhibiting T lymphocyte proliferation, ouabain does not affect natural killer (NK) cytotoxic activity nor lymphokine-activated killer (LAK) cytotoxicity.[30,32] However, the generation of LAK activity by IL-2 is inhibited by ouabain.[32]

Antigen or mitogen-activated lymphocytes control their number through a physiologic mechanism, known as activation-induced cell death (AICD), occurring at the end of immune responses. Activated lymphocytes exposed to ouabain follow the apoptotic pathway[31,43] similar to what has been observed with the human T lymphocyte cell line Jurkat,[44] and it has been suggested that this represents an exacer-

bation of AICD.[43] Stimulation of the Fas receptor leads to inhibiton of K^+ uptake,[45] and a central role for K^+ ions in apoptosis has been advanced as normal concentrations of this ion inhibit caspase and nuclease activity.[46–49]

A similar mechanism could be proposed to explain the increased production induced by ouabain of the cytokine IL-1.[50] The enzyme capable of cleaving pro-IL-1β to the biologically active form is the caspase ICE (IL-1β-converting enzyme), and its activation was reported to be enhanced by K^+ depletion.[51,52]

In addition to IL-1,[50,53–55] the production of tumor necrosis factor (TNF)-α is also increased by ouabain.[53,54] Not only cytokine production is modulated by ouabain but also the production of nitric oxide by rat peritoneal macrophages[56] and the expression of CD14 at the plasma membrane of macrophages derived from human peripheral blood monocytes (R.C. Valente, C.R. Nascimento, E.G. Araujo (from Universidade Federal do Rio de Janeiro and Universidade Federal Fluminense, Brazil), and V.M. Rumjanek, unpublished observations).

The modulation of cytokine levels produced by ouabain may also affect hematopoietic progenitor cells. Incubation of mouse bone marrow cells with ouabain had a dual effect depending on the concentration used. However, the response of progenitor cells differed as there was a tendency to inhibit the formation of CFU-S (pluripotent stem cells) and CFU-C (granulocyte progenitor cells) while it increased the proliferation of erythroid progenitor cells (both BFU-E and CFU-E).[57,58]

Receptors for Ouabain in the Immune System

Mature peripheral lymphocytes are reported to have approximately 43,000 ouabain-binding sites per cell.[59] At present the only known receptor for ouabain is the enzyme Na,K-ATPase. This enzyme promotes the active transport system that is responsible for maintenance of the gradients of Na^+ and K^+ across the plasma membrane. This transport protein is present in all animal cells where it is responsible for various cellular functions. The Na–K pump is a transmembrane protein composed of three subunits: α, β, and γ.[60,61] The α subunit has 10 transmembrane segments, an intracellular nucleotide-binding site, and the phosphorylation domain. The β subunit has a single transmembrane segment and a large extracellular domain.[62] The Na,K-ATPase α and β subunits may also associate with a third subunit known as the γ subunit.[63] The α subunit of the Na,K-ATPase is responsible for the catalytic and transport properties of the enzyme. Its structure provides binding sites for cations, ATP, and digitalis-like compounds.[64] There are also suggestions that the α subunit has binding domains capable of interaction with the actin cytoskeleton.[65] Furthermore, this subunit appears to be a substrate for kinase-mediated phosphorylation, and there is evidence that phosphorylation of the α subunit of the Na,K-ATPase may inhibit the activity of the enzyme[66,67] or induce its internalization,[68] thus contributing to a reduction in the activity of the Na,K-ATPase.

The β subunit is essential for the activity of the enzyme and is involved in the occlusion of K^+ and the affinity modulation for Na^+ and K^+ ions. In addition, the β subunit acts a chaperone to the α subunit, allowing its delivery to the plasma membrane.[62] The $\beta 2$ isoform has adhesion molecule properties that appear to be independent of the structure and function of the Na,K-ATPase complex.[69]

The γ subunit[70] modulates the transport function of Na,K-ATPase[71] and may contribute to the formation of the site-binding cardiac glycosides, such as ouabain.[70,72,73]

Several isoforms of the α and β subunits of Na,K-ATPase have been described, whereas only one γ isoform subunit has been identified so far. There are four α and three β subunits and their pattern of expression is specific for different tissues and different stages of development.

The α subunit is encoded by a multigene family, and four genes for different α subunit isoforms have been described. Differences in cation affinity, ATP affinity, and other kinetic parameters of the enzymatic activity have been reported. The three isoforms also vary according to their sensitivity to ouabain: $\alpha 3$ displaying high, $\alpha 2$ intermediate, and $\alpha 1$ low sensitivity to cardiac glycosides.[69] As a result of variations in the distribution of the isoforms, the inhibitory effect of ouabain varies for different species and, for a given species, for different tissues. In rodents the affinity of the $\alpha 2$ and $\alpha 3$ isoforms for ouabain is 1000-fold greater than the $\alpha 1$ isoform.[74,75]

Differences in the distribution of α isoforms may account for the sensitivity of different tissues to ouabain. Little is known, however, regarding the isozyme distribution in the immune system. Our group investigated the expression of the different isoforms $\alpha 1$, $\alpha 2$, $\alpha 3$, and $\alpha 4$ in cells obtained from murine thymus, lymph nodes, and spleen and compared their expression in kidney and spermatozoa. As observed in Figure 1, using RT-PCR, $\alpha 1$, $\alpha 2$, and $\alpha 3$ isoforms were expressed in thymus, lymph nodes, and spleen, whereas $\alpha 4$ was only seen in the testis.

When Na,K-ATPase activity sensitive to ouabain was compared between cells obtained from rat thymus, lymph nodes, spleen, and peripheral blood, it was observed that thymocytes presented the highest activity, peripheral blood the lowest, and spleen and lymph node an intermediate activity.[76]

Ouabain and Plasma Membrane Depolarization of Lymphoid Cells

Having established that lymphoid cells also express α isoforms with high affinity for ouabain, the possibility was raised that the various effects produced by ouabain on cells from the immune system were dependent on the inhibition of the Na,K-ATPase. In lymphocytes the plasma membrane potential is maintained predominantly by the electrogenic action of this pump, which is responsible for the maintenance

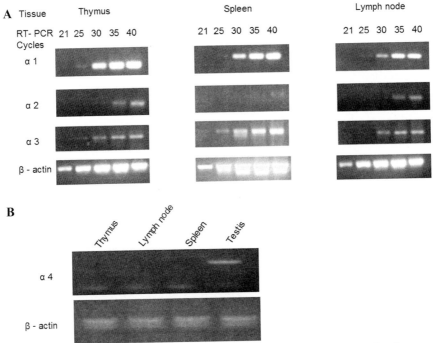

Figure 1. Expression of Na,K-ATPase α subunit isoforms in murine lymphoid tissue. (**A**) Expression of Na,K-ATPase α subunit isoforms in thymus, spleen, and lymph node estimated by RT-PCR. Different PCR cycles, namely 21, 25, 30, 35, and 40 were tested using cDNA samples. β-actin was used for standardization. (**B**) Expression of Na,K-ATPase α4 isoform. Amplification for α4 isoform was estimated after 40 RT-PCR cycles. Mouse testis cDNA was used as a positive control. PCR amplification was carried out with cDNA obtained from total RNA from fresh tissue (spleen, thymus, lymph node, testis, and kidney) of adult male mouse C57/Bl6. Primer sequences were obtained from GenBank (accession number of each gene available at http://www.ncbi.nlm.nih.gov). During PCR amplification of the different isoforms of the α subunit, at the times indicated in the legend, equal volumes of PCR mixtures were collected and the products fractionated in agarose gel electrophoresis. The mRNA expression of the isoforms was normalized by calculating the ratio of the several amplicons to that of β-actin of each sample.

of high potassium and low sodium levels within the cell. However, inhibition of this enzyme leading to plasma membrane depolarization was only obtained when micromolar concentrations of ouabain were used (Fig. 2). Despite the absence of effect on the plasma membrane potential of thymocytes, nanomolar concentrations of ouabain were capable of inducing the expression of CD69 in these cells.[77]

This resistance to depolarization has already been described in murine thymocytes[78,79] and human lymphocytes.[43,80] However, ouabain is capable of increasing glucocorticoid-induced plasma membrane depolarization in thymocytes[79] and other lymphoid cells (Fig. 3).

Ouabain synergizes with hydrocortisone *in vivo* in the induction of thymic atrophy. Although ouabain by itself does not affect total viability or thymocyte subpopulations, the combined treatment with corticoid leads to a decrease in the cellularity of the thymus that reflects an increased apoptosis of the double-positive population.[81]

Intracellular Pathways Activated by Ouabain

Despite only affecting plasma membrane potential at the micromolar range, nanomolar

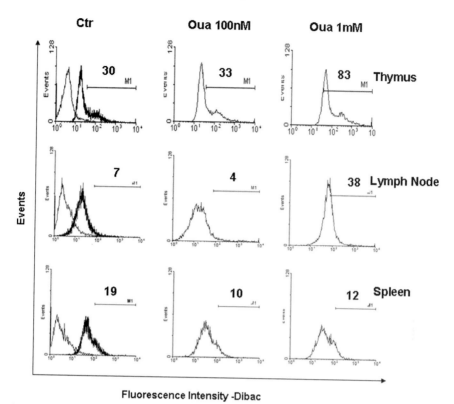

Figure 2. Ouabain (OUA) depolarizes lymphocyte plasma membrane in a dose-dependent manner. Acute changes in plasma membrane potential were measured by flow cytometry, using bis-(1,3-dibutilbarbiturate) trimethine oxonol – DiBAC$_4$. Lymphocytes at 1 × 10^6 cells/mL isolated from thymus, lymph nodes, and spleen were exposed to 100 nmol/L or 1 mmol/L OUA for 6 h. Cells were incubated with oxonol to evaluate plasma membrane potential. Representative DiBAC$_4$ fluorescence histograms are shown for each treatment.

concentrations of ouabain are capable of regulating a number of parameters in thymocytes and lymphocytes, and there is evidence that inhibition of macromolecular synthesis occurs at an ouabain concentration one order of magnitude lower than that affecting K$^+$ transport and Na,K-ATPase activity.[82] Furthermore, in some systems, ouabain seems to have opposing effects depending on the concentration used, with results that indicate that the mechanism of action of ouabain is not restricted to a global inhibition of the Na,K-ATPase activity.[57,83]

In a vascular smooth muscle cell system 1 nmol/L ouabain was capable of increasing intracellular calcium levels.[84] In the murine thymocyte model, concentrations as low as 30 nmol/L were capable of eliciting Ca^{2+} mobilization.[78] It seems unlikely that the observed

intracellular increase in Ca^{2+} levels was a result of the classical view of calcium accumulation being dependent on pump inhibition.

It has been suggested that low concentrations of ouabain may be able to interact with Na,K-ATPase and elicit a signaling cascade of events that is independent of changes in intracellular Na$^+$ and K$^+$ concentrations and that activates gene transcription.[85] Different intracellular pathways are activated that involve the Ras/Raf/mitogen-activated protein kinase (MAPK) cascade,[86] transactivation of epidermal growth factor receptor (EGFR),[87] and protein kinase C.[88]

In an attempt to define possible signaling pathways independent of ionic changes, our group looked at the MAPK pathways. The family of MAPK consists of four

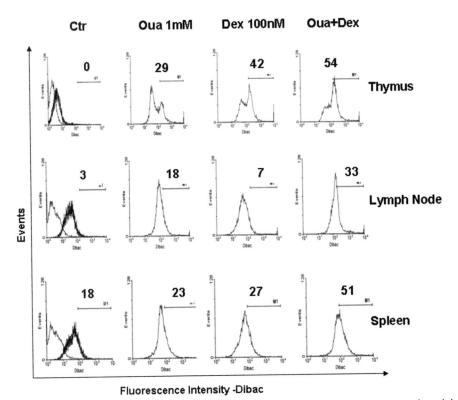

Figure 3. OUA (1 mmol/L) increases plasma membrane depolarization induced by 100 nmol/L dexamethasone. Acute changes in plasma membrane potential were measured by flow cytometry, using bis-(1,3-dibutilbarbiturate) trimethine oxonol – DiBAC$_4$. Lymphocytes at 1×10^6 cells/mL isolated from thymus, lymph nodes, and spleen were exposed to 100 nmol/L dexamethasone for 6 h in the presence or absence of 1 mmol/L OUA. Representative DiBAC$_4$ fluorescence histograms are shown for each treatment.

members: ERK (extracellular signal-regulated kinase)1/2, JNK (c-Jun N-terminal kinase)/ SAPK (stress-activated protein kinase), p38, and ERK5/big mitogen-activated kinase 1. In culture, ouabain did not induce ERK phosphorylation or modified the phosphorylation of this MAPK induced by Con A despite the fact that NFATc was inhibited (Fig. 4). Activation of lymphocytes via the T cell receptor leads to activation of ZAP-70, which phosphorylates both p38 and the MAPK cascade upstream of ERK. The fact that NFAT is one of the major targets of p38 in mature T lymphocytes[89] led us to study this pathway in mitogen-activated thymocytes in the presence of ouabain.[41] As shown in Figure 5A ouabain *per se* did not induce p38 activation but decreased the levels of phosphorylated p38 induced by Con A. Fur-

thermore, concentrations as low as 10 nmol/L ouabain produced an effect.[41] The mechanism involved is still unclear. The p38 kinase pathway is classically activated by stress[90] and inflammatory cytokines.[91] Ouabain induces changes in cellular volume (shrinkage), and this could be recognized by the cell as a stress signal. However, no increase in p38 was observed despite the fact that these cells responded to another stress inducer, UV, enhancing the levels of p38 (Fig. 5B).

Alternatively, the effect produced by ouabain on P-p38 could result from an increase in phosphatase activity leading to dephosphorylation and not by the lack of p38 activation. There is evidence that glucocorticoids increase the levels of MAPK phosphatase 1,[92] and an equivalent mechanism could be operating with ouabain.

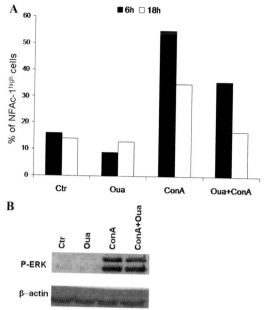

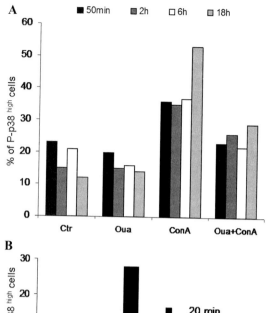

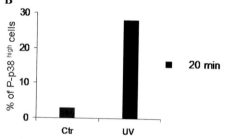

Figure 4. Effect of OUA on concanavalin A (Con A)-induced activation of nuclear factor of activated T cells transcription complex (NFATc)1 and extracellular signal-regulated kinase (ERK) mitogen-activated protein kinase (MAPK). Thymocytes at 1×10^6 cells/mL were incubated for 20 min (for phosphorylated (P)-ERK), 6 and 18 h (for P-p38) in RPMI medium and 10% fetal calf serum (FCS) in the presence or absence of 100 nmol/L OUA and/or 2.5 μg/mL Con A. (**A**) NFATc1 expression was studied by flow cytometry analysis after 6 and 18 h. The numbers represent the percentage of NFATc1^{high} cells. (**B**) P-ERK expression was studied by Western blot analysis. The bands were visualized with the enhanced chemiluminescence system (Amersham, Buckinghamshire, England). One representative of four experiments (**A**) and one representative of three independent experiments (**B**) are shown. (In color in *Annals* online.)

Figure 5. Activation of p38 and the effect of OUA. Thymocytes at 1×10^6 cells/mL were treated for different times or were subjected to UV radiation in phosphate-buffered saline solution, and P-p38 expression was studied by flow cytometry analysis. (**A**) Cells were incubated for 50 min, 2, 6, and 18 h in RPMI medium and 10% FCS in the presence or absence of 100 nmol/L OUA and/or 2.5 μg/mL Con A. (**B**) Cells were subjected to UV radiation for 10 min. The numbers represent the percentage of P-p38^{high} cells. One representative of five experiments (**A**) and one representative of four independent experiments (**B**) are shown.

Conclusion

Ouabain is capable of regulating mature and immature lymphocytes, modulating monocytes, modifying cytokine levels and, consequently, could be considered an immunomodulatory molecule. Some of the effects observed in the immune system can be produced by ouabain at the nanomolar range and seem to result from a mechanism different from the traditional inhibition of the Na,K-ATPase.

Taking into account that ouabain can also be released from the adrenal under the stimu-

lus of ACTH, similar to what is observed with glucocorticoids, the role of ouabain on the immune system should also be considered when studying a stress response.

Acknowledgments

This work was supported by grants from Conselho Nacional de Desenvolvimento Científico e Tecnológico (CNPq) and Fundação de Amparo à Pesquisa do Estado do Rio de Janeiro (FAPERJ).

Conflicts of Interest

The authors declare no conflicts of interest.

References

1. Goto, A., K. Yamada, N. Yagi, *et al*. 1992. Ouabain as endogenous digitalis-like factor in animals? *Clin. Chem.* **38:** 161–162.
2. Hamlyn, J.M., M.P. Blaustein, S. Bova, *et al*. 1991. Identification and characterization of a ouabain-like compound from human plasma. *Proc. Natl. Acad. Sci. USA* **88:** 6259–6263.
3. Ferrandi, M., P. Manunta, S. Balzan, *et al*. 1997. Ouabain-like factor quantification in mammalian tissues and plasma: comparison of two independent assays. *Hypertension* **30:** 886–896.
4. Doris, P.A. & D.M. Stocco. 1989. An endogenous digitalis-like factor derived from the adrenal gland: studies of adrenal tissue from various sources. *Endocrinology* **125:** 2573–2579.
5. Ludens, J.H., M.A. Clark, F.G. Robinson & D.W. DuCharme. 1992. Rat adrenal cortex is a source of a circulating ouabainlike compound. *Hypertension* **19:** 721–724.
6. Boulanger, B.R., M.P. Lilly, J.M. Hamlyn, *et al*. 1993. Ouabain is secreted by the adrenal gland in awake dogs. *Am. J. Physiol.* **264:** 413–419.
7. Laredo J., B.P. Hamilton & J.M. Hamlyn. 1994. Ouabain is secreted by bovine adrenocortical cells. *Endocrinology* **135:** 794–797.
8. Beck, M., K.S. Szalay, G.M. Nagy, *et al*. 1996. Production of ouabain by rat adrenocortical cells. *Endocr. Res.* **22:** 845–849.
9. Hinson, J.P., S. Harwood & A.B. Dawnay. 1998. Release of ouabain-like compound (OLC) from the intact perfused rat adrenal gland. *Endocr. Res.* **24:** 721–724.
10. Goto, A., K. Yamada, H. Nagoshi, *et al*. 1995. Stress-induced elevation of ouabainlike compound in rat plasma and adrenal. *Hypertension* **26:** 1173–1176.
11. Schoner, W., N. Bauer, J. Müller-Ehmsen, *et al*. 2003. Ouabain as a mammalian hormone. *Ann. N. Y. Acad. Sci.* **986:** 678–684.
12. Sophocleous, A., I. Elmatzoglou & A. Souvatzoglou. 2003. Circulating endogenous digitalis-like factor(s) (EDLF) in man is derived from the adrenals and its secretion is ACTH-dependent. *J. Endocrinol. Invest.* **26:** 668–674.
13. Laredo J., J.R. Shah, Z.R. Lu, *et al*. 1997. Angiotensin II stimulates secretion of endogenous ouabain from bovine adrenocortical cells via angiotensin type 2 receptors. *Hypertension* **29:** 401–407.
14. Shah, J.R., J. Laredo, B.P. Hamilton & J.M. Hamlyn. 1998. Different signaling pathways mediate stimulated secretions of endogenous ouabain and aldosterone from bovine adrenocortical cells. *Hypertension* **31:** 463–468.
15. Tymiak, A.A., J.A. Norman, M. Bolgar, *et al*. 1993. Physicochemical characterization of a ouabain isomer isolated from bovine hypothalamus. *Proc. Natl. Acad. Sci. USA* **90:** 8189–8193.
16. Zhao, N., L.C. Lo, N. Berova, *et al*. 1995. Na,K-ATPase inhibitors from bovine hypothalamus and human plasma are different from ouabain: nanogram scale CD structural analysis. *Biochemistry* **34:** 9893–9896.
17. Yamada, K., A. Goto & M. Omata. 1995. Modulation of the levels of ouabain-like compound by central catecholamine neurons in rats. *FEBS Lett.* **360:** 67–69.
18. Kawamura, A., J. Guo, Y. Itagaki, *et al*. 1999. On the structure of endogenous ouabain. *Proc. Natl. Acad. Sci. USA* **96:** 6654–6659.
19. Huang, B.S., E. Harmsen, H. Yu & F.H. Leenen. 1992. Brain ouabain-like activity and the sympathoexcitatory and pressor effects of central sodium in rats. *Circ. Res.* **71:** 1059–1066.
20. Yamada, K., A. Goto, H. Nagoshi, *et al*. 1994. Role of brain ouabainlike compound in central nervous system-mediated natriuresis in rats. *Hypertension* **23:** 1027–1031.
21. Budzikowski, A.S. & F.H. Leenen. 1997. Brain 'ouabain' in the median preoptic nucleus mediates sodium-sensitive hypertension in spontaneously hypertensive rats. *Hypertension* **29:** 599–605.
22. Monteith, G.R. & M.P. Blaustein. 1998. Different effects of low and high dose cardiotonic steroids on cytosolic calcium in spontaneously active hippocampal neurons and in co-cultured glia. *Brain Res.* **795:** 325–340.
23. de Wardener, H.E. 2001. The hypothalamus and hypertension. *Physiol. Rev.* **81:** 1599–1658.
24. Xiao, A.Y., L. Wei, S. Xia, *et al*. 2002. Ionic mechanism of ouabain-induced concurrent apoptosis and necrosis in individual cultured cortical neurons. *J. Neurosci.* **22:** 1350–1362.
25. de Rezende Corrêa, G., A.A. dos Santos, C.F.L. Fontes & E.G. Araujo. 2005. Ouabain induces an increase of retinal ganglion cell survival in vitro: the involvement of protein kinase C. *Brain Res.* **1049:** 89–94.
26. Fimbel, S.M., J.E. Montgomery, C.T. Burket & D.R. Hyde. 2007. Regeneration of inner retinal neurons after intravitreal injection of ouabain in zebrafish. *J. Neurosci.* **27:** 1712–1724.
27. Echevarria-Lima, J. & V. M. Rumjanek. 2006. Effect of ouabain on the immune system. *Curr. Hypertens. Rev.* **2:** 83–95.

28. Quastel, M. R. & J. G. Kaplan. 1968. Inhibition by ouabain of human lymphocyte transformation induced by phytohaemagglutinin in vitro. *Nature* **219:** 198–200.

29. Szamel, M., S. Schneider & K. Resch. 1981. Functional interrelationship between (Na+ + K+)-ATPase and lysolecithin acyltransferase in plasma membranes of mitogen-stimulated rabbit thymocytes. *J. Biol. Chem.* **256:** 9198–9204.

30. de Moraes, V.L., B. Olej, L. de la Rocque & V.M. Rumjanek. 1989. Lack of sensitivity to ouabain in natural killer activity. *FASEB J.* **3:** 2425–2429.

31. Olej, B., N.F. dos Santos, L. Leal & V.M. Rumjanek.1998. Ouabain induces apoptosis on PHA-activated lymphocytes. *Biosci. Rep.* **18:** 1–7.

32. Olej, B., L. de La Rocque, F.P. Castilho, *et al*. 1994. Effect of ouabain on lymphokine-activated killer cells. *Int. J. Immunopharmacol.* **16:** 769–774.

33. Brodie, C., A. Tordai, J. Saloga, *et al*. 1995. Ouabain induces inhibition of the progression phase in human T-cell proliferation. *J. Cell. Physiol.* **165:** 246–253.

34. Szamel, M., H. Leufgen, R. Kurrle & K. Resch. 1995. Differential signal transduction pathways regulating interleukin-2 synthesis and interleukin-2 receptor expression in stimulated human lymphocytes. *Biochim. Biophys. Acta* **1235:** 33–42.

35. Jensen, P., L. Winger, H. Rasmussen & P. Nowell.1977. The mitogenic effect of A23187 in human peripheral lymphocytes. *Biochim. Biophys. Acta* **496:** 374–383.

36. Redondo, J.M., A. López Rivas & M. Fresno. 1986. Activation of the Na+/K+-ATPase by interleukin-2. *FEBS Lett.* **206:** 199–202.

37. Pires, V., R.C. Harab, B. Olej & V.M. Rumjanek. 1997. Ouabain effects on activated lymphocytes: augmentation of CD25 expression on TPA-stimulated cells and of CD69 on PHA-and TPA-stimulated cells. *Int. J. Immunopharmacol.* **19:** 143–148.

38. Stoeck, M., H. Northoff & K. Resch. 1983. Inhibition of mitogen-induced lymphocyte proliferation by ouabain: interference with interleukin 2 production and interleukin 2 action. *J. Immunol.* **131:** 1433–1437.

39. Lillehoj, H. & E.M. Shevach. 1985. A comparison of the effects of cyclosporin A, dexamethasone, and ouabain on the interleukin-2 cascade. *J. Immunopharmacol.* **7:** 267–284.

40. Dornand, J., J. Favero, J.C. Bonnafous & J.C. Mani. 1986. Mechanism whereby ouabain inhibits human T lymphocyte activation: effect on the interleukin 2 pathway. *Immunobiology* **171:** 436–450.

41. Rodrigues-Mascarenhas, S., F.F. Bloise, J. Moscat & V.M. Rumjanek. 2008. Ouabain inhibits p38 activation in thymocytes. *Cell Biol. Int.* **32:** 1323–1328.

42. Chow, C.W., M. Rincón & R.J. Davis. 1999. Requirement for transcription factor NFAT in interleukin-2 expression. *Mol. Cell Biol.* **19:** 2300–2307.

43. Esteves, M.B., L.F. Marques-Santos, O.R. Affonso-Mitidieri & V.M. Rumjanek. 2005. Ouabain exacerbates activation-induced cell death in human peripheral blood lymphocytes. *An. Acad. Bras. Cienc.* **77:** 281–292.

44. Orlov, S.N., N. Thorin-Trescases, S.V. Kotelevtsev, *et al*. 1999. Inversion of the intracellular Na+/K+ ratio blocks apoptosis in vascular smooth muscle at a site upstream of caspase-3. *J. Biol. Chem.* **274:** 16545–16552.

45. Gómez-Angelats, M., C.D. Bortner & J.A. Cidlowski. 2000. Protein kinase C (PKC) inhibits fas receptor-induced apoptosis through modulation of the loss of K+ and cell shrinkage. A role for PKC upstream of caspases. *J. Biol. Chem.* **275:** 19609–19619.

46. Bortner, C.D., F.M. Hughes, Jr. & J.A. Cidlowski. 1997. A primary role for K+ and Na+ efflux in the activation of apoptosis. *J. Biol. Chem.* **272:** 32436–32442.

47. Hughes, F.M., Jr., C.D. Bortner, G.D. Purdy & J.A. Cidlowski. 1997. Intracellular K+ suppresses the activation of apoptosis in lymphocytes. *J. Biol. Chem.* **272:** 30567–30576.

48. Kroemer, G., B. Dallaporta & M. Resche-Rigon. 1998. The mitochondrial death/life regulator in apoptosis and necrosis. *Annu. Rev. Physiol.* **60:** 619–642.

49. Penning, L.C., G. Denecker, D. Vercammen, *et al*. 2000. A role for potassium in TNF-induced apoptosis and gene-induction in human and rodent tumour cell lines. *Cytokine* **12:** 747–750.

50. Dornand, J., J. Favero, J.C. Bonnafous & J.C. Mani. 1984. Paradoxical production of mouse thymocyte activating factor by ouabain-treated human mononuclear cells. *Cell Immunol.* **83:** 351–359.

51. Perregaux, D. & C.A. Gabel. 1994. Interleukin-1 beta maturation and release in response to ATP and nigericin. Evidence that potassium depletion mediated by these agents is a necessary and common feature of their activity. *J. Biol. Chem.* **269:** 15195–15203.

52. Walev, I., K. Reske, M. Palmer, A. Valeva & S. Bhakdi. 1995. Potassium-inhibited processing of IL-1 beta in human monocytes. *EMBO J.* **14:** 1607–1614.

53. Foey, A.D., A. Crawford & N.D. Hall. 1997. Modulation of cytokine production by human mononuclear cells following impairment of Na, K-ATPase activity. *Biochim. Biophys. Acta* **1355:** 43–49.

54. Matsumori, A., K. Ono, R. Nishio, *et al*. 1997. Modulation of cytokine production and protection against lethal endotoxemia by the cardiac glycoside ouabain. *Circulation* **96:** 1501–1506.

55. Matsumori, A., K. Ono, R. Nishio, *et al.* 2000. Amilodipine inhibits the production of cytokines induced by ouabain. *Cytokine* **12:** 294–297.

56. Sowa, G. & R. Przewłocki. 1997. Ouabain enhances the lipopolysaccharide-induced nitric oxide production by rat peritoneal macrophages. *Immunopharmacology* **36:** 95–100.

57. Spivak, J.L., J. Misiti, R. Stuart, *et al.* 1980. Suppression and potentiation of mouse hematopoietic progenitor cell proliferation by ouabain. *Blood* **56:** 315–317.

58. Gallicchio, V.S. & M.J. Murphy, Jr. 1981. Erythropoiesis in vitro. IV. Effects of ouabain on erythroid stem cells (CFU-e and BFU-e). *Stem Cells* **11:** 30–37.

59. Pedersen, K.E. & N.A. Klitgaard. 1983. The characteristics of [3H]-ouabain binding to human lymphocytes. *Br. J. Clin. Pharmacol.* **15:** 657–665.

60. Blanco, G. & R.W. Mercer. 1998. Isozymes of the Na-K-ATPase: heterogeneity in structure, diversity in function. *Am. J. Physiol.* **275:** 633–650.

61. Kaplan J.H. 2002. Biochemistry of Na,K-ATPase. *Annu. Rev. Physiol.* **71:** 511–535.

62. Chow, D.C. & J.G. Forte. 1995. Functional significance of the beta-subunit for heterodimeric P-type ATPases. *J. Exp. Biol.* **198:** 1–17.

63. Therien, A.G. & R. Blostein. 2000. Mechanisms of sodium pump regulation. *Am. J. Physiol. Cell Physiol.* **279:** 541–566.

64. Lingrel J.B., M.L. Croyle, A.L. Woo & J.M. Arguello. 1998. Ligand binding sites of Na,K-ATPase. *Acta Physiol. Scand.* **643:** 69–77.

65. Cantiello H.F. 1995. Actin filaments stimulate the Na(+)-K(+)-ATPase. *Am. J. Physiol.* **269:** 637–643.

66. Bertorello, A.M., A. Aperia, S.I. Walaas, *et al.* 1991. Phosphorylation of the catalytic subunit of Na+,K(+)-ATPase inhibits the activity of the enzyme. *Proc. Natl. Acad. Sci. USA* **88:** 11359–11362.

67. Middleton, J.P., W.A. Khan, G. Collinsworth, *et al.* 1993. Heterogeneity of protein kinase C-mediated rapid regulation of Na/K-ATPase in kidney epithelial cells. *J. Biol. Chem.* **268:** 15958–15964.

68. Chibalin, A.V., G. Ogimoto, C.H. Pedemonte, *et al.* 1999. Dopamine-induced endocytosis of Na+,K+-ATPase is initiated by phosphorylation of Ser-18 in the rat alpha subunit and Is responsible for the decreased activity in epithelial cells. *J. Biol. Chem.* **274:** 1920–1927.

69. Mobasheri, A., J. Ávila, I. Cózar-Castellano, *et al.* 2000. Na+, K+-ATPase isozyme diversity; comparative biochemistry and physiological implications of novel functional interactions. *Biosci. Rep.* **20:** 51–91.

70. Mercer, R.W., D. Biemesderfer, D.P. Bliss, Jr., *et al.* 1993. Molecular cloning and immunological characterization of the gamma polypeptide, a small protein associated with the Na,K-ATPase. *J. Cell Biol.* **121:** 579–586.

71. Béguin, P., X. Wang, D. Firsov, *et al.* 1997. The gamma subunit is a specific component of the Na,K-ATPase and modulates its transport function. *EMBO. J.* **16:** 4250–4260.

72. Forbush, B., 3rd, J.H. Kaplan & J.F. Hoffman. 1978. Characterization of a new photoaffinity derivative of ouabain: labeling of the large polypeptide and of a proteolipid component of the Na, K-ATPase. *Biochemistry* **17:** 3667–3676.

73. Fontes, C.F.L., F.E.V. Lopes, H.M. Scofano, *et al.* 1999. Stimulation of ouabain binding to Na,K-ATPase in 40% dimethyl sulfoxide by a factor from Na,K-ATPase preparations. *Arch. Biochem. Biophys.* **366:** 215–223.

74. Erdmann, E., K. Werdan & L. Brown. 1984. Evidence for two kinetically and functionally different types of cardiac glycoside receptors in the heart. *Eur. Heart. J.* **5:** 297–302.

75. Sweadner, K.J. 1985. Enzymatic properties of separated isozymes of the Na,K-ATPase. Substrate affinities, kinetic cooperativity, and ion transport stoichiometry. *J. Biol. Chem.* **260:** 11508–11513.

76. Spach, C. & A. Aschkenasy. 1973. Na and K levels and ATP-ase activity in lymph node, spleen and blood lymphocytes as compared with thymocytes in the male rat. *J. Physiol.* **66:** 585–592.

77. Rodrigues Mascarenhas, S., J. Echevarria-Lima, N.F. dos Santos & V.M. Rumjanek. 2003. CD69 expression induced by thapsigargin, phorbol ester and ouabain on thymocytes is dependent on external Ca2+ entry. *Life Sci.* **73:** 1037–1051.

78. Echevarria-Lima, J., E.G. de Araújo, L. de Meis & V.M. Rumjanek. 2003. Ca2+ mobilization induced by ouabain in thymocytes involves intracellular and extracellular Ca2+ pools. *Hypertension* **41:** 1386–1392.

79. Mann, C.L., C.D. Bortner, C.M. Jewel & J.A. Cidlowski. 2001. Glucocorticoid-induced plasma membrane depolarization during thymocyte apoptosis: association with cell shrinkage and degradation of the Na(+)/K(+)-adenosine triphosphatase. *Endocrinology* **142:** 5059–5068.

80. Wilson, H.A. & T.M. Chused. 1985. Lymphocyte membrane potential and Ca2+-sensitive potassium channels described by oxonol dye fluorescence measurements. *J. Cell. Physiol.* **125:** 72–81.

81. Rodrigues-Mascarenhas, S., N.F. dos Santos & V.M. Rumjanek. 2006. Synergistic effect between ouabain and glucocorticoids for the induction of thymic atrophy. *Biosci. Rep.* **26:** 159–169.

82. Segel, G.B. & M.A. Lichtman. 1980. The apparent discrepancy of ouabain inhibition of cation transport and of lymphocyte proliferation is explained by

time-dependency of ouabain binding. *J. Cell. Physiol.* **104:** 21–26.

83. Saunders, R. & G. Scheiner-Bobis. 2004. Ouabain stimulates endothelin release and expression in human endothelial cells without inhibiting the sodium pump. *Eur. J. Biochem.* **271:** 1054–1062.

84. Zhu, Z., M. Tepel, M. Neusser & W. Zidek. 1996. Low concentrations of ouabain increase cytosolic free calcium concentration in rat vascular smooth muscle cells. *Clin. Sci.* **90:** 9–12.

85. Xie, Z. & A. Askari. 2002. Na(+)/K(+)-ATPase as a signal transducer. *Eur. J. Biochem.* **269:** 2434–2439.

86. Kometiani, P., J. Li, L. Gnudi, *et al.* 1998. Multiple signal transduction pathways link Na$^+$/K$^+$ATPase to growth-related genes in cardiac myocytes—The roles of Ras and mitogen-activated protein kinases. *J. Biol. Chem.* **273:** 15249–15256.

87. Haas, M., A. Askari & Z. Xie. 2000. Involvement of Src and epidermal growth factor receptor in the signal-transducing function of Na$^+$/K$^+$-ATPase. *J. Biol. Chem.* **275:** 27832–27837.

88. Mohammadi, K., P. Kometiani, Z. Xie & A. Askari. 2001. Role of protein kinase C in the signal pathways that link Na$^+$/K$^+$-ATPase to ERK1/2. *J. Biol. Chem.* **276:** 42050–42056.

89. Wu, C.C., S.C. Hsu, H.M. Shih & M.Z. Lai. 2003. Nuclear factor of activated T cells c is a target of p38 mitogen-activated protein kinase in T cells. *Mol. Cell Biol.* **23:** 6442–6454.

90. Jinlian, L., Z. Yingbin and W. Chunbo. 2007. p38 MAPK in regulating cellular responses to ultraviolet radiation. *J. Biomed. Sci.* **14:** 303–312.

91. Raingeaud, J., S. Gupta, J. Roger, *et al.* 1995. Pro-inflammatory cytokines and environmental stress cause p38 MAP kinase activation by dual phosphorylation on tyrosine and threonine. *J. Biol. Chem.* **270:** 7420–7426.

92. Lasa, M., S.M. Abraham, C. Boucheron, *et al.* 2002. Dexamethasone causes sustained expression of mitogen-activated protein kinase (MAPK) phosphatase 1 and phosphatase-mediated inhibition of MAPK p38. *Mol. Cell Biol.* **22:** 7802–7811.

Nutrition, Inflammation, and Cognitive Function

Julia Wärnberg,[a,b] **Sonia Gomez-Martinez,**[a] **Javier Romeo,**[a]
Ligia-Esperanza Díaz,[a] **and Ascensión Marcos**[a]

[a]*Immunonutrition Research Group, Department of Nutrition and Metabolism,
Institute of Food Science, Technology and Nutrition (ICTAN), Instituto del Frio,
Spanish National Research Council (CSIC), Madrid, Spain*

[b]*Unit for Preventive Nutrition, Department of Biosciences and Nutrition, Karolinska
Institutet, Stockholm, Sweden*

Inflammation, particularly low-grade chronic inflammation, appears to affect several brain functions, from early brain development to the development of neurodegenerative disorders and perhaps some psychiatric diseases. On the other hand, nutrition and dietary components and patterns have a plethora of anti- and pro-inflammatory effects that could be linked to cognitive function. Even a modest effect of nutrition on cognitive decline could have significant implications for public health. This paper summarizes the available evidence regarding inflammation as a key mechanism in cognitive function and nutritional pro- or anti-inflammatory effects with the purpose of linking the apparent disparate disciplines of nutrition, immunity, and neurology.

Key words: low-grade chronic inflammation; C-reactive protein; cytokines; neurodegenerative disorders; dementia; anti-inflammatory diet; polyunsaturated fatty acids; antioxidants; phytochemicals; Mediterranean diet

Introduction

Inflammation is a key function in the process by which the body responds to an injury or an infection. It limits the survival and proliferation of invading pathogens; promotes tissue survival, repair, and recovery; and is generally beneficial to the organism. Pro-inflammatory pathways are highly regulated by an extensive array of anti-inflammatory processes, and the acute phase of inflammation normally results in recovery from infection and to healing and a return to normal values within a few days. However, if the response is not properly controlled, the process can persist and lead to a state of chronic low-grade inflammation. This is detrimental and may trigger the development of several diseases. Prospective studies have shown that chronic low-grade inflammation may contribute to the pathogenesis of diseases, such as atherosclerosis,[1–3] type I and type II diabetes,[4] autoimmune diseases,[5] cancer,[6] and those that will be the focus of this review—several types of neurodegenerative disorders.[7–12]

C-reactive protein (CRP) concentrations are easily, accurately, and fairly inexpensively measured in blood. CRP is an acute-phase reactant and a very sensitive marker of inflammation. High CRP levels have no specificity in differentiating disease entities from one another, but despite its lack of specificity, CRP has now emerged as one of the most powerful predictors of cardiovascular risk.[1,3,13] In a direct comparison of a panel of inflammatory and lipid markers in their ability to predict cardiovascular events in adults, CRP surpassed other classical risk markers, including low-density lipoprotein cholesterol.[14,15] The American Heart Association and the Center for Disease Control and Prevention in the United States issued a joint statement confirming

Address for correspondence: Julia Wärnberg, Grupo Inmunonutricion, Dpto. Metabolismo y Nutricion, ICTAN, Instituto del Frio, CSIC, Calle José Antonio Novais, 10. 28040 Madrid, Spain. julia.warnberg@immunonutrition.info

Neuroimmunomodulation: Ann. N.Y. Acad. Sci. 1153: 164–175 (2009).
doi: 10.1111/j.1749-6632.2008.03985.x © 2009 New York Academy of Sciences.

that CRP is the best and most clinically useful of the markers of inflammation currently available, with the following cutoff points for assessing cardiovascular disease risk: low risk (CRP < 1.0 mg/L), average risk (1.0–3.0 mg/L), and high risk (>3.0 mg/L).[13] There is now great interest in elucidating how dietary and lifestyle factors can modulate inflammation. A wide range of anti-inflammatory dietary and lifestyle remedies are being suggested, while scientific publications are quickly responding to the demand for evidence to support these recommendations.

Much evidence also supports the concept that lifestyle factors, such as diet and exercise, can improve learning and memory, delay age-related cognitive decline, reduce the risk of neurodegeneration, and play a part in alleviating psychiatric diseases, such as depression. Corroborative evidence on the association between low-grade inflammation and cognitive decline has also accumulated from a series of epidemiological studies, supporting the assumption that higher CRP levels either directly or indirectly promote cognitive attrition.[7–12,16]

Our hypothesis is that healthy diets have a dual effect on both reducing inflammation and meliorating neurodegenerative disorders. This paper reviews the evidence for inflammation as the key mechanism in cognitive function and dietary approaches that are anti-inflammatory, with the purpose of unifying the disciplines of nutrition, immunity, and neurology.

Diet and Inflammation

It is evident that macronutrients and micronutrients in the diet are essential for maintaining the function of immune cells. Nutrient deficiencies adversely affect the immune system. Conversely, one could speculate that a dietary pattern rich in nutrients with favorable anti-inflammatory properties and poor in proinflammatory nutrients may protect against inflammatory chronic diseases and, of special interest for this review, neurodegenerative disorders.

The beneficial effects of polyunsaturated omega-3 fatty acids (omega-3 PUFAs) intake on human health, especially on cardiovascular disease, are well established.[17,18] At sufficiently high intakes, long-chain omega-3 PUFAs decrease the production of inflammatory eicosanoids, cytokines, reactive oxygen species, and the expression of adhesion molecules.[19] Eicosapentaenoic acid (EPA; 20:5) and docosahexaenoic acid (DHA; 22:6) are found in oily fish and fish oils, and alpha-linolenic acid, the precursor of EPA and DHA of plant origin, is principally found in walnuts. EPA and DHA act both directly [e.g., by replacing arachidonic acid (AA; 20:4, omega-6) as an eicosanoid substrate and inhibiting AA metabolism] and indirectly (e.g., by altering the expression of inflammatory genes through effects on transcription factor activation). They also give rise to a family of anti-inflammatory mediators termed *resolvins*. Thus, omega-3 PUFAs are potentially potent anti-inflammatory agents. As such, they may be of therapeutic use in a variety of acute and chronic inflammatory settings.

While inflammatory cells produce reactive oxygen species, oxidative stress *per se* may have pro-inflammatory effects.[20] Specific antioxidant nutrients, which act mechanistically to decrease levels of hydrogen peroxide and lipid peroxides, may play an important role in suppressing inflammation.[21] Many potent dietary antioxidants occur in plant fruiting bodies, seeds, or roots and contain one or more phenol groups that contribute to potent antioxidant activities presumably selected to protect the plant germ line. Grapes, apples, many types of berries, pomegranates, green tea, and many other plant sources are rich in these antioxidant compounds that often have potent antioxidant and anti-inflammatory properties and related health benefits.[22] Although studies are limited in number, the available evidence strongly indicates that a high consumption of vegetables and fruits or a diet rich in antioxidants, serum carotenoids, vitamins, fiber, and magnesium are beneficial in terms of reducing inflammation and in particular CRP levels.[21,23–25]

Dietary Patterns and Lifestyle

More important than single nutrients or any specific phytochemicals are the foods that are eaten and the dietary and lifestyle pattern as a whole. Obesity is undoubtedly related to low-grade chronic inflammation,[4] even at early ages.[26,27] Adipocytes and monocyte-derived macrophages in adipose tissue secrete pro-inflammatory cytokines, such as interleukin (IL)-6 and tumor necrosis factor-alpha (TNF-α), and these in turn induce hepatic synthesis of acute-phase proteins, such as CRP.[4] Smoking is also related to increased levels of inflammation[28]; this positive association may be a reflection of underlying atherosclerotic lesions or from systemic or nonvascular local inflammation. Low-grade inflammation is also noted in the presence of the metabolic syndrome, which is a constellation of metabolic abnormalities, such as glucose intolerance, hypertriglyceridemia, and hypertension, that increase the risk of cardiovascular disease as well as type II diabetes, with central obesity as a core component.[4] It is alarming to note that inflammation and features of the metabolic syndrome are already present in childhood, suggesting that the development of inflammation-related chronic diseases is occurring faster than ever.[29] Although further studies are needed to determine the relationship of physical activity to low-grade inflammation, it is hypothesized that some of the benefits of regular physical activity are from its anti-inflammatory effects.[30] It is obviously necessary to take all these factors into consideration when investigating the relation to disease risk as well as dietary determinants of low-grade inflammation. The imbalance that results from obesity and other features of the metabolic syndrome, smoking, and physical inactivity together with an unhealthy dietary pattern may favor the creation of a pro-inflammatory milieu, which could promote disease development or progression.

Western dietary patterns are characterized as high in refined starches, sugar, and saturated and trans-fatty acids and poor in natural antioxidants and fiber from fruits, vegetables, and whole grains. This Western dietary pattern has been found to be positively associated with pro-inflammatory markers of oxidative stress.[31,32] Furthermore, the modern eating patterns of Western societies generate an almost continuous postprandial phase that could be accompanied by a possible chronic activation of the innate immune system throughout most of the day.[33]

A prudent dietary pattern would be one that satisfies several if not all strategies for reducing inflammation and oxidative stress, that is a lifestyle characterized by no tobacco use, moderate physical activity, and a higher intake of fruits, vegetables, legumes, whole grains, olive oil, and fish. One such healthy dietary pattern is the Mediterranean diet, which has been associated with a lower risk of several forms of cancer, obesity, dyslipidemia, hypertension, diabetes, coronary heart disease, and overall mortality.[34-39] As expected, observational studies have shown reduced levels of inflammatory markers in adults adhering to the Mediterranean diet in comparison to those following a Western dietary pattern.[40-42] The effects of the Mediterranean diet may be the composite effect of the dietary antioxidants, such as complex phenols, and many other substances with important antioxidant properties, such as olive oil, wine, fruits and vegetables, vitamins C and E, and carotenoids, that are found in high concentrations in this dietary pattern.[43]

Nutrition and Brain Function

As with any other organ, the brain needs nutrients to build and maintain its structure, both to function harmoniously and to be protected from diseases or premature aging. However, for many years it was not fully accepted that food can have an influence on brain structure and thus on its functions, including cognitive, intellectual, and mental. Most micronutrients (vitamins, minerals, essential amino acids, and essential fatty acids, including omega-3 PUFAs) have been directly evaluated with regard to cerebral functioning.[44,45] In fact, the full genetic potential of the child for physical growth and mental development may be compromised in the presence of dietary deficiencies (even subclinical). Children and adolescents with poor nutritional status are prone to alterations of mental and behavioral functions that can, to a certain extent, be corrected by dietary measures. Indeed, nutrient composition and meal pattern can exert either immediate or long-term effects, beneficial or adverse.[44–46]

Long-chain omega-3 PUFAs, in particular, have been associated with the integrity of the central nervous system (CNS) and are essential for neurocognitive development and normal brain functioning. Because of the cellular composition of the brain, the lipid content is high (60%), and long-chain PUFAs are especially essential in the formation of new tissue, including neurons and glial cells. Long-chain PUFAs are also involved in axonal myelination and are key components in synaptic function where they serve as secondary messengers.[47] DHA is hypothesized to be particularly important for brain function because it maintains an optimal state of neural membranes, ensuring membrane fluidity and thickness that in turn affects cell signaling.[47] Omega-3 PUFAs also affect neurotransmitter actions, particularly the dopaminergic systems of the frontal lobes.[48] Thus appropriate prenatal and postnatal supplies of these long-chain PUFAs seem to be essential for normal fetal and neonatal growth, neurological development, and functional maturation, including learning and behavior.[46,49] Several studies have shown a positive correlation between breast feeding and cognitive development and several functional neurological outcomes, including improved attention spans and mental processing in children. One explanation for these results is that breast milk provides nutrients required for development of the brain, particularly DHA.[50] As long-chain omega-3 PUFAs are also protective against vascular disease, one of the major causes of age-related dementia, it is interesting to note that childhood IQ seems to be related to

cardiovascular events, heart disease and stroke events during adulthood and up to the age of 65.[51]

Inflammation and Brain Function

For many years the brain was regarded as an "immune-privileged" organ, which was not susceptible to inflammation or immune activation and was thought to be largely unaffected by systemic inflammatory and immune responses. This view has now been revised significantly. The rapidly expanding area of research known as neuroimmunomodulation explores the way in which the nervous system interacts with the immune system via neural, hormonal, and paracrine actions.

It has long been known that multiple sclerosis is an inflammatory disease of the brain, but it is only in recent years that it has been suggested that inflammation may significantly contribute to diseases, such as stroke, traumatic brain injury, HIV-related dementia, Alzheimer's disease (AD), and prion disease.[52] Inflammation in the brain and its contribution to CNS injury is a relatively new area of research and clinical interest but is now the focus of extensive investigation, and several excellent reviews have been published in recent years.[9,52] It is now clear that the brain does respond to peripheral inflammatory stimuli (through neural and humoral afferent signals), it integrates and regulates many aspects of the acute-phase response, and it exhibits many local inflammatory responses. However, this does not necessarily indicate a causal role, and it is important to investigate the functional consequences of increased systemic inflammatory markers in the CNS.

Inflammation is present in diverse acute and chronic disorders of the CNS. Acute neurodegenerative conditions, such as cerebral ischemia (e.g., stroke) and traumatic brain injury, are characterized by rapid and (usually) severe insults to the brain that lead to a substantial loss of nerve cells with associated functional deficits.

There are substantial data demonstrating the active involvement of inflammatory processes in these diseases. Chronic CNS diseases have a more complex etiology than acute injuries and are generally multifactorial, with environmental factors and genetic background contributing to the development and progression of the disease.[9,52–54] All these factors also contribute to CNS inflammation, which is further exacerbated by aging.

CRP has been shown to be directly neurotoxic.[55] Neurons can generate CRP and other pentraxins, which will promote induction of neuronal pro-apoptotic pathways and play a role in neurodegenerative disorders.[56–58] In addition to the pro-inflammatory response that may cause direct neuronal damage, raised CRP concentrations indirectly, by acting as a cardiovascular risk factor causing cerebral atherosclerosis, may result in cerebral macro-angiopathy (i.e., large observable stroke) or cerebral micro-angiopathy (i.e., leukoaraiosis). Both types of lesions disrupt the integrity of frontal-subcortical circuits and are responsible for the development of cognitive impairment, dementia, and probably also depressive disorders.[59–61] Among other markers of chronic inflammation, specific cytokines (most notably IL-1β but also IL-6 and TNF-α), α1 antichymotrypsin, or white blood cell counts have been implicated in acute neurodegeneration, such as head injury and stroke,[52,62] and have been associated with dementia and depression.[63,64]

Cognitive Decline and Dementia

Inflammation has been found to play a key role in different types of dementia, especially of the AD type. AD is characterized by the progressive inability to form new memories and access existing ones as a result of neuronal cell death in the hippocampus and frontal cortex. CNS inflammation in AD and similarly in vascular dementia is characterized by reactive microglia and elevated IL-1β and complement factors as well as CRP, IL-6, and TNF-α.[8,16,53,56,65]

"Normal" aging accompanies chronic low-grade inflammation as well as many behavioral changes do, including both motor and cognitive declines. This could support the hypothesis that higher inflammatory markers are associated with greater atrophy than expected for age.[66,67] There is a growing body of literature assessing the associations between CRP and cognitive performance. The occurrence of elevated systemic inflammatory markers in patients in comparison to healthy peers suggests that inflammation at least participates in the amplification of the disease state. A meta-analysis of six studies examining CRP and cognition concluded that higher levels of CRP were predictive of cognitive decline and dementia.[9]

Growing evidence also implicates oxidative damage in the pathogenesis of AD, with neurons at risk for AD degeneration having increased lipid peroxidation, nitration, free carbonyls, and nucleic acid oxidation.[68] Both oxidative damage and inflammation begin early in AD, accompanying amyloid accumulation and neurodegeneration, and it has been suggested that increased plasma levels of inflammatory proteins are present before the clinical onset of dementia, AD, and vascular dementia.[63,69]

If increases in sensitivity to oxidative stress and inflammation in the aged brain lead to motor and cognitive deficits and under certain circumstances can lead to alterations in brain morphology and cognitive diseases, such as AD, the problem becomes one of reducing the vulnerability of the brain to these processes. One approach to preventing or reversing these would be through improved nutrition.

Dietary Prevention of Cognitive Decline

Of interest when proposing the possible role of anti-inflammatory components in the diet for the prevention of AD is the fact that the risk of developing AD is reduced by antioxidants[70,71] and by nonsteroidal anti-inflammatory drugs.[16,72] In epidemiological studies of human populations and experiments in animal models of neurodegenerative disorders, the plethora of natural antioxidants found in plant food matrices possess neuroprotective as well as cardioprotective and chemoprotective properties.[73–78] Many articles have been published reporting the neuroprotective effects of fruits (especially berry fruits), vegetables, and grains, which are rich sources of antioxidant compounds and phytochemicals, including α-tocopherol, vitamin E, selenium, lycopene, resveratrol, bilobalide, and ginsenosides.[75,76,79]

The neuroprotective effects of various phytochemicals are most probably from their ability to reduce oxidative stress levels. Notable among these are resveratrol from red wine, the green tea catechins, and the turmeric extract curcumin, which have been intensively studied for their potential to prevent or treat disease and are worthy of consideration in relation to AD.[80]

Neurons and synapses are highly enriched in long-chain PUFAs, the most vulnerable of these being DHA. Because DHA is heavily concentrated in neurons, its oxidation products are a good index of neuronal oxidative damage. Based on the observation that low serum levels of DHA could be a risk factor for AD and that PUFAs protect neurons directly by preventing neuronal apoptosis and suppressing the production of neurotoxic TNF, a large number of studies have demonstrated that these fatty acids might be beneficial in AD and other dementias.[81–85] It is also known that long-chain PUFAs are protective against vascular disease, one of the other major causes of age-related dementia, which suggests that supplementation of these fatty acids is a potential primary prevention measure. Of special interest is a study suggesting that AA and DHA supplementation can improve the cognitive dysfunction that is caused by organic brain damage or aging (not AD).[86]

Greater adherence to the Mediterranean diet has been associated with a lower risk of developing AD and with reducing mortality in AD.[87,88] The Mediterranean diet is a composite of dietary antioxidant and dietary anti-inflammatory compounds, and this could, at least partially, explain the association with these outcomes. Another possible mechanism is that the Mediterranean diet may be exerting its protective effect against AD through cardiovascular–cerebrovascular mechanisms and hence lower disease risk.[89]

It is important to note that it is not only dietary changes that may be important in reducing risk and consequences of disease. Avoiding chronic stress situations and increasing physical activity and exercise (including mental exercise) are also important and can modify the course of cognitive decline and delay mortality.[90–93]

The Metabolic Syndrome, Diabetes, and Obesity

Of the various aspects of the metabolic syndrome (including abdominal obesity, hypertension, hyperglycemia, insulin insensitivity, and dyslipidemia), those most likely to adversely affect cognitive function seem to be hypertension and glucose intolerance.[94] A common feature of many of these conditions is systemic inflammation, which contributes to most, if not all, of the conditions of the metabolic syndrome. Several lines of mechanistic evidence implicate insulin and glucose metabolism in the risk of developing dementia, including AD. One of the mechanisms might be that inflammation promotes atherothrombosis and attenuates nitric oxide production, thereby inhibiting angiogenesis.[3] This has important implications given that the frontal lobes have less collateral circulation than the rest of the brain and therefore would be more susceptible to microvascular disease. Vascular dementia and hypertension are two conditions associated with frontal lobe dysfunction.[95–97] Data examining the association between CRP and stroke, although available, are relatively sparse in comparison with coronary heart disease or combined vascular events. A systematic review assessing the association between CRP and stroke, cognitive disorders, and depression[9] concluded that high concentrations of CRP are associated with increased risk of stroke and cognitive impairment. In this context, the ability of specific CRP-lowering aspects of lifestyle changes, such as diet and exercise, to synergistically modulate cardiovascular disease risk and cognitive impairment is becoming increasingly recognized.

The cognitive problems associated with diabetes have been traditionally assumed to be a result of atherosclerosis. There are, however, many mechanisms through which diabetes could increase the risk of dementia, including glycemia, insulin resistance, oxidative stress, advanced glycation end products, inflammatory cytokines, and microvascular and macrovascular disease.[98,99] Given the high vulnerability of the hippocampus, low-grade metabolic insults may, in the long run, lead to damage and volume loss, especially in the presence of elevated cortisol levels. The fact that juvenile diabetics have cognitive deficits, even after accounting for hypoglycemic episodes and years of diabetes prior to any evidence of cardiovascular disease,[100] suggests that diabetes itself may have a direct role in contributing to memory impairments. Furthermore, prospective studies of diabetics have demonstrated that improvements in glucose tolerance were associated with cognitive improvements.[101] Interestingly, there is now an expanding body of literature linking cognitive deficits with obesity, independent of the other metabolic dysregulations previously mentioned,[102–106] although not all studies confirm these results.[107]

Psychiatric Disorders and Personal Traits

More recently some psychiatric disorders, such as depression and anxiety, have been added to the list of diseases that have inflammation as a possible factor in disease development, progression, and/or prevention.[108–115] It is accepted that the brain coordinates and regulates many aspects of the host defense response, which may begin to explain the behavioral responses to disease, such as fatigue and depression, and how psychological states can influence susceptibility to disease and subsequent recovery.[52] It has even been proposed that pro-inflammatory cytokines might cause depressive illness.[82,116] Nevertheless, we should bear in mind that the relationships are not consistent across all existing population-based cross-sectional studies and a causal process cannot be concluded.[9] Interestingly, antipsychotic drugs have long been known to be immunomodulatory, targeting cytokine networks, and raising the possibility of an alternative mechanistic explanation for the actions of these agents.[52,108]

Dietary supplementation with DHA and EPA has long been used for the treatment or amelioration of several psychiatric disorders.[82,117,118] The potential mechanism behind this is the restoration of plasma concentrations of PUFAs in postpartum-depressed patients to the levels of healthy controls.[119,120] Nevertheless, only a few large studies have reported an inverse relationship between dietary omega-3 PUFAs or fish intake and depression or personality traits, such as anxiety or hostility[121–124] (with stronger associations seen among women), while other studies have not shown any significant differences.[125,126] There is a need for further large longitudinal studies that include both men and women to assess the potential protective role of fish and omega-3 consumption against depression.

Summary

Epidemiological evidence indicates that increased inflammation, and in particular CRP concentrations, are associated with neurodegenerative disorders and perhaps also some psychiatric diseases as well as indices of metabolic and cardiovascular health. Nevertheless, proof of causality can only be established by showing that lowering inflammatory markers can prevent these problems. Although a healthy dietary pattern significantly correlates with lower CRP concentrations, the question of whether a direct CRP-lowering effect from such preventive measures can prevent stroke, cognitive decline, or depression can only be answered if the study is multidisciplinary in design. The apparent convergence of the disciplines of nutrition, inflammation, and neurology/psychology urgently show the need for greater research collaboration and cross-disciplinary exchange of ideas if we are to understand the common mechanisms underlying many diseases as well as to propose methods for their prevention or treatment. Prospective, cross-disciplinary, controlled trials are needed to fully understand how dietary prescription can be used as an effective tool to prevent, halt the progression of, or even reverse, inflammatory neurogenerative disorders.

Conflicts of Interest

The authors declare no conflicts of interest.

References

1. Hansson, G.K. 2001. Regulation of immune mechanisms in atherosclerosis. *Ann. N. Y. Acad. Sci.* **947:** 157–165; discussion 165–156.
2. Libby, P. 2006. Inflammation and cardiovascular disease mechanisms. *Am. J. Clin. Nutr.* **83:** 456S-460S.
3. Hansson, G.K. 2005. Inflammation, atherosclerosis, and coronary artery disease. *N. Engl. J. Med.* **352:** 1685–1695.
4. Hotamisligil, G.S. 2006. Inflammation and metabolic disorders. *Nature* **444:** 860–867.
5. Vogt, B. *et al.* 2007. CRP and the disposal of dying cells: consequences for systemic lupus erythematosus and rheumatoid arthritis. *Autoimmunity* **40:** 295–298.
6. de Visser, K.E., A. Eichten & L.M. Coussens. 2006. Paradoxical roles of the immune system during cancer development. *Nat. Rev. Cancer* **6:** 24–37.
7. Teunissen, C.E. *et al.* 2003. Inflammation markers in relation to cognition in a healthy aging population. *J. Neuroimmunol.* **134:** 142–150.
8. Britschgi, M. & T. Wyss-Coray. 2007. Immune cells may fend off Alzheimer disease. *Nat. Med.* **13:** 408–409.
9. Kuo, H.K. *et al.* 2005. Relation of C-reactive protein to stroke, cognitive disorders, and depression in the general population: systematic review and meta-analysis. *Lancet Neurol.* **4:** 371–380.
10. Gunstad, J. *et al.* 2006. C-reactive protein, but not homocysteine, is related to cognitive dysfunction in older adults with cardiovascular disease. *J. Clin. Neurosci.* **13:** 540–546.
11. Dimopoulos, N. *et al.* 2006. Indices of low-grade chronic inflammation correlate with early cognitive deterioration in an elderly Greek population. *Neurosci. Lett.* **398:** 118–123.
12. Ravaglia, G. *et al.* 2005. Serum C-reactive protein and cognitive function in healthy elderly Italian community dwellers. *J. Gerontol. A Biol. Sci. Med. Sci.* **60:** 1017–1021.
13. Pearson, T.A. *et al.* 2003. Markers of inflammation and cardiovascular disease: application to clinical and public health practice: a statement for healthcare professionals from the Centers for Disease Control and Prevention and the American Heart Association. *Circulation* **107:** 499–511.
14. Ridker, P.M. *et al.* 2003. C-reactive protein, the metabolic syndrome, and risk of incident cardiovascular events: an 8-year follow-up of 14 719 initially healthy American women. *Circulation* **107:** 391–397.
15. Ridker, P.M., M.J. Stampfer & N. Rifai. 2001. Novel risk factors for systemic atherosclerosis: a comparison of C-reactive protein, fibrinogen, homocysteine, lipoprotein(a), and standard cholesterol screening as predictors of peripheral arterial disease. *JAMA* **285:** 2481–2485.
16. Pratico, D. & J. Trojanowski. 2000. Inflammatory hypotheses: novel mechanisms of Alzheimer's neurodegeneration and new therapeutic targets? *Neurobiol. Aging* **21:** 441–445.
17. Din, J.N., D.E. Newby & A.D. Flapan. 2004. Omega 3 fatty acids and cardiovascular disease – fishing for a natural treatment. *BMJ* **328:** 30–35.
18. Kris-Etherton, P.M. *et al.* 2003. Fish consumption, fish oil, omega-3 fatty acids, and cardiovascular disease. *Arterioscler. Thromb. Vasc. Biol.* **23:** e20–30.
19. Calder, P.C. 2006. n-3 polyunsaturated fatty acids, inflammation, and inflammatory diseases. *Am. J. Clin. Nutr.* **83:** S1505–S1519.
20. Abramson, J.L. *et al.* 2005. Association between novel oxidative stress markers and C-reactive protein among adults without clinical coronary heart disease. *Atherosclerosis* **178:** 115–121.
21. Hughes, D.A. 2000. Dietary antioxidants and human immune function. *Nutr. Bull.* **25:** 35–41.
22. Maron, D.J. 2004. Flavonoids for reduction of atherosclerotic risk. *Curr. Atheroscler. Rep.* **6:** 73–78.

23. van Herpen-Broekmans, W.M. *et al.* 2004. Serum carotenoids and vitamins in relation to markers of endothelial function and inflammation. *Eur. J. Epidemiol.* **19:** 915–921.

24. Brighenti, F. *et al.* 2005. Total antioxidant capacity of the diet is inversely and independently related to plasma concentration of high-sensitivity C-reactive protein in adult Italian subjects. *Br. J. Nutr.* **93:** 619–625.

25. Ajani, U.A., E.S. Ford & A.H. Mokdad. 2004. Dietary fiber and C-reactive protein: findings from national health and nutrition examination survey data. *J. Nutr.* **134:** 1181–1185.

26. Wärnberg, J. *et al.* 2006. Inflammatory proteins are related to total and abdominal adiposity in a healthy adolescent population: the AVENA Study. *Am. J. Clin. Nutr.* **84:** 505–512.

27. Wärnberg, J. *et al.* 2007. Lifestyle-related determinants of inflammation in adolescence. *Br. J. Nutr.* **98:** S116–120.

28. Bazzano, L.A. *et al.* 2003. Relationship between cigarette smoking and novel risk factors for cardiovascular disease in the United States. *Ann. Intern. Med.* **138:** 891–897.

29. Wärnberg, J. & A. Marcos. 2008. Low-grade inflammation and the metabolic syndrome in children and adolescents. *Curr. Opin. Lipidol.* **19:** 11–15.

30. Petersen, A.M. & B.K. Pedersen. 2005. The anti-inflammatory effect of exercise. *J. Appl. Physiol.* **98:** 1154–1162.

31. Lopez-Garcia, E. *et al.* 2004. Major dietary patterns are related to plasma concentrations of markers of inflammation and endothelial dysfunction. *Am. J. Clin. Nutr.* **80:** 1029–1035.

32. Schulze, M.B. *et al.* 2005. Dietary pattern, inflammation, and incidence of type 2 diabetes in women. *Am. J. Clin. Nutr.* **82:** 675–684.

33. Giugliano, D., A. Ceriello & K. Esposito. 2006. The effects of diet on inflammation: emphasis on the metabolic syndrome. *J. Am. Coll. Cardiol.* **48:** 677–685.

34. Trichopoulou, A. *et al.* 2003. Adherence to a Mediterranean diet and survival in a Greek population. *N. Engl. J. Med.* **348:** 2599–2608.

35. Trichopoulou, A. *et al.* 2000. Cancer and Mediterranean dietary traditions. *Cancer Epidemiol. Biomarkers Prev.* **9:** 869–873.

36. Trichopoulou, A. *et al.* 2005. Modified Mediterranean diet and survival: EPIC-elderly prospective cohort study. *BMJ* **330:** 991.

37. Alonso, A. & M.A. Martinez-Gonzalez. 2005. Mediterranean diet, lifestyle factors, and mortality. *JAMA* **293:** 674.

38. Martinez-Gonzalez, M.A. *et al.* 2008. Mediterranean Diet Inversely Associated With the Incidence of Metabolic Syndrome: the SUN Prospective Cohort: Response to Giugliano, Ceriello, and Esposito. *Diabetes Care* **31:** e37.

39. Martinez-Gonzalez, M.A. *et al.* 2008. Adherence to Mediterranean diet and risk of developing diabetes: prospective cohort study. *BMJ* **336:** 1348–1351.

40. Salas-Salvado, J. *et al.* 2008. Components of the Mediterranean-type food pattern and serum inflammatory markers among patients at high risk for cardiovascular disease. *Eur. J. Clin. Nutr.* **62:** 651–659.

41. Chrysohoou, C. *et al.* 2004. Adherence to the Mediterranean diet attenuates inflammation and coagulation process in healthy adults: The ATTICA Study. *J. Am. Coll. Cardiol.* **44:** 152–158.

42. Esposito, K. *et al.* 2004. Effect of a mediterranean-style diet on endothelial dysfunction and markers of vascular inflammation in the metabolic syndrome: a randomized trial. *JAMA* **292:** 1440–1446.

43. Martinez-Gonzalez, M.A. *et al.* 2003. What is protective in the Mediterranean diet? *Atherosclerosis* **166:** 405–407.

44. Bourre, J.M. 2006. Effects of nutrients (in food) on the structure and function of the nervous system: update on dietary requirements for brain. Part 2: macronutrients. *J. Nutr. Health Aging* **10:** 386–399.

45. Bourre, J.M. 2006. Effects of nutrients (in food) on the structure and function of the nervous system: update on dietary requirements for brain. Part 1: micronutrients. *J. Nutr. Health Aging* **10:** 377–385.

46. Bryan, J. *et al.* 2004. Nutrients for cognitive development in school-aged children. *Nutr. Rev.* **62:** 295–306.

47. Uauy, R., F. Calderon & P. Mena. 2001. Essential fatty acids in somatic growth and brain development. *World Rev. Nutr. Diet.* **89:** 134–160.

48. Wainwright, P. 2000. Nutrition and behaviour: the role of n-3 fatty acids in cognitive function. *Br. J. Nutr.* **83:** 337–339.

49. Birberg-Thornberg, U. *et al.* 2006. Nutrition and theory of mind—The role of polyunsaturated fatty acids (PUFA) in the development of theory of mind. *Prostaglandins Leukot Essent Fatty Acids* **75:** 33–41.

50. Eilander, A. *et al.* 2007. Effects of n-3 long chain polyunsaturated fatty acid supplementation on visual and cognitive development throughout childhood: a review of human studies. *Prostaglandins Leukot Essent Fatty Acids* **76:** 189–203.

51. Hart, C.L. *et al.* 2004. Childhood IQ and cardiovascular disease in adulthood: prospective observational study linking the Scottish Mental Survey 1932 and the Midspan studies. *Soc. Sci. Med.* **59:** 2131–2138.

52. Lucas, S.-M., N.J. Rothwell & R.M. Gibson. 2006. The role of inflammation in CNS injury and disease. *Br. J. Pharmacol.* **147:** S232-S240.

53. McGeer, P.L., K. Yasojima & E.G. McGeer. 2001. Inflammation in Parkinson's disease. *Adv. Neurol.* **86:** 83–89.

54. Campbell, A. 2004. Inflammation, neurodegenerative diseases, and environmental exposures. *Ann. N. Y. Acad. Sci.* 117–132.

55. Duong, T., P.J. Acton & R.A. Johnson. 1998. The in vitro neuronal toxicity of pentraxins associated with Alzheimer's disease brain lesions. *Brain Res.* 303–312.

56. McGeer, P.L., E.G. McGeer & K. Yasojima. 2000. Alzheimer disease and neuroinflammation. *J. Neural. Transm. Suppl.* **59:** 53–57.

57. Yasojima, K. *et al.* 2000. Human neurons generate C-reactive protein and amyloid P: upregulation in Alzheimer's disease. *Brain Res.* **887:** 80–89.

58. Duong, T., M. Nikolaeva & P.J. Acton. 1997. C-reactive protein-like immunoreactivity in the neurofibrillary tangles of Alzheimer's disease. *Brain Res.* **749:** 152–156.

59. Mast, B.T. 2004. Cerebrovascular disease and late-life depression: a latent-variable analysis of depressive symptoms after stroke. *Am. J. Geriatr. Psychiatry* **12:** 315–322.

60. Lowery, K. *et al.* 2002. Cognitive decline in a prospectively studied group of stroke survivors, with a particular emphasis on the >75's. *Age Ageing* **31:** S24–27.

61. Stephens, S. *et al.* 2004. Neuropsychological characteristics of mild vascular cognitive impairment and dementia after stroke. *Int. J. Geriatr. Psychiatry* **19:** 1053–1057.

62. Lindsberg, P.J. & A.J. Grau. 2003. Inflammation and infections as risk factors for ischemic stroke. *Stroke* 2518–2532.

63. Engelhart, M.J. *et al.* 2004. Inflammatory proteins in plasma and the risk of dementia: the rotterdam study. *Arch. Neurol.* **61:** 668–672.

64. Licinio, J. & M.L. Wong. 1999. The role of inflammatory mediators in the biology of major depression: central nervous system cytokines modulate the biological substrate of depressive symptoms, regulate stress-responsive systems, and contribute to neurotoxicity and neuroprotection. *Mol. Psychiatry* **4:** 317–327.

65. Wyss-Coray, T. 2006. Inflammation in Alzheimer disease: driving force, bystander or beneficial response? *Nat. Med.* **12:** 1005–1015.

66. Ahluwalia, N. 2004. Aging, nutrition and immune function. *J. Nutr. Health Aging* **8:** 2–6.

67. Bruunsgaard, H. *et al.* 2003. Elevated levels of tumor necrosis factor alpha and mortality in centenarians. *Am. J. Med.* **115:** 278–283.

68. Pratico, D. 2002. Alzheimer's disease and oxygen radicals: new insights. *Biochem. Pharmacol.* **63:** 563–567.

69. Pappolla, M.A. *et al.* 2002. Cholesterol, oxidative stress, and Alzheimer's disease: expanding the horizons of pathogenesis. *Free Radic. Biol. Med.* **33:** 173–181.

70. Morris, M.C. *et al.* 2002. Dietary intake of antioxidant nutrients and the risk of incident Alzheimer disease in a biracial community study. *JAMA* **287:** 3230–3237.

71. Zandi, P.P. *et al.* 2004. Reduced risk of Alzheimer disease in users of antioxidant vitamin supplements: the Cache County Study. *Arch. Neurol.* **61:** 82–88.

72. in t' Veld, B.A. *et al.* 2001. Nonsteroidal antiinflammatory drugs and the risk of Alzheimer's disease. *N. Engl. J. Med.* **345:** 1515–1521.

73. Bokov, A., A. Chaudhuri & A. Richardson. 2004. The role of oxidative damage and stress in aging. *Mech. Ageing Dev.* **125:** 811–826.

74. Galli, R.L. *et al.* 2002. Fruit polyphenolics and brain aging: nutritional interventions targeting age-related neuronal and behavioral deficits. *Ann. N. Y. Acad. Sci.* **959:** 128–132.

75. Joseph, J.A., B. Shukitt-Hale & G. Casadesus. 2005. Reversing the deleterious effects of aging on neuronal communication and behavior: beneficial properties of fruit polyphenolic compounds. *Am. J. Clin. Nutr.* **81:** 313S–316S.

76. Joseph, J.A., B. Shukitt-Hale & F.C. Lau. 2007. Fruit polyphenols and their effects on neuronal signaling and behavior in senescence. *Ann. N. Y. Acad. Sci.* **1100:** 470–485.

77. Lau, F.C., B. Shukitt-Hale & J.A. Joseph. 2005. The beneficial effects of fruit polyphenols on brain aging. *Neurobiol. Aging* **26**(Suppl 1): 128–132.

78. Liu, R.H. 2003. Health benefits of fruit and vegetables are from additive and synergistic combinations of phytochemicals. *Am. J. Clin. Nutr.* **78:** S517–520.

79. Ikeda, K., H. Negishi & Y. Yamori. 2003. Antioxidant nutrients and hypoxia/ischemia brain injury in rodents. *Toxicology* **189:** 55–61.

80. Mancuso, C. *et al.* 2007. Natural antioxidants in Alzheimer's disease. *Expert Opin. Investig. Drugs* **16:** 1921–1931.

81. Cole, G.M. *et al.* 2005. Prevention of Alzheimer's disease: omega-3 fatty acid and phenolic anti-oxidant interventions. *Neurobiol. Aging* **26:** S133–136.

82. Das, U.N. 2008. Folic acid and polyunsaturated fatty acids improve cognitive function and prevent depression, dementia, and Alzheimer's disease–but

how and why? *Prostaglandins Leukot Essent Fatty Acids* **78:** 11–19.

83. Morris, M.C. 2006. Docosahexaenoic acid and Alzheimer disease. *Arch. Neurol.* **63:** 1527–1528.

84. Morris, M.C. *et al.* 2003. Dietary fats and the risk of incident Alzheimer disease. *Arch. Neurol.* **60:** 194–200.

85. Morris, M.C. *et al.* 2003. Consumption of fish and n-3 fatty acids and risk of incident Alzheimer disease. *Arch. Neurol.* **60:** 940–946.

86. Kotani, S. *et al.* 2006. Dietary supplementation of arachidonic and docosahexaenoic acids improves cognitive dysfunction. *Neurosci. Res.* **56:** 159–164.

87. Scarmeas, N. *et al.* 2007. Mediterranean diet and Alzheimer disease mortality. *Neurology* **69:** 1084–1093.

88. Scarmeas, N. *et al.* 2006. Mediterranean diet and risk for Alzheimer's disease. *Ann. Neurol.* **59:** 912–921.

89. Scarmeas, N. *et al.* 2006. Mediterranean diet, Alzheimer disease, and vascular mediation. *Arch. Neurol.* **63:** 1709–1717.

90. Larson, E. *et al.* 2006. Exercise is associated with reduced risk for incident dementia among persons 65 years of age and older. *Ann. Intern. Med.* **144:** 73–81.

91. Rolland, Y. *et al.* 2007. Exercise program for nursing home residents with Alzheimer's disease: a 1-year randomized, controlled trial. *J. Am. Geriatr. Soc.* **55:** 158–165.

92. Romeo, J. *et al.* 2008. Nutrition, stress and neuroimmunomodulation. *Neuroimmunomodulation* **15**(3): 165–169.

93. Pukay-Martin, N.D. *et al.* 2003. The relationship between stressful life events and cognitive function in HIV-infected men. *J. Neuropsychiatry Clin. Neurosci.* **15:** 436–441.

94. Yaffe, K. *et al.* 2007. Metabolic syndrome and cognitive decline in elderly Latinos: findings from the Sacramento Area Latino Study of Aging study. *J. Am. Geriatr. Soc.* **55:** 758–762.

95. Gold, S.M. *et al.* 2005. Hypertension and hypothalamo-pituitary-adrenal axis hyperactivity affect frontal lobe integrity. *J. Clin. Endocrinol. Metab.* **90:** 3262–3267.

96. Bombois, S. *et al.* 2007. Prevalence of subcortical vascular lesions and association with executive function in mild cognitive impairment subtypes. *Stroke* **38:** 2595–2597.

97. Frisoni, G.B. *et al.* 2002. Mild cognitive impairment with subcortical vascular features: clinical characteristics and outcome. *J. Neurol.* **249:** 1423–1432.

98. Convit, A. 2005. Links between cognitive impairment in insulin resistance: an explanatory model. *Neurobiol. Aging* **26:** S31–35.

99. Starr, V.L. & A. Convit. 2007. Diabetes, sugar-coated but harmful to the brain. *Curr. Opin. Pharmacol.* **7:** 638–642.

100. Bjorgaas, M. *et al.* 1997. Cognitive function in type 1 diabetic children with and without episodes of severe hypoglycaemia. *Acta Paediatr.* **86:** 148–153.

101. Ryan, C.M. *et al.* 2006. Improving metabolic control leads to better working memory in adults with type 2 diabetes. *Diabetes Care* **29:** 345–351.

102. Elias, M.F. *et al.* 2005. Obesity, diabetes and cognitive deficit: The Framingham Heart Study. *Neurobiol. Aging* **26:** S11–16.

103. Sweat, V. *et al.* 2008. C-reactive protein is linked to lower cognitive performance in overweight and obese women. *Inflammation* **31:** 198–207.

104. Gunstad, J. *et al.* 2007. Elevated body mass index is associated with executive dysfunction in otherwise healthy adults. *Compr. Psychiatry* **48:** 57–61.

105. Jeong, S.K. *et al.* 2005. Interactive effect of obesity indexes on cognition. *Dement Geriatr. Cogn. Disord.* **19:** 91–96.

106. Cournot, M. *et al.* 2006. Relation between body mass index and cognitive function in healthy middle-aged men and women. *Neurology* **67:** 1208–1214.

107. Sakakura, K. *et al.* 2008. Association of body mass index with cognitive function in elderly hypertensive Japanese. *Am. J. Hypertens.* **21:** 627–632.

108. Maes, M. *et al.* 1997. Acute phase proteins in schizophrenia, mania and major depression: modulation by psychotropic drugs. *Psychiatry Res.* **66:** 1–11.

109. Maes, M. *et al.* 1992. Disturbances in acute phase plasma proteins during melancholia: additional evidence for the presence of an inflammatory process during that illness. *Prog. Neuropsychopharmacol. Biol. Psychiatry* **16:** 501–515.

110. Panagiotakos, D.B. *et al.* 2004. Inflammation, coagulation, and depressive symptomatology in cardiovascular disease-free people; the ATTICA study. *Eur. Heart J.* **25:** 492–499.

111. Papageorgiou, C. *et al.* 2006. Association between plasma inflammatory markers and irrational beliefs; the ATTICA epidemiological study. *Prog. Neuropsychopharmacol. Biol. Psychiatry* **30:** 1496–1503.

112. Pitsavos, C. *et al.* 2006. Anxiety in relation to inflammation and coagulation markers, among healthy adults: the ATTICA study. *Atherosclerosis* **185:** 320–326.

113. Ford, D.E. & T.P. Erlinger. 2004. Depression and C-reactive protein in US adults: data from the Third

National Health and Nutrition Examination Survey. *Arch. Intern. Med.* **164:** 1010–1014.

114. Liukkonen, T. *et al.* 2006. The Association Between C-Reactive Protein Levels and Depression: Results from the Northern Finland 1966 Birth Cohort Study. *Biol. Psychiatry* **60:** 825–830.

115. Danner, M. *et al.* 2003. Association between depression and elevated C-reactive protein. *Psychosom. Med.* **65:** 347–356.

116. Das, U.N. 2007. Is depression a low-grade systemic inflammatory condition? *Am. J. Clin. Nutr.* **85:** 1665–1666; author reply 1666.

117. Kidd, P.M. 2007. Omega-3 DHA and EPA for cognition, behavior, and mood: clinical findings and structural-functional synergies with cell membrane phospholipids. *Altern. Med. Rev.* **12:** 207–227.

118. Logan, A. 2003. Neurobehavioral aspects of omega-3 fatty acids: possible mechanisms and therapeutic value in major depression. *Altern. Med. Rev.* **8:** 410–425.

119. Otto, S.J., R.H. de Groot & G. Hornstra. 2003. Increased risk of postpartum depressive symptoms is associated with slower normalization after pregnancy of the functional docosahexaenoic acid status. *Prostaglandins Leukot Essent Fatty Acids* **69:** 237–243.

120. De Vriese, S.R., A.B. Christophe & M. Maes. 2003. Lowered serum n-3 polyunsaturated fatty acid (PUFA) levels predict the occurrence of postpartum depression: further evidence that lowered n-PUFAs are related to major depression. *Life Sci.* **73:** 3181–3187.

121. Iribarren, C. *et al.* 2004. Dietary intake of n-3, n-6 fatty acids and fish: relationship with hostility in young adults—the CARDIA study. *Eur. J. Clin. Nutr.* **58:** 24–31.

122. Green, P. *et al.* 2006. Red cell membrane omega-3 fatty acids are decreased in nondepressed patients with social anxiety disorder. *Eur. Neuropsychopharmacol.* **16:** 107–113.

123. Tanskanen, A. *et al.* 2001. Fish consumption and depressive symptoms in the general population in Finland. *Psychiatr. Serv.* **52:** 529–531.

124. Timonen, M. *et al.* 2004. Fish consumption and depression: the Northern Finland 1966 birth cohort study. *J. Affect. Disord.* **82:** 447–452.

125. Sanchez-Villegas, A. *et al.* 2007. Long chain omega-3 fatty acids intake, fish consumption and mental disorders in the SUN cohort study. *Eur. J. Nutr.* **46:** 337–346.

126. Hakkarainen, R. *et al.* 2004. Is low dietary intake of omega-3 fatty acids associated with depression? *Am. J. Psychiatry* **161:** 567–569.

Early Maternal Deprivation in Rats

A Proposed Animal Model for the Study of Developmental Neuroimmunoendocrine Interactions

M. De la Fuente, R. Llorente, I. Baeza, N. M. De Castro, L. Arranz, J. Cruces, and M. P. Viveros

Department of Animal Physiology, Faculty of Biology, Complutense University of Madrid, Madrid, Spain

Adult animals that had been subjected to a single prolonged episode of maternal deprivation (MD) [24 h, postnatal day (PND) 9–10] show long-term behavioral alterations that resemble specific symptoms of schizophrenia. Moreover, at adolescence MD rats showed depressive-like behavior and altered motor responses. According to the neurodevelopmental hypothesis, certain behavioral abnormalities observed in MD animals may be related to altered neurodevelopmental processes triggered by MD-induced elevated glucocorticoids in relevant specific brain regions. We review here these neuroendocrine effects and show new data indicating that the MD procedure induces diverse detrimental effects on the immune system that are already revealed in the short term (PND 13) and persist into adulthood. These long-lasting effects might be related to altered hypothalamus–pituitary–adrenal axis activity and to social as well as nutrition-related factors. In fact, MD induces long-lasting decreases in body weight. In view of our findings we propose the present MD procedure as a potentially useful model to analyze developmental interactions between early psychophysiological stress and immunodeficient states.

Key words: maternal deprivation; immune system; behavioral changes; corticosterone

Maternal Deprivation, a Potential Animal Model for Schizophrenia and Other Neuropsychiatric Disorders

There is evidence indicating that traumatic experiences during early developmental periods might be associated with psychopathology later in life. Thus, parental loss during childhood has been reported to significantly increase the likelihood of developing major depression[1] and psychosis.[2] Early maternal deprivation (MD) in rodents has been proposed as an interesting animal model for certain aspects of schizophrenia. Thus, maternally deprived rats [deprived from their mothers for a single period of 24 h shortly after birth, typically on postnatal day (PND) 9] showed, in adulthood, a series of behavioral abnormalities that resemble psychotic-like symptoms, such as disturbances in prepulse inhibition, latent inhibition, and auditory sensory gating and startle habituation.[3,4]

One of the most prevalent hypotheses for the pathogenesis of schizophrenia states that the disease is a neurodevelopmental disorder associated with early brain developmental abnormalities.[5–7] It has been hypothesized that certain deficits observed in maternally deprived animals may be related to neurodegenerative processes triggered by stress-induced increases in corticosterone levels.[8] In fact,

Address for correspondence: María-Paz Viveros and Mónica De la Fuente, Departamento de Fisiología (Fisiología Animal II), Facultad de Ciencias Biológicas, Universidad Complutense, Ciudad Universitaria, C/Jose Antonio Novais, 2, 28040-Madrid, Spain. Voice: 34-91-3944993; fax: 34-91-3944935. pazviver@bio.ucm.es or mondelaf@bio.ucm.es

Neuroimmunomodulation: Ann. N.Y. Acad. Sci. 1153: 176–183 (2009).
doi: 10.1111/j.1749-6632.2008.03979.x © 2009 New York Academy of Sciences.

TABLE 1. Summary of the Most Relevant Results Regarding Maternal Deprivation Effects in the Peri-Adolescent Period Responses

Corticosterone assay	
(basal corticosterone levels)	Decreased corticosterone levels in female rats
Behavioral tests	
Holeboard	Decreased vertical activity in male rats
Elevated plus maze	Decreased locomotor activity in male rats
Forced swimming test	Depressive-like behavior in both genders
Immunological parameters	
in different lymphoid organs	
Spleen	Reduced ConA–lymphoproliferation in both genders
Axillary nodes	Reduced ConA–lymphoproliferation and chemotaxis index in both genders
Thymus	Reduced ConA–lymphoproliferation and chemotaxis index in both genders

The rats were submitted to 24-h maternal deprivation in postnatal day (PND) 9 or left undisturbed. Animals were sacrificed at PND 40 when blood samples and tissues were collected.
ConA, concanavalin A.

long-lasting changes in brain-derived neurotrophic factor[9] as well as immediate cell loss[10] have been related to MD procedures. Moreover, we have recently found that 13-day-old rats subjected to 24 h of MD at PND 9 showed significantly increased plasma corticosterone levels that, in male rats, were accompanied by hippocampal alterations,[11,12] further supporting a neurodevelopmental basis for MD-induced behavioral abnormalities.

Psychoimmunoendocrine Characterization of MD Animals in the Adolescent Period

Adolescence represents a critical developmental period during which some major neuropsychiatric disorders may become evident, including schizophrenia.[13–15] We carried out a series of experiments in order to further characterize the above-described animal model by evaluating the psychoimmunoendocrine status of MD animals in the peri-adolescent period. We analyzed behavioral symptoms of anxiety and depression, relevant immunological parameters, and corticosterone levels as an indication of hypothalamus–pituitary–adrenal (HPA) function in adolescent male and female rats[16]

(see Table 1 for a summary of the results). We used a battery of tests that have been validated for the assessment of different behavioral aspects: the holeboard, which provides independent measures of general motor activity and directed exploration,[17,18] the elevated plus maze, a useful animal model for the assessment of anxiety-related responses based on the natural aversion of rodents to height and open spaces,[19] and the forced swimming test (FST),[20] a paradigm for the assessment of the depressive phenotype. In this latter test, MD, adolescent, male rats showed a significantly reduced latency to reach a passive floating posture, and both male and female rats showed a significant increase in floating behavior. According to the classic interpretation of this test, these data indicate that early MD may reduce the ability of animals to cope with a stressful situation. In a previous study it was shown that adult mice deprived of their mother during 24 h at PND 12 showed a reduced latency to reach the floating posture in the FST.[21] Data from our laboratory are in agreement with this conclusion and extend the results, indicating that early MD might precipitate the emergence of depressive symptoms in the adolescent period. In addition, our experiments indicate that maternally deprived male rats show a significant reduction in rearing behavior (vertical activity). Previous data from Ellenbroek *et al.*[22] showed that MD significantly decreased rearing behavior in infant rats (PND 12–18). Our data confirm the MD-induced impairment of rearing behavior until adolescence. A delayed development of the dopaminergic system[22] and possible stress-induced damage in cerebellar structures allowing full display of vertical activity[23] might account for this specific behavioral alteration.

Corticosterone determinations showed the frequently observed sexual dimorphism in control nondeprived animals, which is in agreement with previous results showing higher corticosterone levels in female rats. In fact, this sex difference appears to be present in adult,[24] adolescent,[25] and neonatal[26] rats. MD appeared to decrease baseline hormone concentration in adolescent female rats but not male rats. We have found that the same deprivation procedure induces short-term significant increases in plasma corticosterone concentration in both sexes measured at PND 13.[11,12] It seems that the HPA axis, which is clearly affected by the stress of MD, shows dynamic (possibly compensatory) changes throughout development that may be sex dependent. Previous studies indicate that MD effects on corticosterone secretion are long lasting and become evident differently at different ages. In experiments by Suchecki and Tufik[27] in which the 24-h MD stress took place at PND 11, they determined the corticosterone response to a saline injection. At PND 12, the response of the deprived pups was higher than that of nondeprived pups. No group differences were observed at PND 16 and 22. On PND 30, the adrenal response to stress of deprived rats was smaller than that of nondeprived pups. Workel *et al.*[28] used a 24-h MD protocol at PND 3 in male rats and determined the corticosterone levels at 3, 12, and 30–32 months. At 3 months there was a rise in basal hormone levels, whereas the corticosterone output in response to novelty was attenuated in the deprived rats. In contrast, a striking surge in novelty stress-induced corticosterone output occurred at midlife while, at

senescence, the corticosterone responses were attenuated again in the deprived animals, particularly after the more severe restraint stressor. Other authors have found that adult (60 PND) male rats that were maternally deprived for 24 h at PND 3 showed elevated basal plasma corticosterone concentrations when compared to nondeprived rats.[29]

Persistent Immunological Alterations Induced by MD

Immunological abnormalities have long been described in diverse psychiatric disorders.[30–32] In particular, some relevant functions of the immune system, such as lymphoproliferation in response to mitogens[33] or directed chemotactic capacity[34] have been shown to be impaired in schizophrenic patients. Because the rat MD procedure described above is considered an animal model of that illness, we hypothesized that an impaired immune function might be found in the MD animals. To confirm this hypothesis, lymphoid organs (spleen, thymus, and axillary nodes) from maternally deprived male and female adolescent rats were removed and immunological parameters evaluated, namely mitogen-induced lymphoproliferation and chemotaxis.[16] As summarized in Table 1, MD adolescent animals showed an impaired immunological function as revealed by the general decrease in the analyzed immunological parameters: a significant decrease in concanavalin A (ConA)-induced proliferative activity of lymphocytes in the three lymphoid organs and a diminished chemotaxis index in the thymus and the axillary nodes. In order to provide a more complete dynamic picture of MD immunological changes, we further analyzed the effects of MD at PND 13 and in adulthood (PND 75), and the results of these experiments are shown in this review article as original data. Figure 1 shows the changes observed in MD 13-day-old rats. In both male and female neonatal animals, MD caused significant decreases in the natural killer (NK) activity

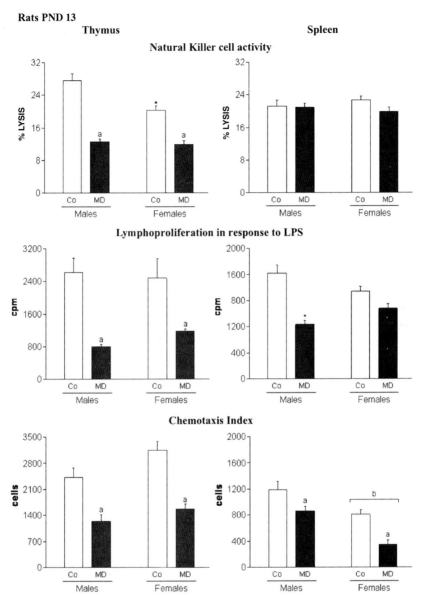

Figure 1. Effects of early maternal deprivation (MD) on immunological parameters in the thymus and spleen of 13-day-old rats. The animals were submitted to 24-h MD from postnatal day (PND) 9 to PND 10 or left undisturbed (Co). At PND 13 the animals were sacrificed and the lymphocytes isolated from the thymus and the spleen. Histograms represent the mean ± SEM of natural killer cell activity (% lysis) (five to eight animals per experimental group), lymphoproliferation in response to lipopolysaccharide (LPS) (count per minute) (six to eight animals per experimental group), and chemotaxis index (eight to 10 animals per experimental group). ANOVA and Tukey ($P < 0.05$): a, significant overall effects of MD (see text for details); b, significant overall effects of gender (see text for details); * versus male Co.

of cells from thymus as well as in the proliferative response to lipopolysaccharide (LPS) and in the chemotaxis of lymphocytes from thymus and spleen. In adulthood (Fig. 2), both male and female MD animals showed marked reductions in the NK activity and lymphoproliferative responses of cells obtained from thymus and spleen as well as a reduced

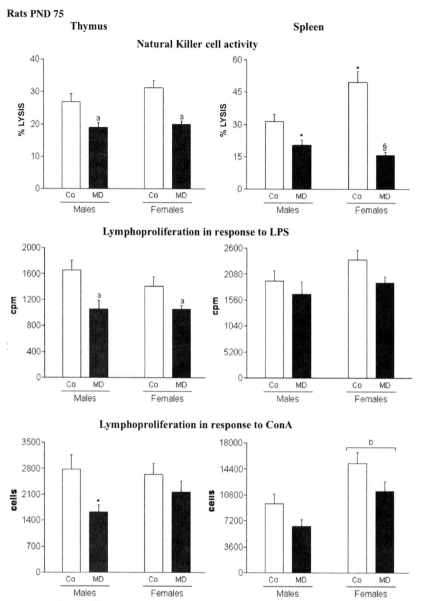

Figure 2. Effects of early MD on immunological parameters in the thymus and spleen of 75-day-old rats. The animals were submitted to 24-h MD from PND 9 to PND 10 or left undisturbed (Co). At PND 75 the animals were sacrificed and the lymphocytes isolated from the thymus and the spleen. Histograms represent the mean ± SEM (seven to 10 animals per experimental group) of natural killer cell activity (% lysis), lymphoproliferation in response to LPS, and chemotaxis index. ANOVA and Tukey ($P < 0.05$): a, significant overall effects of MD (see text for details); b, significant overall effects of gender (see text for details); * versus male Co; § versus female Co.

lymphoproliferation in response to ConA that, in the thymus, was significant in male animals. It is worth noting that, whereas immunohistochemical[11,12] and behavioral[16] parameters tend to be gender dependent, with male rats being more affected, the immunological parameters analyzed are clearly decreased in the two genders.

There is substantial evidence for the importance of interacting neuroendocrine–immune networks in physiological homeostatic mechanisms. In this context, glucocorticoids, the end products of the HPA axis, appear to play a pivotal role in coordinating the development of the immune system functions.[35] As indicated above, the present MD protocol induces a short-term increase in plasma corticosterone levels of male and female rats (measured at PND 13). This abnormally enhanced glucocorticoid level at such an early age may account, at least partially, for the long-lasting impaired immune function observed in the maternally deprived animals. In line with our findings, Groër *et al.*[36] have reported that a 3 h daily MD from PND 6–10 caused a decrease of splenocyte proliferative response to ConA at PND 15. This effect could be reversed by maternal tactile stimulation, further supporting the important role of maternal care in the maintenance of homeostasis during postnatal development. However, the present 24-h MD procedure appears to be particularly severe in terms of its effects on the immune system; the presence of the mother until PND 22, when weaning took place, does not seem to be able to improve the immune status of the MD animals, at least as regards the parameters analyzed in these experiments. By using the same MD protocol of the present study, Teunis *et al.*[37] showed that MD rats suffered an increased severity of experimental autoimmune encephalomyelitis at 9 weeks of age.

Malnutrition in critical developmental periods, including neonatal maturation, impairs the development and differentiation of a normal immune system. Therefore, infections are more frequent and more often become chronic in the malnourished child. Since the immune system is immature at birth, malnutrition in childhood might have long-term effects on health.[38] For example, exposure to bacteria from the mother's skin and the provision of immunological factors of breast milk seem to be key events that promote maturation of the gut of infants and gut-associated systemic immune system.[39] Our results indicate that MD rats show significantly decreased body weights.[16] Using the same model other authors have shown that early MD results in a significant reduction in body weight in neonatal (PND 9–24)[22] and adult rats.[40] The fact that the reduced weight of maternally deprived rats has been observed extending into adulthood suggests that it might be not only a result of the lack of milk ingestion during the 24-h deprivation period. It is likely that MD results in long-term altered interactions with the dam throughout the pre-weaning period. In fact, there are data suggesting that maternal separation may affect maternal behavior (and possibly milk production), which may result in altered mother–pup interactions.[8] Thus, social and nutritional factors may be implicated in the long-lasting detrimental effects on the immune system. It has been proposed that nutrition early in life might affect later immune competence, including the ability to mount an appropriate immune response upon infection, the ability to develop a tolerance response to "self" and to benign environmental antigens, and the development of immunological disorders.[39] The present MD model deserves further analyses of additional immunological indices and specific vulnerabilities, such as those related to the gastrointestinal immune system.

In conclusion, the present results indicate that a single episode of 24 h of MD (PND 9–10) induces clear signs of impaired lymphocyte function that were evident as early as PND 13 and persisted into adulthood. The endocrine and immune systems are interrelated via a bidirectional network in which hormones affect immune function and, in turn, immune responses are reflected in neuroendocrine changes.[41] In this context, the primary hormonal pathway by which the central nervous system regulates the immune system is the HPA axis through the hormones of the neuroendocrine stress response,[42] and these interactions may be particularly relevant during the critical neonatal and peri-adolescent periods.[43,44] It is also important to consider the long-lasting impact that the acute (but long 24-h) episode of milk restriction and lack of mother contact may have on the developing immune system.[45] The impaired immune function of maternally deprived rats further supports the view that this animal model may represent a useful model of schizophrenia. In fact it has been proposed that schizophrenia could have as its base a dysregulated immune function.[32]

Summing it up, our findings in relation to the MD procedure suggest that this form of neonatal stress may provide a useful model to investigate neurodevelopmental psychoneuroimmunoendocrine interactions that may underlie certain neuropsychiatric disorders.

Acknowledgments

Supported by Ministerio de Educación y Ciencia ref: SAF2006-07523 and BFU2005-06777 and Red de Trastornos Adictivos RD06/0001/1013 and Red de Envejecimiento y Fragilidad (RD06/0013/0003). R.L. is a predoctoral fellow of the Universidad Complutense and L.A. is a predoctoral fellow of the Ministerio de Educación y Ciencia.

Conflicts of Interest

The authors declare no conflicts of interest.

References

1. Kendler, K.S. *et al.* 2002. Childhood parental loss and risk for first-onset of major depression and alcohol dependence: the time-decay of risk and sex differences. *Psychol. Med.* **32:** 1187–1194.
2. Morgan, C. *et al.* 2007. Parental separation, loss and psychosis in different ethnic groups: a case-control study. *Psychol. Med.* **37:** 495–503.
3. Ellenbroek, B.A. *et al.* 2004. The effects of early maternal deprivation on auditory information processing in adult Wistar rats. *Biol. Psychiatry* **55:** 701–707.
4. Ellenbroek, B.A. & M.A. Riva. 2003. Early maternal deprivation as an animal model for schizophrenia. *Clin. Neurosci. Res.* **3:** 297–302.
5. Lewis, D.A. & P. Levitt. 2002. Schizophrenia as a disorder of neurodevelopment. *Annu. Rev. Neurosci.* **25:** 409–432.
6. Marek, G. & K. Merchant. 2005. Developing therapeutics for schizophrenia and other psychotic disorders. *NeuroRx.* **2:** 579–589.
7. Weinberger, D.R. 1987. Implications of normal brain development for the pathogenesis of schizophrenia. *Arch. Gen. Psychiatry* **44:** 660–669.
8. Ellenbroek, B.A. & A.R. Cools. 2002. Early maternal deprivation and prepulse inhibition: the role of the postdeprivation environment. *Pharmacol. Biochem. Behav.* **73:** 177–184.
9. Roceri, M. *et al.* 2002. Early maternal deprivation reduces the expression of BDNF and NMDA receptor subunits in rat hippocampus. *Mol. Psychiatry* **7:** 609–616.
10. Zhang, L.X. *et al.* 2002. Maternal deprivation increases cell death in the infant rat brain. *Brain Res. Dev. Brain Res.* **133:** 1–11.
11. Llorente, R. *et al.* 2008. Gender-dependent cellular and biochemical effects of maternal deprivation on the hippocampus of neonatal rats: a possible role for the endocannabinoid system. *Dev. Neurobiol.* **68:** 1334–1347.
12. Viveros, M.P. *et al.* 2008a. Early maternal deprivation in rats induces sex-dependent neurodegenerative changes in the hippocampus. [Abstract] *FENS* **4:** 177.13.
13. Adriani, W. & G. Laviola. 2004. Windows of vulnerability to psychopathology and therapeutic strategy in the adolescent rodent model. *Behav. Pharmacol.* **15:** 341–352.
14. Andersen, S.L. 2003. Trajectories of brain development: point of vulnerability or window of opportunity? *Neurosci. Biobehav. Rev.* **27:** 3–18.
15. Kessler, R.C. *et al.* 2007. Age of onset of mental disorders: a review of recent literature. *Curr. Opin. Psychiatry* **20:** 359–364.
16. Llorente, R. *et al.* 2007. Early maternal deprivation and neonatal single administration with a cannabinoid agonist induce long-term sex-dependent psychoimmunoendocrine effects in adolescent rats. *Psychoneuroendocrinology* **32:** 636–650.
17. File, S.E. 1992. Behavioral detection of anxiolytic action. In *Experimental Approaches to Anxiety and Depression.* J.M. Elliot, D.J. Heal & C.A. Marsden, Eds.: 25–44. Wiley. New York.
18. File, S.E. & A.G. Wardill. 1975. Validity of head-dipping as a measure of exploration in a modified hole-board. *Psychopharmacologia* **44:** 53–59.
19. Pellow, S. *et al.* 1985. Validation of open:closed arm entries in an elevated plus-maze as a measure of anxiety in the rat. *J. Neurosci. Methods* **14:** 149–167.
20. Porsolt, R.D. 2000. Animal models of depression: utility for transgenic research. *Rev. Neurosci.* **11:** 53–58.

21. Macri, S. & G. Laviola. 2004. Single episode of maternal deprivation and adult depressive profile in mice: interaction with cannabinoid exposure during adolescence. *Behav. Brain Res.* **154:** 231–238.

22. Ellenbroek, B.A., N. Derks & H.J. Park. 2005. Early maternal deprivation retards neurodevelopment in Wistar rats. *Stress* **8:** 247–257.

23. Viveros, M.P. *et al.* 2008. Sex-dependent degenerative changes in the cerebellar cortex of maternally deprived rats. modulatory effects of two inhibitors of endocannabinoid inactivation. *Presented at 18th symposium of the International Cannabinoid Research Society*, Aviemore, Scotland, June 2008. Book of Abstract, P56.

24. Viveros, M.P. *et al.* 1988. Effects of social isolation and crowding upon adrenocortical reactivity and behavior in the rat. *Rev. Esp. Fisiol.* **44:** 315–321.

25. Romero, E.M. *et al.* 2002. Antinociceptive, behavioural and neuroendocrine effects of CP 55,940 in young rats. *Brain Res. Dev. Brain Res.* **136:** 85–92.

26. Borcel, E. *et al.* 2004. Functional responses to the cannabinoid agonist WIN 55,212-2 in neonatal rats of both genders: influence of weaning. *Pharmacol. Biochem. Behav.* **78:** 593–602.

27. Suchecki, D. & S. Tufik. 1997. Long-term effects of maternal deprivation on the corticosterone response to stress in rats. *Am. J. Physiol.* **273:** R1332–1338.

28. Workel, J.O. *et al.* 2001. Differential and age-dependent effects of maternal deprivation on the hypothalamic-pituitary-adrenal axis of brown norway rats from youth to senescence. *J. Neuroendocrinol.* **13:** 569–580.

29. Rots, N.Y. *et al.* 1996. Neonatal maternally deprived rats have as adults elevated basal pituitary-adrenal activity and enhanced susceptibility to apomorphine. *J. Neuroendocrinol.* **8:** 501–506.

30. Muller, N. *et al.* 2000. The immune system and schizophrenia. An integrative view. *Ann. N. Y. Acad. Sci.* **917:** 456–467.

31. Schwarz, M.J. *et al.* 2001. T-helper-1 and T-helper-2 responses in psychiatric disorders. *Brain. Behav. Immun.* **15:** 340–370.

32. Strous, R.D. & Y. Shoenfeld. 2006. Schizophrenia, autoimmunity and immune system dysregulation: a comprehensive model updated and revisited. *J. Autoimmun.* **27:** 71–80.

33. Moises, H.W. *et al.* 1985. Decreased production of interferon alpha and interferon gamma in leucocyte cultures of schizophrenic patients. *Acta Psychiatr Scand.* **72:** 45–50.

34. Cosentino, M. *et al.* 1996. Assessment of lymphocyte subsets and neutrophil leukocyte function in chronic psychiatric patients on long-term drug therapy. *Prog. Neuropsychopharmacol. Biol. Psychiatry* **20:** 1117–1129.

35. Marchetti, B. *et al.* 2001. Stress, the immune system and vulnerability to degenerative disorders of the central nervous system in transgenic mice expressing glucocorticoid receptor antisense RNA. *Brain Res. Brain Res. Rev.* **37:** 259–272.

36. Groër, M.W. *et al.* 2002. Effects of separation and separation with supplemental stroking in BALb/c infant mice. *Biol. Res. Nurs.* **3:** 119–131.

37. Teunis, M.A. *et al.* 2002. Maternal deprivation of rat pups increases clinical symptoms of experimental autoimmune encephalomyelitis at adult age. *J. Neuroimmunol.* **133:** 30–38.

38. Cunningham-Rundles, S., D.F. McNeeley & A. Moon. 2005. Mechanisms of nutrient modulation of the immune response. *J. Allergy Clin. Immunol.* **115:** 1119–1128; quiz 1129.

39. Calder, P.C. *et al.* 2006. Early nutrition and immunity — progress and perspectives. *Br. J. Nutr.* **96:** 774–790.

40. Husum, H. *et al.* 2002. Early maternal deprivation alters hippocampal levels of neuropeptide Y and calcitonin-gene related peptide in adult rats. *Neuropharmacology* **42:** 798–806.

41. Gaillard, R.C. 2001. Interaction between the hypothalamo-pituitary-adrenal axis and the immunological system. *Ann. Endocrinol. (Paris)* **62:** 155–163.

42. Eskandari, F. & E.M. Sternberg. 2002. Neural-immune interactions in health and disease. *Ann. N. Y. Acad. Sci.* **966:** 20–27.

43. Charmandari, E. *et al.* 2003. Pediatric stress: hormonal mediators and human development. *Horm. Res.* **59:** 161–179.

44. Charmandari, E., C. Tsigos & G. Chrousos. 2005. Endocrinology of the stress response. *Annu. Rev. Physiol.* **67:** 259–284.

45. Bjorksten, B. 2008. Environmental influences on the development of the immune system: consequences for disease outcome. *Nestle Nutr Workshop Ser Pediatr Program* **61:** 243–254.

Leptin and the Immune Response

An Active Player or an Innocent Bystander?

Anna Carla Goldberg,[a,b] **Freddy Goldberg-Eliaschewitz,**[a,c] **Mari Cleide Sogayar,**[a,d] **Julieta Genre,**[e] **and Luiz Vicente Rizzo**[b,e,f,g,h]

[a] *Cell and Molecular Therapy Center, University of São Paulo, São Paulo, Brazil*

[b] *Institute for Investigation in Immunology (iii), Institutos do Milênio, Brazilian Science and Technology Ministry, Brazil*

[c] *Department of Internal Medicine, Hospital Heliópolis, São Paulo, Brazil*

[d] *Department of Biochemistry, Chemistry Institute, University of São Paulo, São Paulo, Brazil*

[e] *Department of Immunology, Biomedical Sciences Institutes, University of São Paulo, São Paulo, Brazil*

[f] *Division of Clinical Immunology and Allergy, University of São Paulo Medical School General Hospital, São Paulo, Brazil*

[g] *Laboratory of Medical Investigation-60, Department of Internal Medicine, University of São Paulo Medical School, São Paulo, Brazil*

[h] *Heart Institute, Fundação Zerbini, São Paulo, Brazil*

Leptin is involved in the control of energy storage by the body. Low serum leptin levels, as seen in starvation, are associated with impaired inflammatory T cell responses that can be reversed by exogenous leptin. Common variable immunodeficiency (CVID) is characterized by hypogammaglobulinemia and recurrent infections. Several defects in T cell function have also been described, and allergy, autoimmune disease, and lymphomas or other malignancies can be present. Previous studies in Brazilian CVID patients have shown that, in contrast with mononuclear cells from healthy controls, CVID cells cultured with phytohemagglutinin and added leptin increased the proliferative response and decreased activation-induced apoptosis. Interleukin (IL)-2 and especially IL-4 production also increased significantly, although the effects of exposure to leptin were not observed uniformly in CVID patients. The majority, however, responded in some degree, and some exhibited completely restored values of the four parameters. These remarkable results indicate leptin could be used to improve immune function in these patients. On the other hand, we found no specific correlation between serum leptin levels and the number of infectious events over a 24-month period, presence of autoimmunity, allergies, or cancer in these patients. The results suggest that the absolute value of serum leptin does not determine the clinical behavior of patients or responses to leptin *in vitro*. Of note is the divergence between serum leptin, response to leptin *in vitro*, and the presence of autoimmunity, indicating the need to identify the cellular and molecular players involved in the regulation of the immune response by leptin in CVID.

Key words: common variable immunodeficiency; leptin; autoimmunity; T cell response

Address for correspondence: Luiz Vicente Rizzo, Clinical Immunology Lab., Dept. Immunology, Biomedical Sciences Institute, University of Sao Paulo, Av. Prof. Lineu Prestes 1730, 05508-900, Sao Paulo – SP, Brazil. Voice: 55 11 3091 7430; fax: 55 11 3091 7394. lvrizzo@icb.usp.br

Neuroimmunomodulation: Ann. N.Y. Acad. Sci. 1153: 184–192 (2009).
doi: 10.1111/j.1749-6632.2008.03971.x © 2009 New York Academy of Sciences.

Introduction

Leptin is a 16-kDa cytokine-like molecule traditionally recognized as a hormone produced by white adipose tissue and involved in control of energy storage by the body.[1] Serum levels correlate with body mass index (BMI), but there is heterogeneity in the individual indices, showing that other factors also affect regulation of leptin levels.[2] Leptin is involved in many different body functions, such as reproduction, angiogenesis, and regulation of the hypothalamic–pituitary–adrenal axis.[3] On the other hand, leptin or leptin receptor-deficient mice exhibit the hallmarks of immune deficiency, such as thymus atrophy and reduced lymphocyte function, establishing a link between nutritional status and immune responses.[4] Besides thyroxin and growth and sex hormones, leptin levels are also influenced, for instance, by diet. Malnourishment and/or starvation are associated with thymus atrophy in mice and humans.[4–6] In leptin-deficient mice, replacement by exogenous leptin is capable of increasing thymic cellularity.[5,7]

It has now been 10 years since the initial description of a clear link between low leptin levels from starvation and hindered inflammatory T cell responses.[8] In their paper, Lord and collaborators showed increased *in vitro* T helper (TH)1 responses and suppression of TH2 cytokine production induced by leptin both in human and mouse assays. Furthermore, leptin reversed starvation-induced inhibition of T cell responses. Two important models, namely the ob/ob and the db/db mouse, carrying functional knockout mutations for leptin and the leptin receptor, respectively, have since been used to clarify the role of leptin in immune responses. Leptin has been shown, in these two experimental models, to impact upon proliferation and effector functions of CD4+ naive but not memory T lymphocytes,[8,9] CD8+ T lymphocytes,[10] monocytes and macrophages,[10] B lymphocytes,[10] dendritic cells,[11] and more recently regulatory T lymphocytes[12] and natural killer (NK) cells[13,14] as well. In a comparison between lean and obese mice, only NK cells from lean animals responded to activation by exogenous leptin.[13] Summarizing, in most studies there is a consensus that leptin acts to induce proliferation, decrease apoptosis, and impart TH1-type inflammatory responses with increased secretion of interleukin (IL)-12, IL-6, tumor necrosis factor (TNF)-α, or interferon (IFN)-γ according to cell type and at the same time diminishes or does not affect IL-4 and IL-10 production.[11] Furthermore, dendritic cells of ob/ob mice were shown to secrete primarily transforming growth factor (TGF)-β1 and to be less capable of stimulating allogeneic T cells.[11]

The association of malnutrition[15] and/or starvation[16] with suppression of T cell immune responses has prompted further studies that showed leptin is capable of restoring proliferation and inflammatory T1-type responses in undernourished individuals.[8,15] In all, in humans, results essentially similar to studies with mice have been obtained *in vitro* for T CD4 lymphocytes,[9] T regulatory lymphocytes,[12,17] dendritic cells,[18] monocytes, and neutrophils.[19,20] All these cell types exhibit leptin receptors, which increase significantly upon cell activation and thus are potential targets for leptin. Some studies show that leptin not only influences T cell function but also induces activation and secretion of IL-6 and TNF-α by peripheral monocytes.[20,21] However, *in vivo* effects are harder to evaluate. A recent study of the immune profile in malnourished infants confirmed lower production of IL-2 and IFN-γ by CD4+ and CD8+ T lymphocytes during resting and after phorbol 12-myristate 13-acetate activation.[22] Addition of leptin augmented production of both cytokines but only in the presence of concomitant activation. In addition, the reverse effects were seen for IL-4 and IL-10 synthesis. In cases of children harboring the human counterpart of the ob mutation, exogenous leptin, in addition to several other benefits, also reversed T lymphocyte dysfunction.[9,23] A family study evidenced a high childhood mortality rate in carriers of the mutation,[23] but some of these patients did survive into adulthood, indicating that other pathways are capable of compensating for leptin deficiency.

The role of leptin in inflammatory, autoimmune, or infectious diseases has also been evaluated. Acute inflammatory conditions, such as cholecystectomy[24] and sepsis,[25] seem to be accompanied by increased serum leptin levels. Furthermore, increased survival from acute sepsis has been associated with increased leptin levels.[26] In human immunodeficiency virus positive children, successful active anti-retroviral therapy not only re-establishes CD4+ T cell count but also serum leptin.[27] However, in other studies of AIDS patients no differences in serum leptin are observed.[28] The most interesting data concerning autoimmune diseases have been obtained in studies of patients diagnosed with relapsing-remitting multiple sclerosis but yet untreated.[17] These patients exhibit increased leptin in serum and, along with increased IFN-γ, in cerebrospinal fluid. Leptin levels correlate inversely with regulatory T lymphocyte number, and leptin production by T cell lines against human myelin basic protein is increased. Neutralizing leptin blocks antigen-specific proliferation of these T cells. In an experimental autoimmune encephalomyelitis animal model,[17] blocking leptin with a soluble leptin receptor fusion protein led to improvement of symptoms. Leptin-deficient mice also show resistance to develop atherosclerosis accompanied by impaired TH1 responses and increased regulatory T cell function.[29] Defective regulatory T lymphocytes have been shown in several other autoimmune diseases and might be targets for therapeutic intervention with leptin blockers. On the other hand, changes in leptin serum levels were not observed either in inflammatory bowel syndrome or in rheumatoid arthritis patients,[30,31] suggesting that the observed effects of leptin in multiple sclerosis may be confined to autoimmunity against targets within the central nervous system where important actions of leptin take place.

Taken together the results indicate that leptin is a pleiotropic cytokine-like molecule that exerts a protective effect on proliferation and/or effector function in a wide variety of immune-response cells.

Leptin in Common Variable Immunodeficiency

Common variable immunodeficiency (CVID) is the most common primary immunodeficiency diagnosed in young adults. The syndrome is characterized by low serum immunoglobulin IgG, IgA, and often IgM. The decreased antibody levels lead to bacterial and viral infections in the respiratory and gastrointestinal tracts. However, there are a number of other symptoms, including inflammatory conditions, allergic reactions, autoimmune disease, and the development of lymphomas and other types of malignancies, that cannot be explained based solely on diminished immunoglobulin levels.[32] A number of defects in T cell function and deficits in the memory B-cell pool have been identified, but the underlying causes remain largely unknown.[27] Prognosis is often hindered by heterogeneity in the clinical manifestations, but established clinical and laboratory criteria allow successful diagnosis of CVID patients.[33]

In normal individuals, B-lymphocyte activation, isotype switching, and differentiation to antibody-secreting plasma cells are dependent on cell-to-cell interactions and rely heavily on signals provided by T lymphocytes, either directly or through professional antigen-presenting cells. Studies have uncovered defects in the expression of CD154 (CD40L)[34] and in the function of T cell co-stimulatory ligands, such as CD28. An *in vitro* study has shown that stimulation through an anti-T cell receptor antibody in the presence of co-stimulatory anti-CD28 was incapable of inducing normal levels of IL-2 and IL-4.[34,35] The interaction between CD27 and CD70, which is critical for plasma cell differentiation, has equally been reported to be affected in CVID patients.[36] In addition, it has been shown that monocytes and

TABLE 1. Clinical Data for the Set of Brazilian Common Variable Immunodeficiency (CVID) Patients and Healthy Controls

Parameter		Mean		Standard deviation		Minimum value		Maximum value		P
		CVID	CTRL	CVID	CTRL	CVID	CTRL	CVID	CTRL	
Age	years	30.32	31.70	15.67	10.70	6	18	63	55	NS
Weight	kg	53.97	67.12	14.12	11.65	20	50	77	103	<0.001
Height	m	1.59	1.69	0.17	0.09	1.10	1.49	1.81	1.90	=0.002
BMI	.....	20.77	23.34	2.97	2.89	14.70	18.72	27.34	28.76	<0.001
Ig G	g/L	467.71	1120	78.82	237	310	NA	713	NA	
Serum leptin	ng/mL	2.38	3.10	1.35	1.19	0.5	1.5	6.5	6.2	<0.001
CD4	10E9/L	869.08	1059.48	181.7	234.88	542	731	1278	1871	=0.002
CD8	10E9/L	619.71	540.13	122.29	141.22	333	289	901	891	=0.01
CD4/CD8	.....	1.47	2.04	0.46	0.54	0.78	0.54	2.01	4.49	<0.001

Brazilian CVID patients ($N = 38$); healthy controls ($N = 40$). BMI, body mass index; CTRL, controls; NA, not applicable; NS, not significant. Statistical analysis used was χ-squared or Student's t-tests.

Epstein–Barr virus-transformed B cells from CVID patients are capable of normal antigen presentation.[37]

B cells are influenced by a variety of cytokines. IL-2, IL-5, and IL-6 enhance proliferation and IL-4 protects B cells against apoptosis. Cytokines, such as IL-6, IL-10, and IL-2, can dictate the outcome of differentiation into memory or plasma cells. Isotype switching is under the control of IL-4, IFN-γ, IL-5, and TGF-β1.[38–40] In fact, previous studies have revealed deficits in the production of IL-2, IL-4, IL-10, and IFN-γ by T cells from patients with CVID,[41] results confirmed in a Brazilian cohort of patients.[42] Furthermore, it has been shown that long-term, low-dose, IL-2 replacement therapy increases T cell proliferative responses to mitogens, antigens, and to IL-2 itself. It was also shown that IL-2 improves antigen-specific antibody synthesis in some of the treated patients and, although statistical significance was not achieved, patients treated with IL-2 recorded fewer days of bronchitis, diarrhea, and joint pain.[43]

Thus, the data in the literature suggest that the primary molecular defects leading to CVID may occur in any step of the B-lymphocyte differentiation to plasma cells in connection with T lymphocyte help to antibody production, in antigen presentation function, or in all

of these combined. In our cohort, over 70% of the patients exhibited some degree of T cell dysfunction in addition to low or almost absent B lymphocytes (P.R. Errante, unpublished results, University of São Paulo, São Paulo, Brazil).

To evaluate the role of leptin in CVID, we conducted a study with a cohort of Brazilian CVID patients[44] from the Clinical Immunology and Allergy Division at the University of São Paulo Medical School, São Paulo, Brazil. The patients were diagnosed according to the criteria defined by the World Health Organization, the Pan American Group for Immunodeficiency, and the Latin American Group for Primary Immunodeficiencies[45] and had a minimum follow-up of 1 year. Control samples ($n = 40$) were obtained from healthy age- and weight-matched individuals referred to the hospital for investigation of ocular toxoplasmosis but cleared of any infection. A summary of the clinical data is shown in Table 1. Of note, CVID patients exhibited lower serum leptin levels and lower BMI than the controls and than the average for the same age and gender in the Brazilian population. However, no correlation between these two parameters was present, reminiscent of similar observations in starved mice.[46] We measured proliferation upon phytohemagglutinin (PHA) activation, percentage of apoptosis by annexin V, and IL-2 and IL-4 production by ELISA assay in samples of peripheral blood mononuclear cells cultivated in the absence or in the presence of 50 ng/mL of recombinant human leptin.

As we were not able to achieve the designed matching from these differences, we excluded some of the patients ($n = 9$) and control samples ($n = 8$) that could not be matched for age and BMI and statistical analysis was applied to this matched subset. The results obtained with the matched set were in all instances comparable to the results of the complete set when the remainder of patients were included. Because these variables showed significant differences between the CVID and control groups, a model was fitted to a general linear model adjusting for sex, age, and BMI. Irrespective of age, weight, and serum leptin levels of patients and controls, the overall comparison of control and patient T cell responses showed significant differences in all parameters analyzed.

As expected, only eight out of 38 CVID patients exhibited lymphocyte proliferative response to PHA, reaching the lower range observed for normal individuals. However, addition of leptin to the tissue culture media resulted in increased [³H]-Thy uptake values by up to 1.5-fold in the proliferative response of lymphocytes from patients with CVID. This increase was observed in the majority of cases, but, in a few instances, counts per minute values were either lower after the addition of the hormone or no variation was observed. The same pattern was observed for annexin V staining. Addition of leptin to lymphocyte cultures from patients with CVID led to a significant decrease in the number of annexin V-stained cells and in eight cases were normalized. It is noteworthy that, in patients where annexin-staining values were close to the normal range, addition of leptin did not induce any change. IL-2 and IL-4 secretion in response to PHA, in the presence or absence of leptin, again showed the same pattern. Mean cytokine values for the patients were mostly below control levels, but both IL-2 and IL-4 production increased notably in the presence of leptin, reaching the lower range of

normal values in 44.7% and 71.0% of patients, respectively. Nevertheless, only six cases showed correction of all parameters when cells were grown in the presence of leptin. In addition, analysis in three patients showed that the low B-lymphocyte count (around 1%) was unchanged in the presence of leptin irrespective of leptin responsiveness. Multivariate analysis, with sex, age, and BMI included as independent variables, confirmed highly significant differences in annexin V binding ($P < 0.001$) and IL-4 production ($P < 0.001$). Thus, our results when studying the effect of leptin on peripheral blood mononuclear cells derived from CVID patients is partially in accordance with published literature on the protective effects of leptin in boosting cell proliferation and diminishing apoptosis rates but contrasts with the general paradigm that leptin favors TH1-type inflammatory responses and blocks IL-4 production.

Although these results are remarkable, and we are proceeding with these studies, which will include a planned clinical trial of the effect of leptin on antibody production *in vivo*, we found no specific correlation between serum leptin levels and the number of infectious events over a 24-month period (Fig. 1A), presence of autoimmunity (Fig. 1B), allergies (Fig. 1C), or cancer (Fig. 1D) in these patients. The results suggest that the absolute value of the serum leptin does not determine either the clinical behavior of patients or the responses to leptin *in vitro*. It is particularly interesting to stress the divergence between serum leptin, response to leptin *in vitro*, and the presence of autoimmunity.[47] The data indicate that although there is a clear *in vitro* response to leptin in some of the patients, low leptin levels *in vivo* are not predictive of a worse outcome in individuals with CVID. Furthermore, it is clear that higher serum leptin levels are not associated with increased susceptibility to inflammation; only one of four patients with clinical autoimmune disease had a leptin level >3 ng/mL. To stress this point we have unpublished data showing that production of IFN-γ by both leptin responders and nonresponders is the same among CVID patients. Furthermore,

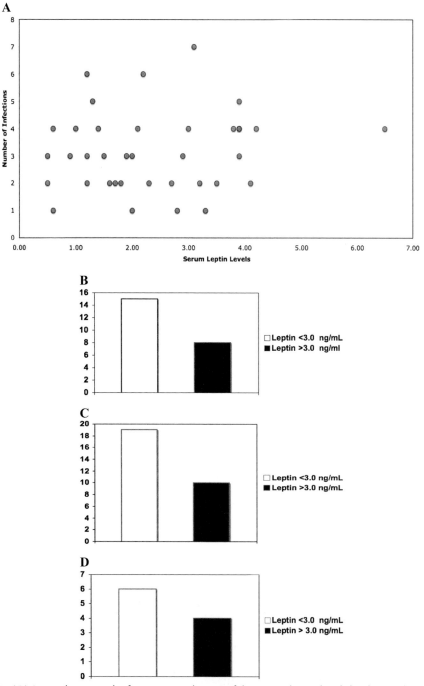

Figure 1. (**A**) Serum leptin and infection. Distribution of the serum leptin levels by the number of infectious events requiring antibiotic treatment in the patient population we studied during a period of 24 months. None of the patients required hospitalization and all but four events were respiratory tract infections. (**B**) Serum leptin and autoimmunity. Percentage of the patients with normal levels of serum leptin (above 3 ng/mL) or low level (below 3 ng/mL) and autoimmune diseases from patients included in this study ($n = 38$). (**C**) Serum leptin and allergy. Percentage of the patients with normal levels of serum leptin (above 3 ng/mL) or low level (below 3 ng/mL) and allergies from patients included in this study ($n = 38$). (**D**) Serum leptin and cancer. Percentage of the patients with normal levels of serum leptin (above 3 ng/mL) or low level (below 3 ng/mL) and cancer from patients included in this study ($n = 38$).

both the *in vitro* data pointing to a response to leptin unassociated with serum leptin levels and the *in vivo* data showing that serum leptin levels do not correlate with clinical outcome suggest that other factors must be studied in order to account for all the effects this hormone seems to have on the immune response.

One should also bear in mind that the effects of exposure to leptin were not observed uniformly in CVID patients, highlighting the complex nature of this disease. The majority, however, do seem to respond to the hormone and some even exhibit a completely restored profile with respect to the response to PHA and cytokine production. It remains to be seen if the effects of leptin on peripheral blood mononuclear cells from CVID patients are capable of rescuing B-lymphocyte function and restoring circulating IgG to normal levels. However, the number of B lymphocytes, measured in three patients, did not increase in the presence of leptin, indicating that leptin alone may not be sufficient to correct for the functional defect in the B-cell compartment.

Scientific literature points at leptin as a major player in the maintenance of inflammatory processes. However, that is clearly not the case in patients with CVID. Because this is a syndrome that may be caused by a variety of gene polymorphisms and/or defects and is triggered by a variety of environmental stimuli, it can be regarded as a interesting target to assess the importance of leptin in human immune response under different conditions. In addition, the data already available point out the need to identify the cellular and molecular players involved in the regulation of the immune response by leptin and the need to establish its cellular targets, not only by learning what regulates the leptin receptor expression in the different cell types but also if the intracellular signaling that follows this hormone/receptor interaction is the same and results in the activation of the same genes. Efforts are being made in our group to address these questions in the CVID population as well as in patients with other diseases.

Acknowledgments

This work was supported by grants from The Foundation for Aid to Research of the State of São Paulo (Fundação de Amparo a Pesquisa do Estado de São Paulo, FAPESP) and the Brazilian Science and Technology Ministry (Institutos do Milênio—MCT). A.C.G. and L.V.R. are recipients of personal grants for scientific achievement from the National Council for Scientific and Technologic Development (CNPq). J.G. is a recipient of a doctoral studentship from FAPESP. We would like to thank the patients and their relatives for their support of our research efforts as well as Drs. Cristina Kokron and Myrthes Toledo-Barros for their clinical help in tending to these and other immunodeficiency patients.

Conflicts of Interest

The authors declare no conflicts of interest.

References

1. Faggioni, R. *et al.* 2001. Leptin regulation of the immune response and the immunodeficiency of malnutrition. *Faseb J.* **15:** 2565–2571.
2. Maffei, M. *et al.* 1995. Leptin levels in human and rodent: measurement of plasma leptin and ob RNA in obese and weight-reduced subjects. *Nat. Med.* **1:** 1155–1161.
3. Otero, M. *et al.* 2005. Leptin, from fat to inflammation: old questions and new insights. *FEBS Lett.* **579:** 295–301.
4. Prentice, A.M. 1999. The thymus: a barometer of malnutrition. *Br. J. Nutr.* **81:** 345–347.
5. Howard, J.K. *et al.* 1999. Leptin protects mice from starvation-induced lymphoid atrophy and increases thymic cellularity in ob/ob mice. *J. Clin. Invest.* **104:** 1051–1059.
6. Savino, W. 2002. The thymus gland is a target in malnutrition. *Eur. J. Clin. Nutr.* **56**(Suppl 3): S46–S49.
7. Hick, R.W. *et al.* 2006. Leptin selectively augments thymopoiesis in leptin deficiency and lipopolysaccharide-induced thymic atrophy. *J. Immunol.* **177:** 169–176.
8. Lord, G.M. *et al.* 1998. Leptin modulates the T-cell immune response and reverses starvation-induced immunosuppression. *Nature* **394:** 897–901.

9. Farooqi, I.S. *et al.* 2002. Beneficial effects of leptin on obesity, T cell hyporesponsiveness, and neuroendocrine/metabolic dysfunction of human congenital leptin deficiency. *J. Clin. Invest.* **110:** 1093–1103.

10. Papathanassoglou, E. *et al.* 2006. Leptin receptor expression and signaling in lymphocytes: kinetics during lymphocyte activation, role in lymphocyte survival, and response to high fat diet in mice. *J. Immunol.* **176:** 7745–7752.

11. Macia, L. *et al.* 2006. Impairment of dendritic cell functionality and steady-state number in obese mice. *J. Immunol.* **177:** 5997–6006.

12. De Rosa, V. *et al.* (2007. A key role of leptin in the control of regulatory T cell proliferation. *Immunity* **26:** 241–255.

13. Nave, H. *et al.* 2008. Resistance of JAK-2 dependent leptin signaling in NK cells-a novel mechanism of NK cell dysfunction in diet-induced obesity. *Endocrinology* **149:** 3370–3378.

14. Tian, Z. *et al.* 2002. Impaired natural killer (NK) cell activity in leptin receptor deficient mice: leptin as a critical regulator in NK cell development and activation. *Biochem. Biophys. Res. Commun.* **298:** 297–302.

15. Palacio, A. *et al.* 2002. Leptin levels are associated with immune response in malnourished infants. *J. Clin. Endocrinol. Metab.* **87:** 3040–3046.

16. Fantuzzi, G. & R. Faggioni. 2000. Leptin in the regulation of immunity, inflammation, and hematopoiesis. *J. Leukoc. Biol.* **68:** 437–446.

17. Matarese, G. *et al.* 2005. Leptin increase in multiple sclerosis associates with reduced number of CD4(+)CD25+ regulatory T cells. *Proc. Natl. Acad. Sci. USA* **102:** 5150–5155.

18. Mattioli, B. *et al.* 2005. Leptin promotes differentiation and survival of human dendritic cells and licenses them for Th1 priming. *J. Immunol.* **174:** 6820–6828.

19. Zarkesh-Esfahani, H. *et al.* 2001. High-dose leptin activates human leukocytes via receptor expression on monocytes. *J. Immunol.* **167:** 4593–4599.

20. Santos-Alvarez, J. *et al.* 1999. Human leptin stimulates proliferation and activation of human circulating monocytes. *Cell Immunol.* **194:** 6–11.

21. Busso, N. *et al.* 2002. Leptin signaling deficiency impairs humoral and cellular immune responses and attenuates experimental arthritis. *J. Immunol.* **168:** 875–882.

22. Rodriguez, L. *et al.* 2007. Effect of leptin on activation and cytokine synthesis in peripheral blood lymphocytes of malnourished infected children. *Clin. Exp. Immunol.* **148:** 478–485.

23. Ozata, M. *et al.* 1999. Human leptin deficiency caused by a missense mutation: multiple endocrine defects, decreased sympathetic tone, and immune system dysfunction indicate new targets for leptin action, greater central than peripheral resistance to the effects of leptin, and spontaneous correction of leptin-mediated defects. *J. Clin. Endocrinol. Metab.* **84:** 3686–3695.

24. Wallace, A.M. *et al.* 2000. The co-ordinated cytokine/hormone response to acute injury incorporates leptin. *Cytokine* **12:** 1042–1045.

25. Torpy, D.J. *et al.* 1998. Leptin and interleukin-6 in sepsis. *Horm. Metab. Res.* **30:** 726–729.

26. Bornstein, S.R. *et al.* 1998. Plasma leptin levels are increased in survivors of acute sepsis: associated loss of diurnal rhythm, in cortisol and leptin secretion. *J. Clin. Endocrinol. Metab.* **83:** 280–283.

27. Salzer, U. & B. Grimbacher. 2006. Common variable immunodeficiency: the power of co-stimulation. *Semin. Immunol.* **18:** 337–346.

28. Grunfeld, C. *et al.* 1996. Serum leptin levels in the acquired immunodeficiency syndrome. *J. Clin. Endocrinol. Metab.* **81:** 4342–4346.

29. Taleb, S. *et al.* 2007. Defective leptin/leptin receptor signaling improves regulatory T cell immune response and protects mice from atherosclerosis. *Arterioscler Thromb. Vasc. Biol.* **27:** 2691–2698.

30. Anders, H.J. *et al.* 1999. Leptin serum levels are not correlated with disease activity in patients with rheumatoid arthritis. *Metabolism* **48:** 745–748.

31. Hoppin, A.G. *et al.* 1998. Serum leptin in children and young adults with inflammatory bowel disease. *J. Pediatr. Gastroenterol. Nutr.* **26:** 500–505.

32. Cunningham-Rundles, C. & C. Bodian. 1999. Common variable immunodeficiency: clinical and immunological features of 248 patients. *Clin. Immunol.* **92:** 34–48.

33. Sneller, M.C. 2001. Common variable immunodeficiency. *Am. J. Med. Sci.* **321:** 42–48.

34. Farrington, M. *et al.* 1994. CD40 ligand expression is defective in a subset of patients with common variable immunodeficiency. *Proc. Natl. Acad. Sci. USA* **91:** 1099–1103.

35. Thon, V. *et al.* 1997. Defective integration of activating signals derived from the T cell receptor (TCR) and costimulatory molecules in both CD4+ and CD8+ T lymphocytes of common variable immunodeficiency (CVID) patients. *Clin. Exp. Immunol.* **110:** 174–181.

36. Brouet, J.C. *et al.* 2000. Study of the B cell memory compartment in common variable immunodeficiency. *Eur. J. Immunol.* **30:** 2516–2520.

37. Thon, V. *et al.* 1997. Antigen presentation by common variable immunodeficiency (CVID) B cells and monocytes is unimpaired. *Clin. Exp. Immunol.* **108:** 1–8.

38. Randall, T.D. *et al.* 1993. Interleukin-5 (IL-5) and IL-6 define two molecularly distinct pathways of B-cell differentiation. *Mol. Cell Biol.* **13:** 3929–3936.

39. Wurster, A.L. *et al.* 2002. Interleukin-4-mediated protection of primary B cells from apoptosis through Stat6-dependent up-regulation of Bcl-xL. *J. Biol. Chem.* **277:** 27169–27175.

40. Arpin, C. *et al.* 1995. Generation of memory B cells and plasma cells in vitro. *Science* **268:** 720–722.

41. North, M.E. *et al.* 1996. Intracellular cytokine production by human CD4+ and CD8+ T cells from normal and immunodeficient donors using directly conjugated anti-cytokine antibodies and three-colour flow cytometry. *Clin. Exp. Immunol.* **105:** 517–522.

42. Kokron, C.M. *et al.* 2004. Clinical and laboratory aspects of common variable immunodeficiency. *An. Acad. Bras. Cienc.* **76:** 707–726.

43. Sneller, M.C. & W. Strober. 1990. Abnormalities of lymphokine gene expression in patients with common variable immunodeficiency. *J. Immunol.* **144:** 3762–3769.

44. Goldberg, A.C. *et al.* 2005. Exogenous leptin restores in vitro T cell proliferation and cytokine synthesis in patients with common variable immunodeficiency syndrome. *Clin. Immunol.* **114:** 147–153.

45. Rosen, F.S. *et al.* 1995. The primary immunodeficiencies. *N. Engl. J. Med.* **333:** 431–440.

46. Ahima, R.S. *et al.* 1996. Role of leptin in the neuroendocrine response to fasting. *Nature* **382:** 250–252.

47. Lopes-da-Silva, S. & L.V. Rizzo. 2008. Autoimmunity in common variable immunodeficiency. *J. Clin. Immunol.* **28:** S46–S55.

The Immune–Pineal Axis

Stress as a Modulator of Pineal Gland Function

Renato Couto-Moraes,[a,b] João Palermo-Neto,[b] and Regina Pekelmann Markus[a]

[a]Laboratory of Chronopharmacology, Department of Physiology, Institute of Bioscience, Universidade de São Paulo, Sao Paulo, Brazil

[b]Laboratory of Neuroimunomodulation, Department of Pathology, School of Veterinary Medicine, Universidade de São Paulo, Sao Paulo, Brazil

The temporal organization of mammals presents a daily adjustment to the environmental light/dark cycle. The environmental light detected by the retina adjusts the central clock in the suprachiasmatic nuclei, which innervate the pineal gland through a polysynaptic pathway. During the night, this gland produces and releases the nocturnal hormone melatonin, which circulates throughout the whole body and adjusts several bodily functions according to the existence and duration of darkness. We have previously shown that during the time frame of an inflammatory response, pro-inflammatory cytokines, such as tumor necrosis factor-α, inhibit while anti-inflammatory mediators, such as glucocorticoids, enhance the synthesis of melatonin, interfering in the daily adjustment of the light/dark cycle. Therefore, injury disconnects the organism from environmental cycling, while recovery restores the light/dark information to the whole organism. Here, we extend these observations by evaluating the effect of a mild restraint stress, which did not induce macroscopic gastric lesions. After 2 h of restraint, there was an increase in circulating corticosterone, indicating activation of the hypothalamus–pituitary–adrenal (HPA) axis. In parallel, an increase in melatonin production was observed. Taking into account the data obtained with models of inflammation and stress, we reinforce the hypothesis that the activity of the pineal gland is modulated by the state of the immune system and the HPA axis, implicating the darkness hormone melatonin as a modulator of defense responses.

Key words: pineal gland; melatonin; corticosterone; stress; restraint

Introduction

The pineal organ is a unique gland located in the wall of the third ventricle. It is part of the circumventricular organs and interacts with molecules present in the blood as well as the cerebrospinal fluid.[1] Its main hormone, melatonin, is produced at night and is therefore known as the chemical transducer of darkness. Mediators of inflammation (cytokines and glucocorticoids) modulate pineal function, leading to the suppression (pro-inflammatory cytokines) or potentiation (glucocorticoids) of nocturnal melatonin synthesis.[2] Stress, the current term for the "general adaptation syndrome" proposed by Hans Selye in 1936,[3] activates the hypothalamus–pituitary (hypophysis)–adrenal (HPA) axis, leading to a sustained tonus of corticosterone release.[4] Stressful conditions that result in increasing glucocorticoid plasma levels should increase the nocturnal melatonin surge. However, the effect of corticosterone on noradrenaline (NA)-induced melatonin production follows a bell-shaped curve,[5] therefore a mild but not severe stress increases corticosterone plasma levels and enhances the production of melatonin.

Address for correspondence: Regina P. Markus, Universidade de São Paulo, Instituto de Biociências, Departamento de Fisiologia, Rua do Matão, travessa 14, 321, sala 323, Sao Paulo, SP, 05508-900, Brazil. Voice: +55-11-3091-7612; fax: +55-11-3091-8095. rpmarkus@usp.br

Neuroimmunomodulation: Ann. N.Y. Acad. Sci. 1153: 193–202 (2009).
doi: 10.1111/j.1749-6632.2008.03978.x © 2009 New York Academy of Sciences.

Pineal and Extra-pineal Sources of Melatonin

Melatonin, a highly soluble hormone, is derived from serotonin (5-HT). It is known as the hormone of darkness because it is synthesized in a rhythmic manner by the pineal gland, with peak levels synthesized at night. Extra-pineal sources that synthesize melatonin in a constitutive or inducible manner do not contribute to pineal diurnal rhythms. They are responsible for increasing melatonin in specific regions and are therefore responsible for the shuttle between the endocrine and paracrine production of melatonin.[2]

In the pineal gland, the synthesis of melatonin is triggered by sympathetic outflow in response to darkness-mediated activation of the suprachiasmatic nuclei, which send information to the paraventricular nucleus (PVN) of the hypothalamus and then to the intermedial lateral column of the spinal cord. NA regulates the activity of the key enzyme that converts 5-HT into N-acetylserotonin (NAS), the immediate precursor of melatonin.[6] The acetylation of 5-HT and the methylation of NAS are catalyzed by the enzymes N-arylalkyltransferase (AA-NAT) and hydroxy-indol-O-methyltransferase (HIOMT), respectively. The transcription of the gene and/or the activity of the enzyme are strictly regulated by activation of $\beta 1$-adrenoceptors[7] and a cyclic adenosine monophosphate (AMP)–protein kinsase A (PKA)–cyclic-AMP response element binding (CREB) pathway and are modulated by the activation of receptors that trigger the Ca/PKC pathway, such as $\alpha 1$-adrenoceptors and P2Y$_1$ purinergic receptors.[8,9] Both NA and ATP are co-released by activation of the neurons that innervate the rat pineal gland.[10] In addition to the sympathetic input, which is responsible for the onset of melatonin synthesis, a neural projection directly from the central structures modulates pineal activity. Several neurotransmitters, such as glutamate, γ-aminobutyric acid, acetylcholine, vasoactive intestinal peptide, pituitary adenylate cyclase-activating peptide, and sub-

stance P, are involved in direct central modulation.[11]

Extra-pineal nonrhythmic synthesis of melatonin can be constitutive or inducible.[2] Melatonin is synthesized in the gastrointestinal tract in a nonrhythmic constitutive manner and plays a role in the protection of the gastric mucosa from its acidic milieu. The level in the jejunum exceeds 500 pg/mL, while the concentration in the plasma at night reaches 40–100 pg/mL.[12] The enterochromaffin cells of the digestive mucosa, which are rich in 5-HT, are the most probable origin of melatonin.

The immune-competent cells are good examples of cells that may be induced to produce melatonin. Activation of mononuclear and polymorphonuclear cells from the blood and the colostrum of humans and rodents induces the synthesis of melatonin.[2] In colostral phagocytes we have shown that the production of melatonin is strictly triggered by the injury stimulus. We incubated cells with *Escherichia coli* enteropatogenic bacteria. The temporal profile of melatonin production follows the phagocytosis and killing of the bacteria (i.e., melatonin production ends after all the bacteria have been phagocytosed).[13]

Pineal Melatonin Production Is Subject to Environmental and Endogenous Control

The classical control of pineal melatonin production by the environmental light/dark cycle is modified during the development of an inflammatory response because the mediators of inflammation found in the plasma interfere with pineal melatonin synthesis.

The rat pineal gland expresses glucocorticoid receptors (GRs), which mediate the potentiation of NA-induced melatonin production in cultured pineal glands[5] and in rats.[14] The effect of corticosterone follows a bell-shaped curve; therefore, while concentrations around 1–10 μmol/L enhance NA-induced melatonin production, a concentration of 100 μmol/L has no effect. With regard to its mechanism of action, corticosterone acts through the GRs and the nuclear factor kappa B (NF-κB) pathway[5] and enhances the transcription of the *aa-nat* gene.[15] In summary, circulating corticosterone could play a role in modulating the nocturnal melatonin surge.

Previous results obtained from mice with chronic inflammation reinforce the idea that increased tonus of adrenal cortex hormone release is of the utmost importance for maintaining the nocturnal melatonin surge. The characteristics of a chronic lesion of a mouse paw induced by a single injection of tuberculosis bacillus (BCG-Calmette-Guérin bacillus) show cyclical daily variations with a reduction of the edema during the night. This daily rhythm is abolished by constant light or pinealectomy and is restored by nocturnal administration of melatonin.[16] Adrenalectomy (surgical or pharmacological by metirapone) also abolishes the diurnal rhythm of the lesion, and this effect is restored by nocturnal administration of melatonin.[17] In order to prove that adrenalectomy abolishes the nocturnal rise in melatonin, we measured the excretion of its main metabolite in the urine. Our results showed that the nocturnal rise in 6-sulfatoximelatonin excretion was abolished by adrenalectomy (i.e., day and night values were not significantly different when a tonus of corticosterone was absent).[17] Therefore, the nocturnal rise of melatonin in the presence of a chronic inflammatory response requires not only sympathetic neural input but also a glucocorticoid tonus.

The nocturnal production of melatonin is also modulated by cytokines that interfere with the NF-κB pathway.[2] Tumor necrosis factor (TNF)-α inhibits the NA-induced transcription of the *aa-nat* gene and the production of NAS. In addition, in women with acute inflammation (mastitis), suppression of the nocturnal melatonin surge is significantly correlated with an increase in circulating TNF-α. At the beginning of inflammation when TNF-α values are high, the nocturnal surge of melatonin is suppressed, and as soon as TNF-α levels return to

values that are below detection, the nocturnal melatonin surge is restored.[13,18]

In summary, both pro- and anti-inflammatory mediators modulate the nocturnal melatonin surge, with pro-inflammatory mediators reducing or even suppressing melatonin production and anti-inflammatory mediators increasing pineal activity, at least within a certain concentration range (Fig. 1).

Pineal Melatonin Imposes a Daily Rhythm in Neural and Defense Responses

The nocturnal rise in melatonin is important for establishing the difference between day and night as well as between the seasons.[6] The nocturnal pineal rise imposes a daily rhythm upon several bodily functions.

Pinealectomy of newborn rats changes the thymus architecture.[19] The reduction in vascular permeability seen at night is not observed after pinealectomy or when the animals are maintained in constant light.[16] This rhythm can be restored by nocturnal administration of melatonin. The reduction in vascular permeability is accompanied by a melatonin-induced reduction of the rolling and adherence of leukocytes to the endothelial layer[20] as a result of a direct effect on endothelial cells.[21] Melatonin is known to block endothelial nitric oxide synthase activation induced by bradykinin,[22] 5-HT, acetylcholine, and activated P2Y$_1$ purinergic receptors.[23]

These effects protect the body against spurious activation of leukocytes. In contrast, when an inflammatory response is mounted, the central production of melatonin is suppressed. This allows full activation of the system, independently of the time of day.

With regard to the nervous system, melatonin imposes a diurnal rhythm in the response to a certain subtype of nicotinic acetylcholine receptors (nAChRs). In all tissues studied (sympathetic nerve terminals, retina, cerebellum, skeletal muscle), the effect of

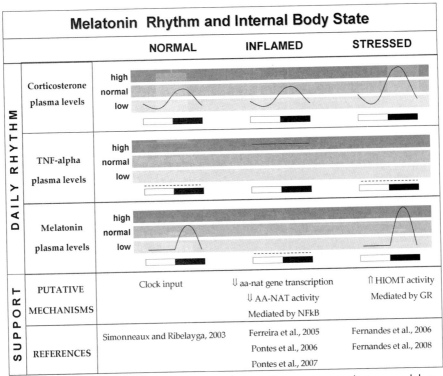

Figure 1. Scheme showing that pro- and anti-inflammatory mediators modulate the nocturnal melatonin surge. The adrenal hormone corticosterone potentiates, while the pro-inflammatory cytokine tumor necrosis factor (TNF)-α inhibits, noradrenaline (NA)-induced melatonin (MEL) production in cultured rat pineal glands.[2] Abbreviations: *aa-nat* gene and AA-NAT enzyme, N-aryl-alkyltransferase; NF-κB, nuclear factor kappa B; HIOMT, hydroxy-indole-O-methyltransferase; GR, glucocorticoid receptor.

melatonin is restricted to the receptors sensitive to α-bungarotoxin.[24–28] These receptors include the classic receptors found in the skeletal muscle end plate and the homomeric receptors in neural tissues. Melatonin increases the release of NA and ATP induced by activation of presynaptic nAChRs located in the extremities of sympathetic nerve terminals,[29,30] the release of glutamate in cerebellum slices,[6] and the activity of cultured retinas.[27]

As melatonin is released at night in almost all living organisms, this hormone is also important for organizing the relationships between species. We have previously shown that the nocturnal melatonin surge synchronizes parasite life cycles in mammalian hosts.[31,32]

Besides being a chronobiotic substance, melatonin has other effects, acting as an antioxidant[33,34] and an anti-apoptotic factor.[35]

Stress

As early as ancient times the Greeks explored the interaction between body and mind. In the Christian era, Galeno (129–200 AD) observed that melancholic women were more susceptible to breast cancer than sanguine women.[36] In the Modern era, Calzolari (1898; cited by Ref. 37) showed that gonadal hormones influence thymic cellularity. In the last century, Hans Selye (1936)[3] established the concept of "general adaptation syndrome," which was more recently termed *stress*.[38] The history surrounding the research examining stress, mainly in the 20th century, has been previously discussed in a review by Lazarus (1993).[39]

Stress can be classified into two main categories: (1) physical (or systemic) stress and (2) psychological (or processive) stress. Physical stress is secondary to noxious stimuli, such as hemorrhage and immune challenge. Psychological stress is caused by stimuli that indicate immediate or future risks; examples include social conflict, an aversive environment, and the presence of or signals of predators, restraint, and noise.[40] The stress response elicits activation of the HPA axis and sympathetic nervous system.[41,42] The basic mechanisms of stress are well conserved along the phylogenetic scale, characterizing a stereotypical response from invertebrates to superior vertebrates.[43]

Briefly, stressful stimuli activate the PVN of the hypothalamus, which produces and releases corticotropin-releasing factor. This molecule stimulates the production and release of adrenocorticotropic hormone by the hypophysis, which acts on the adrenal glands, inducing the production and release of glucocorticoids.[4] The main glucocorticoid in humans is cortisol, while in rats it is corticosterone. Although psychological and physical stresses activate different areas in the central nervous system, the HPA axis is the common output. Therefore, the PVN is the common hypothalamic nucleus for controlling the adrenal and pineal glands.

Corticosterone and cortisol interact with either GRs or mineralocorticoid receptors; however, their low affinity for GRs leads these receptors to be only activated in response to stressful stimuli.[44,45] Immune and neural cells are known to express GRs.[46] It is interesting to note that certain structures that project onto the PVN, such as the hippocampus, amygdala, and limbic system, express detectable amounts of GRs.[47–50] Therefore, glucocorticoids regulate PVN activity either by activating GRs located in this nucleus or by interfering with the input from previous structures that also express GRs.

The Pineal Gland as a Target for Stress

Taking into account the fact that the PVN controls the adrenal and pineal glands, it is pos-sible that glucocorticoids interfere with pineal activity by acting on the PVN. However, it was recently shown that the pineal gland expresses high levels of GRs[5] and is therefore a good target for glucocorticoids increased by stress. In 1993, Del-Bel and colleagues[51] presented the first evidence that stress interferes directly with pineal function by showing that immobilization stress or vibrissae cutting increased the expression of c-FOS in rat pineal glands. More recently, it was shown that restraint stress decreases c-FOS expression in the PVN, and this reduction is observed until 1 week after restraint.[52]

There is no direct evidence to show that the pineal gland plays a role in modulation of the stress response similar to that shown for the inflammatory response.[2] Here, we explored this question by analyzing the effect of restraint stress on the production of NAS and melatonin by rat pineal glands.

Rats (3–4 months old) maintained in a 12 h/12 h light/dark cycle environment with lights on at 06:00 h were restrained in an apparatus for 30 min or 2 h between 15:00 to 17:50 h. The apparatus was ventilated and did not cause physical compression, avoiding hyperthermia and sudoresis. Light was perceived through a transparent lid (Fig. 2). The experimental controls were the so-called naive animals, which were not experimentally manipulated. These isolated animals were individually housed in cages for the same amount of time that the experimental animals were restrained (30 min or 2 h). Animals were euthanized right after (17:00 h) or 6–8 h after (00:30–01:30 h) the stress was applied. The corticosterone serum levels were measured by radioimmunoassay (RIA; animals euthanized at the light phase), and the pineal melatonin and NAS content was measured by HPLC (animals euthanized at the dark phase).

The animals used in this study were maintained in accordance with the guidelines of the Bioethical Committee on Care and Use of Laboratory Animal Resources of the Faculdade de Medicina Veterinária, Universidade de São

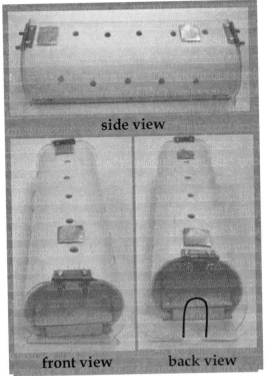

side view

front view back view

Figure 2. The apparatus for rat restraint was constructed according to methods described by Ref. 63. The apparatus has lines of holes in the upper and lateral parts, as can be seen in the side view. This impairs hyperthermia and sudoresis, characterizing the method of restraint as a psychological stress according to Ref. 63. In the front view, a transparent lid for light perception is shown. In the back view, there is a re-entrance that allows a space for freeing the animal's tail. This kind of apparatus is considered to impose a psychological stress that mimics confinement.[64]

Paulo (Number Protocol: 1113/2007), which are similar to those of the National Research Council, Washington, DC.

In order to classify the magnitude of stress, we performed gross examination of the stomachs of the animals. No signs of tissue pathology were observed in any animals in any of the groups. Therefore, this stress model was classified as mild stress.

The levels of corticosterone in the naive animals (177.19 ± 23.51 ng/mL), measured at 17:00 h, were compatible with those found in the literature for the same hour of the day.[53]

Restraint for 2 h resulted in a significant increase in corticosterone levels of 2.14 times the levels of control animals (Fig. 3A).

Pineal NAS content was not different in restrained animals compared to the isolated animals. Pineal melatonin content (ng/pineal) was half the level in animals restrained for 30 min (1.7 ± 0.2) compared to animals restrained for 2 h (3.3 ± 0.6), while no effect of time was detected for the isolated control animals (Fig. 3B).

This data reinforces the hypothesis that body status contributes directly or indirectly to the activity of the pineal gland because we observed a direct correlation between the corticosterone increase right after stress and the nocturnal melatonin surge at midnight.

The Pineal Gland as a Sensor of Different Types of Stress

Although each type of stress (physical or psychological) may result in different changes in the central nervous system,[54] the peripheral response is stereotypical as it is mediated by the activation of the HPA axis.[48] Therefore, the stress response is influenced by cross-talk with the immune system because stress can modulate the immune system; however, the immune system can also modulate the HPA axis (review by Ref. 55).

Here, we show that there is an elevation of corticosterone and melatonin in a model of mild stress, characterized by the lack of induction of gastric ulcers. These data, when compared to those obtained after acute inflammation (i.e., a suppression of the nocturnal melatonin surge)[13,18,56] may at a first glance suggest that there is a conflict between the psychological and physical stresses in terms of the effects on the pineal gland. However, it is important to point out that the restraint stress imposed in this study was unlikely to have increased the levels of TNF-α, which is the cytokine that inhibits NA-induced melatonin production by mechanisms that have previously been explained.[5] Therefore, the magnitude of stress, instead of

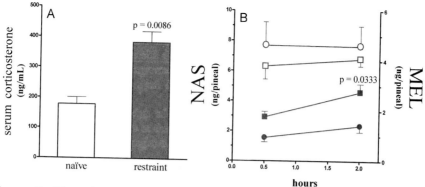

Figure 3. Effect of stress on circulating corticosterone (**A**) and pineal indolamines (**B**). (**A**) Restraint stress increases serum corticosterone levels. Blood collected in plastic tubes maintained on ice just after the introduction of stress (17:00 h) was centrifuged (5000 g, 15 min, 25°C). The serum was stored at −80°C for no more than 1 month before determination of corticosterone levels by radioimmunoassay (RIA) (ImmuChem ^{125}[I] corticosterone RIA; MP Biomedicals, Inc., Costa Mesa, CA). The results are expressed as the mean ± SEM (n = 3 animals per group). The data were analyzed by the Student's *t*-test. (**B**) Restraint stress increases the pineal melatonin (MEL) content. Pineal tissue collected 6–8 h after the introduction of stress (00:30–01:30 h) was stored at −80°C for no more than 1 month before determination of N-acetylserotonin (NAS) and MEL levels by HPLC under specific conditions, as previously described by Ref. 8. The results are expressed as mean ± SEM (n = 5 animals per group). Open symbols refer to NAS, closed symbols refer to MEL, squares refer to restraint animals, and circles refer to isolated animals. Data were analyzed by linear regression. $P = 0.0333$ compared to the restrained animals for 30 min.

the type of stress, appears to be the factor that induces a suppression of the nocturnal pineal melatonin surge.

Other forms of stress, such as immobilization, in addition to activating the HPA axis also lead to an increase in TNF-α in the plasma[57] and central nervous system.[58,59] Similarly, elevated serum levels of TNF-α are also observed in hypothermic conditions.[60] These situations (immobilization and hypothermia) are accompanied by a rise in the adrenal anti-inflammatory hormone corticosterone and in the pro-inflammatory cytokine TNF-α.

Another important factor is that restraint stress induced an increase in melatonin but not in its precursor NAS. Corticosterone increases NA-induced NAS production by inhibiting the transcription factor NF-κB,[5] which is activated by TNF-α.[15] TNF-α inhibits the transcription of the gene and the production of AA-NAT in cultured pineal glands. In the model used in this study, there was no effect of corticosterone on NAS production, reinforcing the suggestion

that the magnitude of the stress was not sufficient to induce TNF-α production.

Regarding the increase in nocturnal melatonin, the intrapineal perfusion of corticosterone, in a dose compatible for mild stress, increased the rise in nocturnal melatonin release. Moreover, cultured pineal glands challenged with the same amount of corticosterone showed an increase in HIOMT with no change in AA-NAT activity,[14] which is in accordance with an increase in melatonin with no change in NAS. Therefore, taking our data, together with those that describe the effects of cytokines and glucocorticoids on pineal function,[2] we suggest that psychological stress in rats may modulate pineal gland function.

In summary, we observed an enhancement in the nocturnal melatonin surge in rats submitted to mild stress induced by restraining the animal in an apparatus. This effect was not accompanied by the development of gastric lesions. The mild stress activated the HPA axis and increased plasma corticosterone levels, which, by acting on HIOMT activity, led to an increase in the nocturnal melatonin level. Therefore, psychological stresses may modulate pineal function.

Conclusion

This study confirmed the existence of an inter-relationship between the adrenal and pineal glands. This communication opens an avenue with the realization that, in addition to indolamine melatonin, the pineal gland can act as a sensor and a player in disease states. We and others have previously shown that melatonin is able to modulate injured areas and control cellular activity as a result of its ability to block the hallmark pathway of inflammation (NF-κB-mediated inflammation),[61] to act as an antioxidant,[33] and to inhibit the migration of immune-competent cells.[20,21] However, we[2] and others[62] have proposed that the pineal gland is a target for signaling molecules of stress and inflammatory processes as well. These findings implicate the pineal gland as a sensor of the state of the organism. This paper reinforces this concept, showing that restraint stress enhances the nocturnal pineal surge.

Acknowledgments

This work was supported by Fundação de Amparo à Pesquisa do Estado de São Paulo (FAPESP, 2002/02957-6) and Conselho Nacional de Desenvolvimento Científico e Tecnológico (CNPq, 484206/2006-0; 301171/2006-8). R.C.-M. is a graduate fellow of FAPESP (2007/01602-3); J.P.-N. and R.P.M. are researcher fellows of CNPq. We gratefully acknowledge the helpful assistance of Professor Zulma S. Ferreira (Institute of Bioscience, Universidade de São Paulo). The technical assistance of Alex A. Monteiro and Débora A. Moura is also gratefully acknowledged.

Conflicts of Interest

The authors declare no conflicts of interest.

References

1. Duvernoy, H.M. & P.Y. Risold. 2007. The circumventricular organs: an atlas of comparative anatomy and vascularization. *Brain Res. Rev.* **56:** 119–147.
2. Markus, R.P., Z.S. Ferreira, P.A. Fernandes & E. Cecon. 2007. The immune-pineal axis: a shuttle between endocrine and paracrine melatonin. *Neuroimmunomodulation* **14:** 126–133.
3. Selye, H. 1936. A syndrome produced by diverse nocuous agents. *Nature* **138:** 32.
4. Herman, J.P., H. Figueiredo, N.K. Mueller, *et al.* 2003. Central mechanisms of stress integration: hierarchical circuitry controlling hypothalamo–pituitary–adrenocortical responsiveness. *Front. Neuroendocrinol.* **24:** 151–180.
5. Ferreira, Z.S., P.A. Fernandes, D. Duma, *et al.* 2005. Corticosterone modulates noradrenaline-induced melatonin synthesis through inhibition of nuclear factor kappa B. *J. Pineal Res.* **38:** 182–188.
6. Markus, R.P. 2003. Ritmos biológicos: entendendo as horas, os dias e as estações do ano. *Einstein* **1:** 140–145.
7. Klein, D.C., D.A. Auerbach & J.L. Weller. 1981. Seesaw signal processing in pineal cells: homologous sensitization of adrenergic stimulation of cyclic GMP accompanies homologous desentization of B-adrenergic stimulation of cycle AMP. *Proc. Natl. Acad. Sci. USA* **78:** 4625–4629.
8. Ferreira, Z.S., J. Cipolla-Neto & R.P. Markus. 1994. Presence of P2-purinoceptors in the rat pineal gland. *Br. J. Pharmacol.* **112:** 107–110.
9. Ferreira, Z.S. & R.P. Markus. 2001. Characterization of P2Y1-like receptor in cultured rat pineal glands. *Eur. J. Pharmacol.* **415:** 151–156.
10. Barbosa E.J.M, Z.S. Ferreira & R.P. Markus. 2000. Purinergic and noradrenergic cotransmission in the rat pineal gland. *Eur. J. Pharmacol.* **401:** 59–62.
11. Simonneaux, V. & C. Ribelayga. 2003. Generation of the melatonin endocrine message in mammals: a review of the complex regulation of melatonin synthesis by norepinephrine, peptides, and other pineal transmitters. *Pharmacol. Ver.* **55:** 325–395.
12. Bubenik, G.A. 2002. Gastrointestinal melatonin: localization, function, and clinical relevance. *Dig. Dis. Sci.* **47:** 2336–2348.
13. Pontes, G.N., E.C. Cardoso, M.M.S. Carneiro-Sampaio & R.P. Markus. 2006. Injury switches melatonin production source from endocrine (pineal) to paracrine (phagocytes)—melatonin in human colostrums and colostrums phagocytes. *J. Pineal Res.* **41:** 136–141.
14. Fernandes, P.A. *et al.* 2008. Local corticosterone infusion enhances nocturnal pineal melatonin production in vivo. *J. Neuroendocrinol.:* Dec 6. [Epub

ahead of print] 10.1111/j.1365-2826.2008.01817.x. PMID: 19076264.

15. Fernandes, P.A., E. Cecon, R.P. Markus & Z.S. Ferreira. 2006. Effect of TNF-α on the melatonin synthetic pathway in the rat pineal gland: basis for a 'feedback' of the immune response on circadian timing. *J. Pineal Res.* **41:** 344–350.

16. Lopes, C., J.L. Delyra, R.P. Markus & M. Mariano. 1997. Circadian rhythm in experimental granulomatous inflammation is modulated by melatonin. *J. Pineal Res.* **23:** 72–78.

17. Lopes, C., M. Mariano & R.P. Markus. 2001. Interaction between the adrenal and the pineal gland in chronic experimental inflammation induced by BCG in mice. *Inflamm. Res.* **50:** 6–11.

18. Pontes, G.N., E.C. Cardoso, M.M.S. Carneiro-Sampaio & R.P. Markus. 2007. Pineal melatonin and the innate immune response: the TNF-alpha increase after cesarean section suppresses nocturnal melatonin production. *J. Pineal Res.* **43:** 365–371.

19. Csaba, G. & P. Barath. 1975. Morphological changes of thymus and the thyroid gland after postnatal extirpation of pineal body. *Endocrinol. Exp.* **9:** 59–67.

20. Lotufo, C.M.C., C. Lopes, M.L. Dubocovich, *et al*. 2001. Melatonin and N-acetylserotonin inhibit leukocyte rolling and adhesion to rat microcirculation. *Eur. J. Pharmacol.* **430:** 351–357.

21. Lotufo, C.M.C., C.E. Yamashita, S.H.P. Farsky & R.P. Markus. 2006. Melatonin effect on endothelial cells reduces vascular permeability increase induced by leukotriene B4. *Eur. J. Pharmacol.* **534:** 258–263.

22. Tamura, E.K., C.L. Silva & R.P. Markus. 2006. Melatonin inhibits endothelial nitric oxide production in vitro. *J. Pineal Res.* **41:** 267–274.

23. Silva, C.L., E.K. Tamura, S.M. Macedo, *et al*. 2007. Melatonin inhibits nitric oxide production by microvascular endothelial cells in vivo and in vitro. *Br. J. Pharmacol.* **151:** 195–205.

24. Carneiro, R.C.G., E.P. Pereira, Cipolla-Neto & R.P. Markus. 1993. Age-related changes in melatonin modulation of sympathetic neurotransmission. *J. Pharmacol. Exp. Ther.* **267:** 1536–1540.

25. Markus, R.P., W.M. Zago & R.C.G. Carneiro. 1996. Melatonin modulation of presynaptic nicotinic acethylcholine receptors in the rat vas deferens. *J. Pharmacol. Exp. Ther.* **27:** 18–22.

26. Reno, L.A.C., W.M. Zago & R.P. Markus. 2004. Release of [(3)H]-l-glutamate by stimulation of nicotinic acetylcholine receptors in rat cerebellar slices. *Neuroscience* **124:** 647–653.

27. Sampaio, L.F.S., D. Hamassaki-Britto & R.P. Markus. 2005. Influence of melatonin on the development of functional nicotinic acetylcholine receptors in cultured chick retinal cells. *Braz. J. Med. Biol. Res.* **38:** 603–613.

28. Almeida-Paula, L.D., L.V. Costa-Lotufo, A.E.G. Monteiro, *et al*. 2005. Melatonin modulates rat myotube-acetylcholine receptors by inhibiting calmodulin. *Eur. J. Pharmacol.* **525:** 24–31.

29. Carneiro, R.C.G. & R.P. Markus. 1990. Presynaptic nicotinic receptors involved in the release of noradrenaline and ATP from the prostatic portion of the rat vas deferens. *J. Pharmacol. Exp. Ther.* **255:** 95–100.

30. Carneiro, R.C.G., J. Cipolla-Neto & R.P. Markus. 1991. Diurnal variation of the rat vas deferens contraction induced by stimulation of presynaptic nicotinic receptors and pineal function. *J. Pharmacol. Exp. Ther.* **259:** 614–619.

31. Hotta, C.T., M.L. Gazarini, F.H. Beraldo, *et al*. 2000. Calcium-dependent modulation by melatonin of the circadian rhythm in malarial parasites. *Nat. Cell Biol.* **2:** 466–468.

32. Garcia, C.R., R.P. Markus & L. Madeira. 2001. Tertian and quartan fevers: temporal regulation in malarial infection. *J. Biol. Rhythms* **16:** 436–443.

33. Cuzzocrea, S. & R.J. Reiter. 2001. Pharmacological action of melatonin in shock, inflammation and ischemia/reperfusion injury injury. *Eur. J. Pharmacol.* **426:** 1–10.

34. Hardeland, R. 2005. Antioxidative protection by melatonin: multiplicity of mechanisms from radical detoxification to radical avoidance. *Endocrine* **27:** 119–130.

35. Srinivasan, V., S.R. Pandi-Perumal, G.J. Maestroni, *et al*. 2005. Role of melatonin in neurodegenerative diseases. *Neutox. Res.* **7:** 293–318.

36. Dunn, A.J. 1988. Nervous system-immune system interactions: an overview. *J. Recept. Res.* **8:** 589–607.

37. Lawrence, D.A. & D. Kim. 2000. Central/peripheral nervous system and immune responses. *Toxicology* **142:** 189–201.

38. Neylan, T.C. 1998. Hans Selye and the field of stress research. *J. Neuropsychiatr.* **10:** 230–231.

39. Lazarus, R.S. 1993. From psychologicals stress to the emotions: history of changing outlooks. *Annu. Rev. Psychol.* **44:** 1–21.

40. Sawchenko, P.E., E.R. Brown, R.K. Chan, *et al*. 1996. The paraventricular nucleus of the hypothalamus and the functional neuroanatomy of visceromotor responses to stress. *Prog. Brain Res.* **107:** 201–222.

41. Lapiz, M.D., Y. Mateo, T. Parker & C. Marsed. 2000. Effects of noradrenaline depletion in the brain on response on novelty in isolation reared rats. *Psychopharmacology* **152:** 312–320.

42. McEwen, B.S. 2000. Effects of adverse experiences for brain structure and function. *Biol. Psychiatry* **48:** 721–731.

43. Ottaviani, E., A. Franchini, E. Caselgrandi, *et al*. 1994. Relationship between corticotropin-releasing

factor and interleukin-2: evolutionary evidence. *FEBS Lett.* **351:** 19–21.

44. Müller, M., F. Holsboer & M.E. Keck. 2002. Genetic modification of corticosteroid receptor signalling: novel insights into pathophysiology and treatment strategies of human affective disorders. *Neuropeptides* **36:** 117–131.

45. Rhen, T. & J.A. Cidlowski. 2005. Antiinflammatory action of glucocorticoids—new mechanisms for old drugs. *N. Engl. J. Med.* **353:** 1711–1723.

46. Marchetti, B., M.C. Morale, N. Testa, *et al.* 2001. Stress, the immune system and vulnerability to degenerative disorders of the central nervous system in transgenic mice expressing glucocorticoid receptor antisense RNA. *Brain Res. Brain Res. Rev.* **37:** 259–272.

47. Davis, M. 1992. The role of the amygdala in fear and anxiety. *Annu. Rev. Neurosci.* **15:** 353–375.

48. Heuser, I. & C.H. Lammers. 2003. Stress and the brain. *Neurobiol. Aging* **24:** 69–76.

49. Herman, J.P. & W.E. Cullinan. 1997. Neurocircitry of stress: central control of the hypothalamo-pituitary-adrenocortical axis. *Trends Neurosci.* **20:** 78–84.

50. Korte, S.M. 2001. Corticosteroids in relation to fear, anxiety and psychopathology. *Neurosci. Biobehav. Rev.* **25:** 117–142.

51. Del-Bel, E.A., R. Titze-De-Almeida, H. Shida, *et al.* 1993. Induction of the c-FOS proto-oncogene in the rat pineal gland during stress. *Braz. J. Med. Biol. Res.* **26:** 975–981.

52. Vallès, A., O. Martí & A. Armario. 2003. Long-term effects of a single exposure to immobilization stress on the hypothalamic-pituitary-adrenal axis: transcriptional evidence for a progressive desensitization process. *Eur. J. Neurosci.* **18:** 1353–1361.

53. Buijs, R.M., A. Kalsbeek, T. Van Der Woude, J.J.V. Heerikhuize & S. Shinn. 1993. Suprachiasmatic nucleus lesion increases corticosterone secretion. *Am. J. Physiol.* **264:** 1186–1192.

54. Dayas, C.V., K.M. Buller, J.W. Crane, *et al.* 2001. Stressor categorization: acute physical and psychological stressors elicit distintictive recruitment patterns in the amygdala and in medullary noradrenergic cell groups. *Eur. J. Neurosci.* **14:** 1143–1152.

55. Besedovsky, H.O. & A. del Rey. 2000. The cytokine-HPA axis feed-back circuit. *Z. Rheumatol.* **59:** 26–30.

56. Carrillo-Vico, A., P.J. Lardone, L. Naji, *et al.* 2005. Beneficial pleiotropic actions of melatonin in an experimental model of septic shock in mice: regulation of pro-/anti-inflammatory cytokine network, protection against oxidative damage and anti-apoptotic effects. *J. Pineal Res.* **39:** 400–408.

57. Viswanathan, K., C. Daugherty & F.S. Dhabhar. 2005. Stress as an endogenous adjuvant: augmentation of the immunization phase of cell-mediated immunity. *Int. Immunol.* **17:** 1059–1069.

58. Madrigal, J.L.M., O. Hurtado, M.A. Moro, *et al.* 2002. The increase in TNF-a levels is implicated in NFkB activation and inducible nitric oxide synthase expression in brain cortex after immobilization stress. *Neurophsychopharmacology* **26:** 155–163.

59. Pawlak, C.R., R.K. Schwarting & A. Bauhofer. 2005. Cytokine mRNA levels in brain and peripheral tissues of the rat: relationships with plus-maze behavior. *Brain Res. Mol. Brain Res.* **137:** 159–165.

60. Kentner, R., F.M. Rollwagen, S. Prueckner, *et al.* 2002. Effects of mild hypothermia on survival and serum cytokines in uncontrolled hemorrhagic shock in rats. *Shock* **17:** 521–526.

61. Gilad, E., H.R. Wong, B. Zingarelli, *et al.* 1998. Melatonin inhibits expression of the inducible isoform of nitric oxide synthase in murine macrophages: role of inhibition of NFkB activation. *FASEB J.* **12:** 685–693.

62. Skwarlo-Sonta, K., P. Majewski, M. Markowska, *et al.* 2003. Bidirectional communication between the pineal gland and the immune system. *Can. J. Physiol. Pharmacol.* **81:** 342–349.

63. Pacak, K., I. Armando, K. Fukuhara, *et al.* 1992. Noradrenergic activation in the paraventricular nucleus during acute and chronic immobilization stress in rats: an in vivo microdialysis study. *Brain Res.* **589:** 91–96.

64. Glavin, G.B., W.P. Paré, T. Sandbak, *et al.* 1994. Restraint stress in biomedical research: an update. *Neurosci. Biobehav. Rev.* **18:** 223–249.

Neuronal Plasticity and Antidepressants in the Diabetic Brain

Juan Beauquis,[a] **Paulina Roig,**[a] **Alejandro F. De Nicola,**[a,b] **and Flavia Saravia**[a,b]

[a]*Neuroendocrine Biochemistry, Institute of Biology and Experimental Medicine, National Research Council, Buenos Aires, Argentina*

[b]*Department of Human Biochemistry, Faculty of Medicine, University of Buenos Aires, Buenos Aires, Argentina*

The hippocampus, a limbic structure linked to higher brain functions, appears vulnerable in diabetic subjects that have a higher risk of stroke, dementia, and cognitive decline. The dentate gyrus (DG) of the hippocampus is one of the limited neurogenic brain areas during adulthood; neurons born in the DG are involved in some types of learning and memory processes. We found a decrease in the ability for proliferation and neuronal differentiation of newborn cells, measured by bromodeoxyuridine incorporation in the DG, from streptozotocin-induced diabetic mice. The hilar region, formed by mature neurons presenting higher sensitivity to brain damage, showed a reduced neuronal density in diabetic mice with respect to vehicle-treated mice. Interestingly, in a spontaneous model of type 1 diabetes, we corroborated a decrease in the rate of neurogenesis in the nonobese diabetic mice compared to control strains, and this reduction was also found during the prediabetic stage. The antidepressant fluoxetine administered over a period of 10 days to diabetic mice was effective in preventing changes in proliferation and differentiation of new neurons. Confocal microscope studies, including using neuronal and glial markers, suggested that differentiation toward a neuronal phenotype was decreased in diabetic animals and was reversed by the antidepressant treatment. In addition, the loss of hilar neurons was avoided by fluoxetine treatment. Several reports have demonstrated that high susceptibility to stress and elevated corticosterone levels are detrimental to neurogenesis and contribute to neuronal loss. These features are common in some types of depression, diabetes, and aging processes, suggesting they participate in the reported hippocampal abnormalities present in these conditions.

Key words: type 1 diabetes; hippocampus; dentate gyrus; neurogenesis; fluoxetine

Brain Complications Associated with Diabetes

Diabetes mellitus is one of the most common metabolic diseases in humans. Type 2 diabetes (T2D), mediated by insulin resistance, is much more frequent than type 1 (T1D), which is caused by insulin deficiency. A result in part to changes in nutritional habits and life style, the incidence of both types of diabetes is increasing throughout the world. Both types have significant short- and long-term consequences. The end organs predominantly damaged by the disease are the kidney, retina, peripheral nervous system, and small and large blood vessels. The central nervous system (CNS) has recently been included among the systems affected by acute and chronic diabetes-associated effects. In this regard, neuroglycopenia and accelerated aging

Address for correspondence: Dr. Flavia Saravia, Institute of Biology and Experimental Medicine, National Research Council (CONICET), Obligado 2490, 1428 Buenos Aires, Argentina. Fax: 54-11-4786-2564. saravia@dna.uba.ar

Neuroimmunomodulation: Ann. N.Y. Acad. Sci. 1153: 203–208 (2009).
doi: 10.1111/j.1749-6632.2008.03983.x © 2009 New York Academy of Sciences.

could be considered among metabolic complications, while stroke and microangiopathy are linked to vascular effects. Brain damage, neurological deficit, and high risk of depression and dementia are some of the related consequences.[1,2]

Aiming to define the status of mild to moderate cognitive impairment in diabetic patients, Mijnhout and co-workers have recently proposed the term "diabetes-associated cognitive decline."[2] In experimental models of this disease, several studies, including ours, agree with the hypothesis of a marked impact of diabetes on the CNS. Working with T1D models, different authors have suggested various mechanisms that operate in diabetic alterations.[3] These include intracellular calcium toxicity, excitotoxic cellular damage associated with excessive glutamate,[4–6] hippocampal astrogliosis, abnormal neural activation,[7,8] and impairment in spatial learning ability.[9–11] Remarkably, the limbic system, including the hippocampus and associated functions, seems to be highly vulnerable to the effects of uncontrolled diabetes.

Hippocampal Neurogenesis Is Impaired in Mice Models of T1D

Adult neurogenesis is the process of generating functionally integrated neurons in two discrete brain regions: the subventricular zone and the dentate gyrus (DG). During the generation of new neurons, some steps are clearly identified in the DG: proliferation, migration through the granular cell layer, maturation, and functional integration into neuronal circuits. The newly generated hippocampal cells have been implicated in learning and memory processes.[12] Several factors and conditions can modulate this event, including gender, hormones, environment, age, early experiences, and physical and mental activity.[13–20] In addition, some pathological conditions can affect the production of new cells in the DG; brain inflammation is linked to a reduced rate of proliferation while

after ischemia, trauma, or seizures a transient increase can be observed.[21]

Using 5-bromo-2'-deoxyuridine (BrdU) detection and specific neural markers, we observed a strong reduction in neurogenesis rate in experimental models of T1D. In diabetic mice induced by streptozotocin (STZ) treatment, which is a well-recognized and characterized pharmacological model, a significant decrease in the number of proliferating cells was clear in both neurogenic areas.[22,23] Remarkably, estradiol treatment was able to restore cell proliferation to normal levels.[23]

However, not only cell proliferation was reduced in STZ-treated mice. We showed a decrease in neuronal differentiation of newborn cells in the DG after administration of BrdU in a special protocol before killing the diabetic animals. The phenotype of these BrdU-positive (BrdU+) cells was corroborated by colocalization with immature neuronal markers, such as β-III tubulin/Tuj-1.[24]

The number of hilar neurons, a heterogeneous population of interneurons especially sensitive to brain damage, was also affected by diabetes. Compared with control mice treated with vehicle, the hilus of STZ-treated animals exhibited fewer neurons stained by the Nissl technique.[24]

In separate studies, we obtained consistent results in nonobese diabetic mice (NOD), a spontaneous T1D model that progressively develops the disease. Compared with two control strains (C57BL/6 and BALB/c), the NOD mice showed a reduced hippocampal cell proliferation at three different ages (5-, 8-, and 12-weeks old). Interestingly, at 5 and 8 weeks of age the NOD mice were still not diabetic, suggesting that potential brain alterations could be present even before overt hyperglycemia.[25] When we explored the survival of the newly generated neurons in the DG, we saw an important decline in NOD mice regardless of diabetic condition compared to control strains, but again the reduction was greater in NOD diabetic rodents that exhibited hyperglycemia.

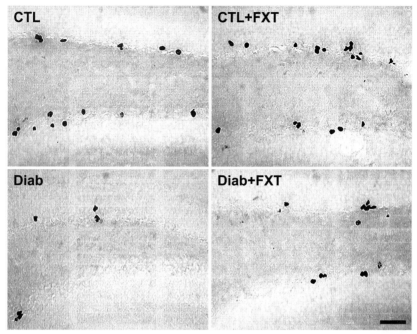

Figure 1. Representative microphotographs corresponding to the cell proliferation protocol of bromodeoxyuridine (BrdU) detection in the dentate gyrus. BrdU-positive cells exhibit darkly stained nuclei and are often distributed in clusters near the subgranular zone. Groups are as follows: vehicle-treated controls (CTL), fluoxetine-treated controls (CTL+FXT), vehicle-treated diabetic mice (Diab), and fluoxetine-treated diabetic mice (Diab+FXT). Note the reduction in the number of BrdU-immunopositive cells in the Diab group compared to the other three groups. Scale bar corresponds to 100 μm.

Antidepressant Treatment Is Able to Recover Reduced DG Neurogenesis in STZ Diabetic Mice

Neurogenesis can be regulated by multiple factors. Stress and some affective-related disorders, such as depression, were associated with high plasma glucocorticoids together with a reduced ability for hippocampal production of new neurons.[15,26,27] Antidepressant treatment was effective in restoring this capability.[27–30]

On the other hand, diabetic subjects present a high prevalence of depression[31–33] and exhibit changes in the serotoninergic system, a feature also found in rodents.[34]

We treated STZ-induced diabetic mice with fluoxetine (a serotonin reuptake inhibitor, 10 mg/kg body weight) over a 10-day period, starting the antidepressant therapy 10 days after diabetes induction, and studied hippocampal cell proliferation and differentiation. The number of BrdU+ cells in the DG significantly increased in diabetic animals after fluoxetine treatment, reaching a rate of proliferation similar to that found in control mice. Interestingly, the experimental control group treated with fluoxetine did not show a significant difference compared to vehicle-treated controls (Fig. 1).

The newly generated cells differentiate mostly into neurons and, to a lesser degree, into glial cells. We performed co-localization studies with neural (Tuj-1) and glial (GFAP) markers in order to establish whether the final phenotype of newborn cells was affected by diabetes. Cellular differentiation was analyzed in fluoxetine-treated diabetic mice injected with BrdU for 7 consecutive days before killing. The proportion of BrdU+ cells also expressing Tuj-1 marker in the DG was increased in diabetic animals under antidepressant treatment compared to

STZ-treated mice treated with vehicle, and it was similar to controls.[24] Our results strongly suggest that not only the number of newborn cells decreased with diabetes but also a decline in the proportion of new cells differentiating into neurons occurred. Fluoxetine administration was able to reverse this situation. The rate of differentiation into GFAP-positive cells was not altered by the diabetic status and was not affected by the antidepressant treatment.[24] Of particular note is that the number of neurons stained with cresyl violet in the hilus of the DG in diabetic mice increased after antidepressant treatment, showing that fluoxetine could be involved in the rescue of these mature neurons.

Concluding Remarks

The hippocampus appears extremely sensitive to the deleterious effects of diabetes. Several reports showed hippocampal alterations in both patients and experimental models. We demonstrated that the diabetic status induced in mice by STZ negatively influences the production of new neurons in both neurogenic brain areas. In the same model, we found a marked reduction in the number of hilar neurons. In the DG of NOD mice, we corroborated a low rate of proliferation that was also, surprisingly, found at prediabetic and diabetic states compared with age-matched control strains. These and other findings are characteristic of an aged or damaged brain and could strongly suggest an accelerated aging process associated with the disease. This finding is in line with those of previously mentioned reports and supports the idea of a diabetic encephalopathy[35] and the more recent concept of diabetes-associated cognitive decline.[36] Interestingly, T2D and obesity could share some brain abnormalities where neuronal systems regulating energy intake and energy expenditure seem to be implicated.[37]

Fluoxetine is a serotonin reuptake inhibitor commonly used with remarkable results in the treatment of depression. In our study we found that fluoxetine treatment during a relatively short period (10 days) was able to prevent some changes in the DG of diabetic mice. Antidepressant treatment effectively increased the proliferation of new cells and the neuronal differentiation of these newborn cells in the DG of STZ-treated mice. In this way, fluoxetine showed efficacy in preventing the loss of hilar density, a neural population especially sensitive to cerebral insult. The lack of effect of fluoxetine treatment on control mice suggests the participation of a mechanism only active during some specific brain alterations or permissive situations.

Several authors have postulated a central role of stress or depression in the atrophy and cell loss in limbic structures associated with higher brain functions.[15,28,38] Reduced birth of new neurons in the adult brain can contribute to this atrophy and/or to a deprived neuronal plasticity, as was observed in experimental models. Diabetes condition is linked to an augmented vulnerability to stress in correlation with a hyperactivity of the HPA axis,[39–42] and this feature, together with high glucocorticoid plasmatic levels, can be intimately involved in adult neurogenesis alterations. Stranahan *et al.* attributed a manifest role to glucocorticoids in the cognitive impairment observed in T1D models,[43] while Revsin *et al.* demonstrated that corticosterone secretion was significantly augmented immediately after diabetes induction in the STZ model but adrenocorticotropic hormone levels were below control levels.[44]

In conclusion, our data have contributed to a better understanding of brain complications associated with a metabolic disease, such as diabetes, and some of these complications are common to depression and accelerated aging. The effectiveness of fluoxetine treatment demonstrated that some of these alterations are not permanent and can be prevented by pharmacological treatment. Further studies are needed to explore the mechanisms and other potential factors involved with the effects of metabolic diseases.

Acknowledgments

We thank the following institutions for financial support: University of Buenos Aires (M022 and M094), Fondo para la Investigación Científica y Tecnológica (FONCYT BID1728-OC-AR PICT 2006 # 1845), Consejo Nacional de Investigaciones Científicas y Técnicas (CONICET PIP 5542). J.B. is recipient of a CONICET PhD fellowship.

Conflicts of Interest

The authors declare no conflicts of interest.

References

1. Selvarajah, D. & S. Tesfaye. 2006. Central nervous system involvement in diabetes mellitus. *Curr. Diab. Rep.* **6:** 431–438.

2. Mijnhout, G.S. *et al.* 2006. Diabetic encephalopathy: A concept in need of a definition. *Diabetologia* **49:** 1447–1448.

3. Northam, E.A., D. Rankins & F. Cameron. 2006. Therapy insight: the impact of type 1 diabetes on brain development and function. *Nat. Clin. Pract. Neurol.* **2:** 78–86.

4. Gardoni, F. *et al.* 2002. Effects of streptozotocin-diabetes on the hippocampal NMDA receptor complex in rats. *J. Neurochem.* **80:** 438–447.

5. Valastro, B. *et al.* 2002. Up-regulation of glutamate receptors is associated with LTP defects in the early stages of diabetes mellitus. *Diabetologia* **45:** 642–650.

6. Revsin, Y. *et al.* 2005. Neuronal and astroglial alterations in the hippocampus of a mouse model for type 1 diabetes. *Brain Res.* **1038:** 22–31.

7. Saravia, F. *et al.* 2002. Increased astrocyte reactivity in the hippocampus of murine models of type 1 diabetes: the nonobese diabetic (NOD) and streptozotocin-treated mice. *Brain Res.* **957:** 345–353.

8. Biessels, G.J. *et al.* 1998. Water maze learning and hippocampal synaptic plasticity in streptozotocin-diabetic rats: effects of insulin treatment. *Brain Res.* **800:** 125–135.

9. Biessels, G.J. & W.H. Gispen. 2005. The impact of diabetes on cognition: what can be learned from rodent models? *Neurobiol. Aging* **26**(Suppl 1): 36–41.

10. Biessels, G. *et al.* 1994. Cerebral function in diabetes mellitus. *Diabetologia* **37:** 643–650.

11. Ming, G.L. & H. Song. 2005. Adult neurogenesis in the mammalian central nervous system. *Annu. Rev. Neurosci.* **28:** 223–250.

12. Cameron, A., T. Hazel & R. McKay. 1998. Regulation of neurogenesis by growth factors and neurotransmitters. *J. Neurobiol.* **36:** 287–306.

13. Cameron, H. & R. McKay. 2001. Adult neurogenesis produces a large pool of new granule cells in the dentate gyrus. *J. Comp. Neurol.* **435:** 406–417.

14. Duman, R., J. Malberg, S. Nakagawa & C. D'Sa. 2000. Neuronal plasticity and survival in mood disorders. *Biol. Psychiatry* **46:** 1181–1191.

15. Gage, F. 2002. Neurogenesis in the adult brain. *J. Neurosci.* 612–613.

16. Gould, E. & H.A. Cameron. 1996. Regulation of neuronal birth, migration and death in the rat dentate gyrus. *Dev. Neurosci.* **18:** 22–35.

17. Kempermann, G., H. Kuhn & F. Gage. 1997. More hippocampal neurons in adult mice living in an enriched environment. *Nature* **386:** 493–495.

18. van Praag, H., G. Kempermann & F. Gage. 1999. Running increases cell proliferation and neurogenesis in the adult mouse dentate gyrus. *Nat. Neurosci.* **2:** 266–270.

19. van Praag, H. *et al.* 2002. Functional neurogenesis in the adult hippocampus. *Nature* **415:** 1030–1034.

20. Saravia, F.E. *et al.* 2007. Neuroprotective effects of estradiol in hippocampal neurons and glia of middle age mice. *Psychoneuroendocrinology* **32:** 480–492.

21. Madsen, T. *et al.* 2000. Increased neurogenesis in a model of electroconvulsive therapy. *Biol. Psychiatry* **47:** 1043–1049.

22. Saravia, F.E. *et al.* 2006. Hippocampal neuropathology of diabetes mellitus is relieved by estrogen treatment. *Cell. Mol. Neurobiol.* **26:** 941–955.

23. Saravia, F. *et al.* 2004. Oestradiol restores cell proliferation in dentate gyrus and subventricular zone of streptozotocin-diabetic mice. *J. Neuroendocrinol.* **16:** 704–710.

24. Beauquis, J. *et al.* 2006. Reduced hippocampal neurogenesis and number of hilar neurones in streptozotocin-induced diabetic mice: reversion by antidepressant treatment. *Eur. J. Neurosci.* **23:** 1539–1546.

25. Beauquis, J. *et al.* 2007. Prominently decreased hippocampal neurogenesis in a spontaneous model of type 1 diabetes, the nonobese diabetic mouse. *Exp. Neurol.* **210:** 359–367.

26. Jacobs, B. 2002. Adult brain neurogenesis and depression. *Brain Behav. Immun.* **16:** 602–609.

27. Kempermann, G. 2002. Regulation of adult hippocampal neurogenesis-implications for novel theories of major depression. *Bipolar Disorders* **4:** 17–33.

28. Duman, R., J. Malberg & S. Nakagawa. 2001. Regulation of adult neurogenesis by psychotropic drugs and stress. *J. Pharmacol. Exp. Ther.* **299:** 401–407.

29. Santarelli, L. *et al*. 2003. Requirement of hippocampal neurogenesis for the behavioral effects of antidepressants. *Science* **301:** 805–809.

30. Malberg, J. 2004. Implications of adult hippocampal neurogenesis in antidepressant action. *Rev. Psychiatric Neurosci.* **29:** 196–205.

31. Katon, W. *et al*. 2004. Behavioral and clinical factors associated with depression among individuals with diabetes. *Diabetes Care* **27:** 914.

32. Lustman, P. *et al*. 1992. Depression in adults with diabetes. *Diabetes Care* **15:** 1631–1639.

33. McEwen, B., A. Magariños & L. Reagan. 2002. Studies of hormone action in the hippocampal formation. Possible relevance to depression and diabetes. *J. Psychosomatic Res.* **53:** 883–890.

34. Barber, M. *et al*. 2003. Diabetes-induced neuroendocrine changes in rats: role of brain monoamines, insulin and leptin. *Brain Res.* **964:** 128–135.

35. Gispen, W. & G. Biessels. 2000. Cognition and synaptic plasticity in diabetes mellitus. *Trends Neurosci.* **23:** 542–549.

36. Mijnhout, G.S. *et al*. 2006. Diabetic encephalopathy: A concept in need of a definition. *Diabetologia* **49:** 1447–1448.

37. Schwartz, M.W. & D. Porte Jr. 2005. Diabetes, obesity, and the brain. *Science* **307:** 375–379.

38. Kempermann, G. & G. Kronenberg. 2003. Depressed new neurons-adult neurogenesis and a cellular plasticity hypothesis of major depression. *Biol. Pychiatry* **54:** 499–503.

39. Kamal, A. 1999. Hippocampal synaptic plasticity in streptozotocin-diabetic rats: interaction of diabetes and ageing. *Neuroscience* **90:** 737–745.

40. Revsin, Y. *et al*. 2008. Adrenal hypersensitivity precedes chronic hypercorticism in streptozotocin-induced diabetes mice. *Endocrinology* **149:** 3531–3539.

41. Magariños, A. & B. McEwen. 2000. Experimental diabetes in rats causes hippocampal dendritic and synaptic reorganization and increased glucocorticoid reactivity to stress. *Proc. Natl. Acad. Sci. USA* **97:** 11056–11061.

42. Homo-Delarche, F. *et al*. 1991. Sex steroids, glucocorticoids, stress and autoimmunity. *J. Steroid Biochem. Mol. Biol.* **40:** 619–637.

43. Stranahan, A.M. *et al*. 2008. Diabetes impairs hippocampal function through glucocorticoid-mediated effects on new and mature neurons. *Nat. Neurosci.* **11:** 309–317.

44. Revsin, Y. *et al*. 2008. Glucocorticoid receptor blockade normalizes hippocampal alterations and cognitive impairment in streptozotocin-induced type 1 diabetes mice. *Neuropsychopharmacology* 1-12 Sept. 10 [Epub ahead of print].

Neuroimmune Interactions in a Model of Multiple Sclerosis

C. Jane Welsh,[a,b] Andrew J. Steelman,[a] Wentao Mi,[a]
Colin R. Young,[a] Ralph Storts,[b] Thomas H. Welsh, Jr.,[a,c]
and Mary W. Meagher[d]

[a]*Department of Veterinary Integrative Biosciences and* [b]*Department of Veterinary Pathobiology, College of Veterinary Medicine and Biomedical Sciences, Texas A&M University, College Station, Texas, USA*

[c]*Department of Animal Science, College of Agriculture and Life Sciences, Texas A&M University, College Station, Texas, USA*

[d]*Department of Psychology, College of Liberal Arts, Texas A&M University, College Station, Texas, USA*

Psychological stress has been implicated in both the onset and exacerbation of multiple sclerosis (MS). Our research has focused on the role of stress at the onset of MS, using the mouse model Theiler's murine encephalomyelitis virus-induced demyelination. Theiler's virus is a natural pathogen of mice that causes a persistent infection of the central nervous system (CNS) and inflammatory immune-mediated demyelination that is very similar to MS. Our research has shown that restraint stress sufficiently increases corticosterone secretion to cause immunosuppression. Stressed mice develop decreased innate and adaptive immune responses, including decreased chemokine and cytokine responses, to virus, which leads to increased viral replication within the CNS. Higher levels of virus then cause increased later demyelinating disease. These findings may have important implications in our understanding of the interactions between stress and the development of autoimmune diseases induced by infectious agents.

Key words: Theiler's virus; multiple sclerosis; demyelination; central nervous system; autoimmunity; viruses; stress; restraint stress; glucocorticoids; corticosterone; HPA axis; immune system; chemokines; cytokines; NK cells; interferon; macrophages; innate immunity; adaptive immunity; Th1; Th2; T cells; CD4[+] T cells; CD8[+] T cells; inflammation

Multiple Sclerosis

Multiple sclerosis (MS) is an autoimmune, inflammatory, demyelinating disease of the central nervous system (CNS) occurring at a prevalence of 350,000 in the United States and an incidence approaching 1/1000.[1,2] Although the etiology of MS is unknown, epidemiological studies have implicated infectious agents as probable initiating factors.[3] For instance, there is an increased risk of developing MS in patients who developed mumps, measles, or Epstein–Barr virus (EBV) infections at an older age.[4] Interestingly, elevated EBV antibody titers occurred 15–20 years prior to MS onset in a 2006 study.[5] In addition, several viruses, such as measles, mumps, parainfluenza type I, and human *Herpes simplex virus*,[6,7] have been isolated from MS brains. Furthermore, exacerbations of MS are frequently preceded by viral infections, such as those caused by rhinoviruses.[8] Interestingly, interferon-beta (IFN-β), an antiviral agent, is currently used to treat relapsing/remitting MS.[9]

Address for correspondence: C. Jane Welsh, Department of Veterinary Integrative Biosciences, College of Veterinary Medicine and Biomedical Sciences, Texas A&M University, College Station, TX 77843-4458. Voice: 979-862-4974; fax: 979-845-9972. jwelsh@cvm.tamu.edu

Neuroimmunomodulation: Ann. N.Y. Acad. Sci. 1153: 209–219 (2009).
doi: 10.1111/j.1749-6632.2008.03984.x © 2009 New York Academy of Sciences.

In animals, viruses are also known to cause demyelination, such as measles virus in rats, visna in sheep, *Herpes simplex* in rabbits, mouse hepatitis virus strain JHM, Semliki Forest virus, and Theiler's virus in mice.[10] Theiler's virus is a natural pathogen of mice that induces a disease that is similar both in disease course and pathology to chronic progressive MS in humans.[11] Theiler's virus infection in mice represents not only an excellent model for the study of the pathogenesis of MS but also a model system for studying disease susceptibility factors, mechanisms of viral persistence within the CNS, and mechanisms of virus-induced autoimmune disease.

Stress and Multiple Sclerosis

Psychological stress has been implicated in the onset and exacerbations of several autoimmune diseases, including MS.[12-14] Anecdotal accounts suggest that significant stressful life events frequently trigger the development of MS symptoms. Psychological stress has been shown to precede both the onset and recurrence of MS symptoms in 70–80% of cases, using standardized assessment of life stressors measures.[15] More recently, stressful life events have been shown to predict the development of new lesions and relapses in MS.[16,17] A meta-analysis of 14 studies concerning stress and MS concluded that there was "a significantly increased risk of exacerbation associated with stressful life events."[18]

Theiler's Virus-induced Demyelination as a Model for MS

Theiler's murine encephalomyelitis virus is a member of the *Picornaviridae* in the cardiovirus genus. Theiler's virus causes an asymptomatic gastrointestinal infection and occasionally paralysis.[19] The persistent Theiler's original strains of Theiler's virus (BeAn, DA, WW, Yale) cause a primary demyelinating disease in susceptible strains of mice that is similar to MS.[20]

Theiler's virus must establish a persistent infection in the CNS in order to cause demyelination.[21] Theiler's virus-induced demyelination (TVID)-resistant strains of mice are able to clear the infection effectively from the CNS. A number of studies have reported that viral persistence and demyelination in susceptible strains of mice are under multigenic control. Major histocompatibility complex (MHC) class I genes, the T cell receptor genes, and a gene locus on chromosome 6 not linked to the T cell receptor locus have been implicated in susceptibility to demyelination.[22,23] Two additional loci, one close to IFN-γ on chromosome 10 and one near Mbp on chromosome 18, have been associated with viral persistence in some strains of mice.[24] Immune recognition of Theiler's virus is clearly an important element in susceptibility to demyelination, as indicated by the genetic association with MHC class I and the T cell receptor, although other undefined factors are also involved.

The Effects of Restraint Stress on the Neuropathogenesis of Acute Theiler's Virus Infection

In order to investigate the psychological effects of stress on the neuropathogenesis of Theiler's virus, we have employed a restraint stress model originally described by Sheridan and colleagues.[25] Restraint stress is both a physiological and psychological stressor and involves placing mice in well-ventilated tubes overnight. Our studies systematically dissected the effects of restraint stress on the various components of the immune response to Theiler's virus. Moreover, we have used three strains of mice with varying degrees of susceptibility to Theiler's virus: (1) SJL mice, which have high susceptibility to TVID; (2) CBA mice, which have intermediate susceptibility to TVID; and (3) C57Bl/6 mice, which are resistant to TVID.

Our first study involved male CBA mice subjected to chronic stress that consisted of five nights (12 h/night) of restraint stress per week for a total of 4 weeks. The experimental groups were: infected/restrained; infected/nonrestrained; infected/food and water deprived; noninfected/restrained; noninfected/nonrestrained and noninfected/food and water deprived. The food- and water-deprived groups were deprived overnight to match the restrained groups and did not differ from the nonrestrained groups and therefore were not included in subsequent studies. Stress had a profound effect on survival; 80% of the stressed-infected mice died during the first 3 weeks of infection. Restraint stress resulted in increases in corticosterone levels, signs of sickness behavior, viral titers in the CNS, circulating neutrophils and adrenal hypertrophy, thymic atrophy, decreased numbers of circulating lymphocytes, and decreased inflammatory cell infiltrates into the CNS.[26–28] Similar results were found in a subsequent study with male and female SJL mice. Chronic restraint stress administered in the first 4 weeks of Theiler's virus infection decreased body weight, increased clinical signs of infection, and increased plasma corticosterone concentration during the acute viral infection. Although all the stressed mice developed significantly increased corticosterone levels, female SJL mice showed higher basal and stress-induced increases in corticosterone.[29]

Clearly stress has a profound impact on the neuropathogenesis of Theiler's virus infection. We proposed the following mechanisms for this phenomenon: stress activates the hypothalamic–pituitary–adrenal (HPA) axis resulting in adrenal hypertrophy and increased production of corticosterone. High levels of corticosterone, in turn, cause thymic atrophy and immunosuppression that reduces both the innate and adaptive immune response to Theiler's virus, thus reducing the effective clearance of virus from the CNS. Evidence for glucocorticoids being the main mediators of increased mortality in Theiler's virus-infected mice were obtained by the replication of the restraint findings by the addition of corticosterone in the drinking water of infected mice.[30]

Effects of Stress on the Innate Immune Response to Theiler's Virus

IFN and Natural Killer Cells in Theiler's Virus Infection

The early host responses, IFN production and natural killer (NK) cell activation, are crucial for the effective clearance of Theiler's virus from the CNS. Failure to clear virus results in the establishment of persistent infection of the CNS and subsequent demyelination.[31,32] Type I IFNs activate NK cells, upregulate MHC class I expression, and induce the antiviral state. Type I IFNs are critical in the early clearance of Theiler's virus from the CNS, as demonstrated by experimentation with IFN-α/β-receptor knockout mice, which die within 10 days of infection with severe encephalomyelitis.[33]

NK cells are activated early in viral infections and play an important role in infection with Theiler's virus. TVID-susceptible SJL mice have a 50% lower NK cell activity when compared to resistant C57Bl/6 mice.[34] The low activity of NK cells in the SJL mice is from a differentiation defect in the thymus that impairs the responsiveness of NK cells to stimulation by IFN-β.[35] Resistant mice depleted of NK cells by monoclonal antibody to NK 1.1 or anti-asialo-GM1 and then infected with Theiler's virus developed severe signs of gray-matter disease.[34] Thus, NK cells are critical in the early clearance of Theiler's virus from the CNS either directly via cytotoxic activity and/or antiviral effects of IFN-γ or indirectly through IFN-γ-mediated activation of signal transducers and activators of transcription (STAT1) protein and polarization of T cells toward a Th1 phenotype.

We examined the effects of stress on the NK cell response to Theiler's virus infection in male CBA mice, using four experimental groups of mice: infected/restrained; infected/nonrestrained; infected/nonrestrained; noninfected/nonrestrained. Restraint stress applied 1 day prior to infection with Theiler's virus resulted in 50% reduction in splenic NK cell activity 24 h post infection (p.i.).[27] Similar results have been obtained with two TVID-resistant strains of mice: C57Bl/6 and BALB/c.[36] Restraint stress did not alter the NK cell response in SJL/J mice infected with Theiler's virus because this strain has a deficiency in NK cell response.[35] However, restraint stress did impact the neuropathogenesis of Theiler's virus infection in SJL/J mice, and therefore stress must mediate its immunosuppressive effects on the other components of the immune response. Stress-induced NK cell suppression may contribute to but is not sufficient to observe the stress-induced exacerbation of acute and chronic Theiler's virus infection.

Stress Reduces Virus Chemokine/Cytokine Expression

CBA mice were subjected to the restraint stress protocol for 7 nights and infected after the first stress session. Then they were euthanized and RNA was isolated from the brains and spleens. Ribonuclease protection analysis (RPA) indicated that infection with Theiler's virus increased the following chemokine mRNA expression in the spleen but not the brain at day 2 p.i.: lymphotactin (Ltn), IFN-induced protein (IP-10), macrophage inflammatory protein-1 (MIP-1), monocyte chemoattractant protein-1 (MCP-1), and T cell activation-3 (TCA-3). Chemokine expression was increased first in the spleen, which provides evidence that the immune response to Theiler's virus is initiated in the periphery. Ltn, regulated upon activation, normal T cell expressed, and secreted (RANTES), and IP-10 were elevated in both the spleen and the brain at day 7 p.i. and were significantly decreased by stress in the brain. These chemokines are responsible for the recruitment of macrophages, NK cells, and CD4$^+$ and CD8$^+$ T cells and thus may account for the diminished inflammatory cell infiltrate in the CNS of stressed mice and subsequently the reduced viral clearance and increased mortality in virus-infected stressed mice.[26,28]

The effects of stress on cytokine production in both the spleen and brain were measured by RPA in CBA mice following seven stress sessions. Theiler's virus infection elevated IFN-γ, lymphotoxin-β (LT-ß), IL-12p40, IL-6, and IFN-β in the brain at day 2 and 7 p.i. Importantly, restraint attenuated the increases in IFN-γ, LT-ß, IL-12p40, and IL-6 but elevated IFN-β. The increased mRNA IFN-β levels may be a result of the increased viral titers stimulating the production of this IFN.[37] In further experiments examining the effect of stress on cytokine expression, mice were subjected to the restraint stress paradigm and, at sacrifice, half the brain taken for measurement of virus titers and the other half for RPA analysis of cytokine mRNA levels. mRNA levels of IFN-γ, LT-ß, and tumor necrosis factor-α (TNF-α) negatively correlated with viral titers in the CNS such that mice with higher cytokine levels had lower virus levels. TNF-α protein levels, as measured by Western blots, gave similar results to the RPA data for this cytokine.[37] These cytokines have multiple immunomodulatory effects, including antiviral activity. Therefore, stress-induced decreased levels of LT-β, IFN-γ, and TNF-α may contribute to increased viral titers in the CNS.

Stress Reduces the Inflammatory Cell Infiltrate in the CNS

CBA mice were restraint stressed and infected with Theiler's virus and their brains examined histologically at either day 7 or 24 p.i.[26] Restraint stress profoundly reduced the inflammatory cell infiltrate into the CNS at day 7 p.i. with Theiler's virus.[26,28] In addition, stress reduced microglial activation. The reduced inflammation may be a result of reduced chemokine expression in the brain, in particular, decreased Ltn, RANTES, and IP-10 levels. In contrast, by day 24 p.i., the stressed mice had increased levels of inflammation in the CNS compared to the unstressed infected mice. This phenomenon may be from recovery of the immune system and increased activation from the increased viral titers in the CNS.[26]

Restraint Stress Facilitates Dissemination of Theiler's Virus during Early Disease

The restraint stress model was used to investigate the effect of stress on the systemic dissemination of Theiler's virus during the early stage of disease in CBA mice.[38] Restraint stress increased viral replication in the CNS and in systemic organs: the spleen, lymph nodes, thymus, lungs, and heart. Restraint stress also resulted in higher titers of virus in the heart that caused granular degeneration of the myocardium, which was not evident in infected unstressed mice. These profound effects may explain the exacerbated clinical symptoms and higher mortality in stressed and infected animals. The fact that stress results in a higher level of viral replication may allow for the increased likelihood of emergence of mutant viruses with altered tissue tropism. Stress may render a virus pathogenic for diverse organs and result in the development of novel diseases.

Restraint Stress Reduces Adaptive Immune Responses to Theiler's Virus

CD8+ and CD4+ T Cells in Theiler's Virus Infection

In early infection with Theiler's virus, both CD8+ and CD4+ T cells have been shown to play an important role in viral clearance.[39–42] However, in later disease these T cell subsets become pathogenic and mediate the demyelinating process.[39,42–44] In early disease, CD4+ T cells activate CD8+ T cells and also assist B cells in the production of antibodies, which are important mediators of picornavirus clearance.[39,45] CD4+ T cells also produce IFN-γ, a potent inhibitor of Theiler's virus infection *in vitro* and *in vivo*.[46–48] CD8+ T cells mediate viral clearance, as demonstrated by *in vivo* depletion experiments and studies with gene knockout mice.[40,49,50] CD8+

T cell–depleted mice fail to clear virus from the CNS and develop more severe demyelinating disease than the immunocompetent infected controls.[40] Similarly, demyelination developed in Theiler's virus-infected, β_2-microglobulin, knockout mice (constructed on a TVID-resistant background). In addition, introduction of resistant H-2D^b or H-2D^d transgene into susceptible strains of mice render these animals resistant to TVID.[51,52] Taken together, these investigations clearly implicate CD8+ T cells in viral clearance and resistance to demyelination. The cytotoxic T cells may function protectively by recognizing viral determinants or by inhibiting delayed-type hypersensitivity (DTH) responses.[40]

Our next series of experiments focused on the effects of stress on the T cell response to Theiler's virus in SJL mice because the immunodominant Theiler's virus-specific T cell epitopes have been identified in this strain of mice.[53–56] SJL mice were assigned to the experimental groups shown in Table 1, with the stressed mice being subjected to eight nights of restraint stress. At termination, splenic and CNS T cell responses to Theiler's virus were measured using an enzyme-linked immunosorbent spot (ELISPOT) assay. Theiler's virus infection increased the number of IFN-γ-producing cells in the periphery in response to either the CD8 epitope (FNFTAPFI corresponding to VP3$_{159–166}$) or the CD4 T cell epitope (QEAFSHIRIPLPH corresponding to VP2$_{74–86}$). Restraint stress significantly decreased both the splenic virus-induced CD4+ and CD8+ T cell response. Furthermore, restraint stress dramatically decreased (50%) the infection-related increase in CD8+ T cell responses within the CNS.[57]

There are reports that stress inhibits Th1 responses and increases Th2 responses. Therefore, we examined the expression of both Th1 and Th2 cytokines in the serum of the experimental animals. Restraint significantly decreased both type 1 [IL-12(p40), IL-12(p70), IFN-γ] and type 2 (IL-4 and IL-5) serum protein concentrations as measured by Bioplex

TABLE 1. The Effects of Stress on the Immune Response to Theiler's Virus

Response	Increases	Decreases
Hormones	Glucocorticoids	
Chemokines	IL-6, KC, and G-CSF	Ltn, RANTES, and IP-10
Cytokines	IFN-β	IFN-γ, LT-ß, IL-12p40, IL-12(p40), IL-12(p70), IL-4, IL-5
Transcription factors		T-bet mRNA
		GATA-3 mRNA
Cellular response	Neutrophils in blood	Lymphocytes in blood
		NK cell activity
		Virus-specific CD4$^+$ T cells
		Virus-specific CD8$^+$ T cells
Virus	Titers in brain, heart, spleen, thymus, and cervical and mesenteric lymph nodes	
CNS pathology	Inflammatory demyelinating disease in late disease	Microgliosis and inflammation in early disease

IL, interleukin; Ltn, lymphotactin; IP-10, interferon-induced protein; LT-β, lymphotoxin-β; RANTES, regulated upon activation, normal T cell expressed, and secreted; KC, keratinocyte-derived chemokine; G-CSF, granulocyte colony stimulating factor; IFN, interferon; NK, natural killer cells.

(Bio-Rad, Inc., Hercules, CA). The transcription factors T-bet and GATA-3 are the drivers of Th1 and Th2 polarization, respectively.[58,59] Therefore, we also measured splenic mRNA expression levels of these factors in the experimental mice and found significant decreases in both when normalized to noninfected/nonrestrained control mice (Steelman *et al.* unpublished observations). Thus our findings do not support the hypothesis that stress selectively inhibits the Th1 response and promotes the Th2 response, rather that stress has a global immunosuppressive effect.

Restraint stress also decreased serum concentrations of RANTES and MCP-1 but increased IL-6, keratinocyte-derived chemokine (KC), and granulocyte colony stimulating factor (G-CSF) protein concentrations. The chemokines RANTES and MCP-1 are involved in the chemoattraction of both memory T cells and monocytes to the site of infection to mediate early viral clearance from the CNS.[57] These findings confirm the previously reported RPA data from the spleen.[28] Interestingly, the chemokine KC (CXCL1) and growth factor G-CSF increased in the serum of stressed mice. KC plays a major role in the trafficking of neu-trophils, and the hematopoetic factor G-CSF is, in part, responsible for the maturation of neutrophils from the bone marrow. The stress-induced increases in KC and G-CSF may explain the increase in neutrophilia that we previously reported.[26,27]

Restraint Stress during Acute Infection Exacerbates the Later Demyelinating Disease Induced by Theiler's Virus

Demyelination induced by Theiler's virus is partly mediated by viral lysis of oligodendrocytes[60]; the continued attempts of the immune system to clear virus, which include bystander demyelination mediated by virus-specific DTH T cells[61]; and also cytotoxic T cell reactivity directed against virus-infected oligodendrocyte[44] autoimmunity[39,42,62,63] and epitope spreading.[64] The autoimmune reactivity seen in TVID may result from viral damage to oligodendrocytes, myelin uptake by macrophage/microglial cells, and subsequent presentation to and activation of autoreactive T cells. These autoimmune T cells have

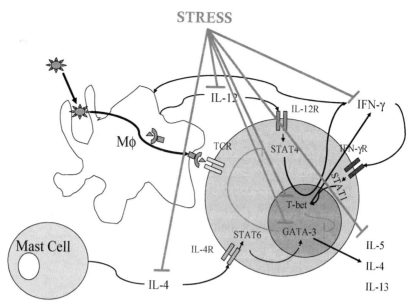

Figure 1. The effects of restraint stress on the immune response to Theiler's virus. Restraint stress causes global immunosuppression of the response to Theiler's virus. Theiler's virus is taken up by macrophages (Mφ) or dendritic cells and presented to T cells via their T cell receptor (TCR) in the context of the major histocompatibility complex (MHC). Natural killer cell activity is reduced by stress and also the production of interferon (IFN)-γ is reduced, which in turn reduces the activation of macrophages and T cells through signal transducers and activators of transcription (STAT)1 signaling. Th1 cells are driven by the transcription factor T-bet and activated by interleukin (IL)-12 through STAT4 signaling pathways. Th2 T cell responses are driven by GATA-3 and activation by IL-4 secretion and STAT6 signaling. Stress reduces the amount of IL-12 secreted by the antigen-presenting cells and then reduces the activation state of the Th1 cells. Stress also reduces mRNA expression of both T-bet and GATA-3 and thereby reduces both Th1 and Th2 responses. (In color in *Annals* online.)

been shown to be pathogenic and are able to demyelinate *in vitro*.[65]

Life stressors have been implicated in the onset of MS, and we have shown that chronic stress during acute infection with Theiler's virus leads to decreased viral clearance from the CNS. Other studies have shown that increased viral load during acute disease leads to increased later demyelinating disease.[40] Thus, we speculated that stress applied during the acute viral infection would result in a higher viral load in the CNS, which would allow the establishment of persistent CNS infection and subsequently lead to increased demyelination. To test this hypothesis we subjected SJL/J mice to restraint stress for 4 weeks (8 h per night for five nights per week) and then monitored the course of disease and assessed the spinal

cord lesions 14 weeks p.i. During early infection, both male and female stressed mice displayed decreased body weights and locomotor activity, with increased behavioral signs of illness and plasma corticosterone levels. During the subsequent demyelinating phase of disease, previously stressed mice had greater behavioral signs of demyelination, worsened rotarod performance, and increased inflammatory demyelinating lesions of the spinal cord.[29]

Interestingly, correlational analysis of the dependent variables revealed that plasma corticosterone levels during stress in the acute phase correlated with disease severity in the chronic disease and thus may be a good predictor of disease course in the chronic phase.[29] This study suggests that restraint-stressed mice develop high levels of corticosterone, which in turn induces immunosuppression and therefore higher viral titers and consequently more severe demyelinating disease.

Summary

Our research into the role of the restraint stress in Theiler's virus infection has clearly demonstrated the importance of the psychological status on the host's immune response to infection and how these interactions contribute to the development of autoimmune disease. In summary, restraint stress affects immune cell development by inducing high levels of corticosterone that reduce circulating lymphocyte numbers and cause thymic atrophy (Table 1). Stress increases KC and G-CSF that leads to increased neutrophils in the circulation. Stress affects the innate immune response to Theiler's virus by reducing NK cell activity and macrophage IL-12 production (Fig. 1). In addition, stress reduces the expression of chemokines in the CNS—Ltn, RANTES, and IP-10—that are responsible for the recruitment of $CD4^+$ and $CD8^+$ T cells, macrophages, and NK cells to the site of infection, and this may explain the reduced inflammation observed during acute infection. Reductions in innate immunity are probably partially responsible for the observed stress-mediated reduction in the acquired immune response to Theiler's virus. Stress-induced decreases in the acquired immune response to Theiler's virus are evidenced by reduced virus-specific $CD4^+$ and $CD8^+$ T cell responses, reduced T-bet and GATA-3 mRNA levels, and decreased virus-induced pro-inflammatory cytokines (TNF-α, IFN-β, and LT-β). As a result of this global immunosuppression, the ability to clear virus from the CNS is diminished and stressed mice subsequently develop more severe demyelinating disease.

Extrapolating these findings to the development of autoimmune diseases in humans, stressful events that occur prior to or during infection may result in immunosuppression and failure to eliminate the pathogen. Persistent infection then may lead to the development of autoimmune disease, such as MS. Stress-induced immunosuppression may also facilitate the emergence of mutant pathogens with enhanced and/or altered pathogenicity, giving rise to novel disease processes.

Acknowledgments

This research was funded by grants to C.J.W. and M.W.M. from the National Multiple Sclerosis Society RG 3128 and National Institutes of Health (NIH)/National Institute of Neurological Disorders and Stroke R01 39569. A.J.S. received support from the Recovery of Function Graduate Training Program at Texas A&M University and NIH/National Research Service Award 5T32AI052072-05.

Conflicts of Interest

The authors declare no conflicts of interest.

References

1. Anderson, D.W., J.H. Ellenberg, C.M. Leventhal, *et al.* 1992. Revised estimate of the prevalence of multiple sclerosis in the United States. *Ann. Neurol.* **31:** 333–336.
2. Hirtz, D., D.J. Thurman, K. Gwinn-Hardy, *et al.* 2007. How common are the "common" neurologic disorders? *Neurology* **68:** 326–337.
3. Acheson, E.D. 1997. Epidemiology of multiple sclerosis. *Brit. Med. Bull.* **33:** 9–14.
4. Hernan, M.A., S.M. Zhang, L. Lipworth, *et al.* 2001. Multiple sclerosis and age at infection with common viruses. *Epidemiology* **12:** 301–306.
5. DeLorenze, G.N., K.L. Munger, E.T. Lennette, *et al.* 2006. Epstein-Barr virus and multiple sclerosis: evidence of association from a prospective study with long-term follow-up. *Arch. Neurol.* **63:** 810–811.
6. Allen, I. & B.J. Brankin. 1993. Pathogenesis of multiple sclerosis-the immune diathesis and the role of viruses. *Neuropathol. Exp. Neurol.* **52:** 95–105.
7. Challoner, P.B., K.T. Smith, J.D. Parker, *et al.* 1995. Plaque-associated expression of human herpesvirus 6 in multiple sclerosis. *P.N.A.S.* **92:** 7440–7444.
8. Sibley, W.A., C.R. Bamford & K. Clark. 1985. Clinical viral infections and multiple sclerosis. *Lancet* **1:** 1313–1315.

9. IFN-β Multiple Sclerosis Study Group. 1993. IFN-β1-β is effective in relapsing remitting multiple sclerosis. I. Clinical results of a multi-center, randomized, double blind, placebo controlled trial. *Neurology* **43:** 655–661.

10. Dal Canto, M.C. & S.G. Rabinowitz. 1982. Experimental models of virus-induced demyelination of the central nervous system. *Ann. Neurol.* **11:** 109–127.

11. Oleszak, E.L., J.R. Chang, H. Friedman, *et al.* 2004. Theiler's virus infection: a model for multiple sclerosis. *Clin. Microbiol. Rev.* **17:** 174–207.

12. Grant, I. 1993. Psychosomatic-somatopsychic aspects of multiple sclerosis. In *Multiple sclerosis: A Neuropsychiatric Disorder*. U. Hailbreich, Ed.: 119–136. American Psychiatric Press. Washington, DC.

13. Golan, A.D., E. Somer, S. Dishon, *et al.* 2008. Impact of exposure to war stress on exacerbations of multiple sclerosis. *Ann. Neurol.* **64**(2): 143–148.

14. Li, J., C. Johansen, H. Brønnum-Hansen, *et al.* 2004. The risk of multiple sclerosis in bereaved parents: a nationwide cohort study in Denmark. *J. Neurol.* **62:** 726–729.

15. Warren, S., S. Greenhill & K.G. Warren. 1982. Emotional stress and the development of multiple sclerosis: case-control evidence of a relationship. *J. Chronic Dis.* **35:** 821–831.

16. Ackerman, K.D., A. Stover, R. Heyman, *et al.* 2003. R. Ader New Investigator award. Relationship of cardiovascular reactivity, stressful life events, and multiple sclerosis disease activity. *Brain Behav. Immun.* **17:** 141–151.

17. Ackerman, K.D., R. Heyman, B.S. Rabin, *et al.* 2002. Stressful life events precede exacerbations of multiple sclerosis. *Psychosom. Med.* **64:** 916–920.

18. Mohr, D.C., S.L. Hart, L. Julian, *et al.* 2004. Association between stressful life events and exacerbation in multiple sclerosis: a meta analysis. *B.M.J.* **328:** 731–735.

19. Theiler, M. 1934. Spontaneous encephalomyelitis of mice—a new virus. *Science* **80:** 122.

20. Lipton, H.L. 1975. Theiler's virus infection in mice: an unusual biphasic disease process leading to demyelination. *Infect. Immun.* **11:** 1147–1155.

21. Chamorro, M., C. Aubert & M. Brahic. 1986. Demyelinating lesions due to Theiler's virus are associated with ongoing central nervous system infection. *J. Virol.* **57:** 992–997.

22. Melvold, R.W., D.M. Jokinen, R.L. Knobler, *et al.* 1987. Variations in genetic control of susceptibility to Theiler's virus (TMEV)-induced demyelinating disease. *J. Immunol.* **138:** 1429–1433.

23. Bureau, J.F., X. Montagutelli, S. Lefebvre, *et al.* 1992. The interaction of two groups of murine genes determines the persistence of Theiler's virus in the central nervous system. *J. Virol.* **66:** 4698–4704.

24. Bureau, J.F., X. Montagutelli, F. Bihl, *et al.* 1993. Mapping loci influencing the persistence of Theiler's virus in the murine central nervous system. *Nat. Genet.* **5:** 82–91.

25. Sheridan, J.F., N. Feng, R.H. Bonneau, *et al.* 1991. Restraint stress differentially affects anti-viral cellular and humoral immune responses in mice. *J. Neuroimmunol.* **31:** 245–255.

26. Campbell, T., M.W. Meagher, A. Sieve, *et al.* 2001. The effects of restraint stress on the neuropathogenesis of Theiler's virus-induced demyelination. I. Acute disease. *Brain Behav. Immun.* **15:** 235–254.

27. Welsh, C.J.R., L. Bustamante, M. Nayak, *et al.* 2004. The effects of restraint stress on the neuropathogenesis of Theiler's virus infection II: NK cell function and cytokine levels in acute disease. *Brain Behav. Immun.* **18:** 166–174.

28. Mi, W., M. Belyavskyi, R.R. Johnson, *et al.* 2004. Alterations in chemokine expression in Theiler's virus infection and restraint stress. *J. Neuroimmunol.* **151:** 103–115.

29. Sieve, A.N., A.J. Steelman, C.R. Young, *et al.* 2004. Chronic restraint stress during early Theiler's virus infection exacerbates the subsequent demyelinating disease in SJL mice. *J. Neuroimmunol.* **155:** 103–118.

30. Young, E.E., T.W. Prentice, D. Satterlee, *et al.* 2008. Glucocorticoid exposure alters the pathogenesis of Theiler's murine encephalomyelitis virus during acute infection. *Physiol. Behav.* **95:** 63–71.

31. Brahic, M., W.G. Stroop & J.R. Baringer. 1981. Theiler's virus persists in glial cells during demyelinating disease. *Cell* **26:** 123–128.

32. Rodriguez, M., K.D. Pavelko, M.K. Njenga, *et al.* 1996. The balance between persistent virus infection and immune cells determines demyelination. *J. Immunol.* **157:** 5699–5709.

33. Fiette, L., C.M. Aubert, M. Ulrike, *et al.* 1995. Theiler's virus infection of 129Sv mice that lack the interferon a/b or IFN-γ receptors. *J. Exp. Med.* **181:** 2069–2076.

34. Paya, C.V., A.K. Patick, P.J. Leibson, *et al.* 1989. Role of natural killer cells as immune effectors in encephalitis and demyelination induced by Theiler's virus. *J. Immunol.* **143:** 95–102.

35. Kaminsky, S.G., I. Nakamura & G. Cudkowicz. 1987. Defective differentiation of natural killer cells in SJL mice. Role of the thymus. *J. Immunol.* **138:** 1020–1025.

36. Welsh, C.J.R., W. Mi, A. Sieve, *et al.* 2006. The effect of restraint stress on the neuropathogenesis of Theiler's virus-induced demyelination, a murine model for multiple sclerosis. In *Neural and Neuroendocrine Mechanisms in Host Defense and Autoimmunity*. C.J. Welsh, M.W. Meagher & E. Sternberg, Eds.: 190–225. Springer. New York.

37. Mi, M., T.W. Prentice, C.R. Young, *et al.* 2006. Restraint stress decreases virus-induced pro-inflammatory cytokine expression during acute Theiler's virus infection. *J. Neuroimmunol.* **178:** 49–61.

38. Mi, W., C.R. Young, R. Storts, *et al.* 2006. Stress alters pathogenecity and facilitates systemic dissemination of Theiler's virus. *Microb. Path.* **41:** 133–143.

39. Welsh, C.J.R., P. Tonks, A.A. Nash, *et al.* 1987. The effect of L3T4 T cell depletion on the pathogenesis of Theiler's murine encephalomyelitis virus infection in CBA mice. *J. Gen. Virol.* **68:** 1659–1667.

40. Borrow, P., P. Tonks, C.J.R. Welsh, *et al.* 1992. The role of CD8+ T cells in the acute and chronic phases of Theiler's virus-induced disease in mice. *J. Gen. Virol.* **73:** 1861–1865.

41. Murray, P.D., K.D. Pavelko, J. Leibowitz, *et al.* 1998. CD4 (+) and CD8 (+) T cells make discrete contributions to demyelination and neurologic disease in a viral model of multiple sclerosis. *J. Virol.* **72:** 7320–7329.

42. Welsh, C.J.R., W.F. Blakemore, P. Tonks, *et al.* 1989. Theiler's murine encephalomyelitis virus infection in mice: a persistent viral infection of the central nervous system which induces demyelination. In *Immune Responses, Virus Infection and Disease.* N. Dimmock, Ed.: 125–147. Oxford University Press. Oxford, UK.

43. Clatch, R.J., H.L. Lipton & S.D. Miller. 1987. Class II-restricted T cell responses in Theiler's murine encephalomyelitis virus (TMEV)-induced demyelinating disease. II. Survey of host immune responses and central nervous system virus titers in inbred mouse strains. *Micro. Path.* **3:** 327–337.

44. Rodriguez, M. & S. Sriram. 1998. Successful therapy of Theiler's virus-induced demyelination (DA strain) with monoclonal anti-Lyt2 antibody. *J. Immunol.* **140:** 2950–2955.

45. Borrow, P., C.J.R. Welsh & A.A. Nash. 1993. Study of the mechanisms by which CD4+ T cells contribute to protection in Theiler's murine encephalomyelitis. *Immunology* **80:** 502–506.

46. Welsh, C.J.R., B.V. Sapatino, B. Rosenbaum, *et al.* 1995. Characteristics of cloned cerebrovascular endothelial cells following infection with Theiler's virus. I. Acute Infection. *J. Neuroimmunol.* **62:** 119–125.

47. Kohanawa, M., A. Nakane & T. Minagawa. 1993. Endogenous gamma interferon produced in central nervous system by systemic infection with Theiler's virus in mice. *J. Neuroimmunol.* **48:** 205–211.

48. Rodriguez, M., K. Pavelko & R.L. Coffman. 1995. Gamma interferon is critical for resistance to Theiler's virus-induced demyelination. *J. Virol.* **69:** 7286–7290.

49. Pullen, L.C., S.D. Miller, M.C. Dal Canto, *et al.* 1993. Class I-deficient resistant mice intracerebrally inoc-

ulated with Theiler's virus show an increased T cell response to viral antigens and susceptibility to demyelination. *Eur. J. Immunol.* **23:** 2287–2293.

50. Fiette, L., C. Aubert, M. Brahic, *et al.* 1993. Theiler's virus infection of β2-microglobulin deficient mice. *J. Virol.* **67:** 589–592.

51. Azoulay, A., M. Brahic & J.F. Bureau. 1994. FVB mice transgenic for the H-2D^b gene become resistant to persistent infection by Theiler's virus. *J. Virol.* **68:** 4049–4052.

52. Rodriguez, M. & C.S. David. 1995. H-2Dd transgene suppresses Theiler's virus-induced demyelination in susceptible strains of mice. *J. Neurovirol.* **1:** 111–117.

53. Kang, B.S., M.A. Lyman & B.S. Kim. 2002. Differences in avidity and epitope recognition of CD8(+) T cells infiltrating the central nervous systems of SJL/J mice infected with BeAn and DA strains of Theiler's murine encephalomyelitis virus. *J. Virol.* **76:** 11780–11784.

54. Gerety, S.J., R.J. Clatch, H.L. Lipton, *et al.* 1991. Class II-restricted T cell responses in Theiler's murine encephalomyelitis virus-induced demyelinating disease IV. Identification of an immunodominant T cell determinant on the N-terminal end of the VP2 capsid protein in susceptible SJL/J mice. *J. Immunol.* **146:** 2401–2408.

55. Gerety, S., W. Karpus & A.R. Cubbon, *et al.* 1994. Class II-restricted T cell responses in Theiler's murine encephalomyelitis virus-induced demyelinating disease V. Mapping of a dominant immunopathological VP2 T cell epitope in susceptible mice. *J. Immunol.* **152:** 908–918.

56. Kang, B.S., M.A. Lyman & B.S. Kim. 2002. The majority of infiltrating CD8 cells in the central nervous system of susceptible SJL/J mice infected with Theiler's virus are virus specific and fully functional. *J. Virol.* **76:** 6577–6585.

57. Welsh, C.J.R., A.J. Steelman, A.N. Sieve, *et al.* 2008. Neuroendocrine-immune interactions in neurotropic viral infections. In *Neurotropic Viral Infections.* C. Shoshkes Reiss, Ed.: 300–314. Cambridge University Press. Cambridge, UK.

58. Zheng, W. & R.A. Flavell. 1997. The transcription factor GATA-3 is necessary and sufficient for Th2 cytokine gene expression in CD 4 T cells. *Cell* **89:** 587–596.

59. Szabo, S.J., S.T. Kim, G.L. Costa, *et al.* 2000. A novel transcription factor, T-bet, directs Th1 lineage commitment. *Cell* **100:** 655–669.

60. Roos, R.P. & R. Wollmann. 1984. DA strain of Theiler's murine encephalomyelitis virus induces demyelination in nude mice. *Ann. Neurol.* **15:** 494–499.

61. Gerety, S.J., W.J. Karpus, A.R. Cubbon, *et al.* 1994. Class II-restricted T cell responses in Theiler's

murine encephalomyelitis virus-induced demyelinating disease. V. Mapping of a dominant immunopathologic VP2 T cell epitope in susceptible SJL/J mice. *J. Immunol.* **152:** 908–918.

62. Welsh, C.J.R., P. Tonks, P. Borrow, *et al.* 1990. Theiler's virus: an experimental model of virus-induced demyelination. *Autoimmunity* **6:** 105–112.

63. Borrow, P., C.J.R. Welsh, D. Dean, *et al.* 1998. Investigation of the role of autoimmune responses to myelin in the pathogenesis of TMEV-induced demyelinating disease. *Immunol.* **93:** 478–484.

64. Miller, S.D., C.L. VanDerlugt, W.S. Begolka, *et al.* 1997. Persistent infection with Theiler's virus leads to CNS autoimmunity via epitope spreading. *Nat. Med.* **3:** 1133–1136.

65. Dal Canto, M.C., M.A. Calenoff, S.D. Miller, *et al.* 2000. Lymphocytes from mice chronically infected with Theiler's murine encephalomyelitis virus produce demyelination of organotypic cultures after stimulation with the major encephalitic epitope of myelin proteolipid protein. Epitope spreading in TMEV infection has functional activity. *J. Neuroimmunol.* **104:** 79–84.

Neuroimmune Regulation in Immunocompetence, Acute Illness, and Healing

Istvan Berczi,[a] Andres Quintanar-Stephano,[b] and Kalman Kovacs[c]

[a] *Department of Immunology, Faculty of Medicine, the University of Manitoba, Winnipeg, Canada*

[b] *Department of Physiology, Universidad Autónoma de Aguascalientes, Aguascalientes, Mexico*

[c] *Department of Laboratory Medicine, St. Michael's Hospital, University of Toronto, Toronto, Ontario, Canada*

Adaptive immunocompetence is maintained by growth hormone (GH), prolactin (PRL), and vasopressin (VP). Innate or natural immunocompetence depends on cytokines, hormones (especially of the hypothalamus–pituitary–adrenal axis), and catecholamines. The acute phase response (APR, or acute febrile illness) is an emergency defense reaction whereby the adaptive, T cell–dependent, immune reactions are suppressed and the innate immune function is dramatically amplified. Infection and various forms of injury induce APR. Cytokines [interleukin (IL)-1β, tumor necrosis factor-α, and IL-6] stimulate corticotropin-releasing hormone (CRH) and VP secretion and cause a "sympathetic outflow." Colony-stimulating factors activate leukocytes. CRH is a powerful activator of the pituitary adrenocortical axis and elevates glucocorticoid (GC) levels. Cytokines, GCs, and catecholamines play fundamental roles in the amplification of natural immune defense mechanisms. VP supports the APR at this stage. However, VP remains active and is elevated for a longer period than is CRH. VP, but not CRH, is elevated during chronic inflammatory diseases. VP controls adaptive immune function and stimulates adrenocorticotropic hormone (ACTH) and PRL secretion. PRL maintains the function of the thymus and of the T cell–dependent adaptive immune system. The ACTH–adrenal axis stimulates natural immunity and of suppressor/regulatory T cells, which suppress the adaptive immune system. VP also has a direct effect on lymphoid cells, the significance of which remains to be elucidated. It is suggested that VP regulates the process of recovery from acute illness.

Key words: immunocompetence; acute illness; healing; growth and lactogenic hormones; HPA axis; glucocorticoids; catecholamines; cytokines; liver; acute phase proteins

Introduction

Considerable information has been accumulated to date on the biological significance of growth and lactogenic hormones (GLH). These closely related hormone families are those of growth hormone (GH), prolactin (PRL), and placental lactogens (PL). All these hormones support numerous and important biological functions in animals and humans.[1] It is beyond the scope of this review to discuss the biology of GLH any further. Rather, we shall concentrate on the role of GH and PRL in immune function. Here again we must be selective and hence we call attention to a book and of

Address for correspondence: Dr. Istvan Berczi, Department of Immunology, Faculty of Medicine, The University of Manitoba, 745 Bannatyne Avenue, Winnipeg, MB, R3E, 0J9, Canada. Voice: 204-789-3320; fax: 204-789-3921. berczii@ms.umanitoba.ca

Neuroimmunomodulation: Ann. N.Y. Acad. Sci. 1153: 220–239 (2009).
doi: 10.1111/j.1749-6632.2008.03975.x © 2009 New York Academy of Sciences.

several recent reviews that have been published on the subject.[1-4] An important recent observation is that B-lymphocyte differentiation into antibody-forming cells is regulated by estradiol (for innate) and PRL (for adaptive immune) B cells.[5]

It is necessary also to point out that the immune system functions in two different ways; it has cells and mediators that exert *innate,* or *natural immunity,* with which we are born and never lose. Monocyte/macrophages, granulocytes, a subset of B lymphocytes producing natural antibodies, natural killer (NK) T cells, gamma-delta T cells, and cells of the "reticuloendothel system" play major roles in innate immunity. Innate immune cells are fully mature and react instantaneously to their specific targets, which are evolutionarily highly preserved homologous epitopes, or *homotopes.* This constant recognition pattern allows for the use of standard receptors encoded by germline genes. They are capable of instantaneous reactions without the requirement of cell growth or differentiation. These cells are also able to function under catabolic conditions.[6,7] On the basis of their metabolic properties and hormonal regulation, one may argue that the suppressor/regulatory T cell (Tsr) is also a member of the innate immune system (see below).

In contrast, the *adaptive* or *acquired immune response* is based on cell proliferation and it is susceptible to senescence and to numerous other factors that influence cell growth.[8] Adaptive immune reactions involve the generation of antigen receptor diversity by gene recombination and clonal selection by the specific antigenic determinants (epitopes), which are very diverse. Bone marrow-derived (B) lymphocytes differentiate in the bone marrow, whereas thymus-derived (T) lymphocytes differentiate in the thymus. Specific epitopes drive the selection process and ensure that the mature cells released in the circulation will recognize the specific foreign antigen. Self-reactive cells are killed by apoptosis in the thymus and bone marrow. Mature, antigen-specific cells enter the bloodstream and recirculate as well as populate the secondary lymphoid organs, which are the spleen, lymph nodes, and mucosal lymphoid tissue.[9]

Cell growth requires anabolic conditions, and considerable time is needed for the development from a few cell clones to a whole army of effector cells during the primary immune response (7–10 days). The secondary response is accelerated by memory cells and thus it may develop within 3–5 days. The adaptive immune system is regulated by antigen and by regulatory T cells, which may act by cell-to-cell contact and by their products, such as cytokines.[9]

We also distinguish *cell-mediated and humoral immunity.* Antibodies secreted by B lymphocytes and of other serum factors, such as complement and acute phase proteins (APPs), constitute humoral immunity. Antibodies may be the result of adaptive or innate immune B cell responses. Thymus-derived (T) cells may be *effector* (Te, e.g., helper, killer), or *suppressor/regulatory* (Tsr) and *innate immune* (T$\gamma\delta$ and NK-T). The adaptive immune system is regulated by Tsr, whereas the innate immune system is regulated *independently of T cells*.[6,9]

All systems are regulated by cytokines, hormones, and neurotransmitters, which are peptides. Today it is clear that the hypothalamus is the ultimate immunoregulator, and its regulatory molecules are delivered to the target cells/tissues by the serum or transported to a specific location by innervation. The availability of an adequate hormonal milieu is fundamental for the maintenance of immune function both in health and disease.[3,7,10,11]

Here we will discuss the evidence that GLH and vasopressin (VP) control adaptive immuocompetence. The hypothalamus–pituitary–adrenal (HPA) axis, jointly with catecholamines (CAT), stimulate Tsr and amplify innate immune function. We hypothesize on the basis of our observations that recovery from acute phase response (APR) as well as normal immune function during physiological (homeostatic) conditions, is regulated by the hypothalamic hormone, VP.

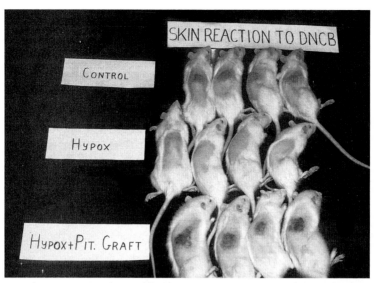

Figure 1. Skin reaction to dinitrochlorobenzene (DNCB). Control animals responded with skin inflammation 5 days after skin painting with DNCB. Hypophysectomized (Hypox) animals did not respond to DNCB challenge. Syngeneic pituitary graft transplanted under the kidney capsule fully restored immune reactivity of Hypox rats.[12] *Note:* Unlike in other species, which need to be sensitized first in order to react to DNCB, rats show natural immunity to DNCB, so they react to the first challenge. (In color in *Annals* online.)

Hormonal Regulation of Immunocompetence

The regulation of adaptive immune function by the pituitary gland was observed by us in 1978. Initial studies revealed that hypophysectomy (Hypox) suppresses the inflammatory response in young rats to dinitrochlorobenzene (DNCB), which may be restored by syngeneic pituitary grafts inserted under the kidney capsule (Fig. 1), and by PRL (Fig. 2).[12] Additional studies indicated that the antibody response is also pituitary dependent, although the secondary response showed partial independence.[13] The rejection of skin allografts and the development of adjuvant-induced arthritis also depends on GLH, e.g., GH, PRL, and PL.[14] The dopamine agonist, bromocriptin, which inhibits pituitary PRL secretion, was as effective in inhibiting adaptive immune function as was Hypox.[15] It was also demonstrated that adrenocorticotropic hormone (ACTH) and glucocorticoids (GC) antagonized the restoration of adaptive immune function by GLH in

Hypox rats.[16,17] In addition it was shown that GH and PRL play an important role in the regulation of bone marrow function.[18]

Passive cutaneous hypersensitivity reactions were not affected by Hypox in rats (unpublished results). Experimental autoimmune encephalomyelitis (EAE) could not be induced in rats 10 days after Hypox as the animals died within 2 days after the injection of antigen (guinea pig brain homogenate) subcutaneously into the right hind paw in complete Freund's adjuvant (unpublished observations). However, if the induction of EAE is carried out at 21 days after Hypox, the animals survive and respond with inflammation in the central nervous system.[19] This difference may be explained by the observation that Hypox rats restore their PRL levels (up to 50% of normal by day 63) and thus become immunocompetent.

Studies on the mechanisms of immunoregulation by pituitary hormones revealed that cell growth and DNA and RNA synthesis in the thymus, spleen, and bone marrow are dependent on GLH. Nucleic acid synthesis in lymphoid

DNCB reaction   Hypox+DNCB   Hypox + PRL + DNCB

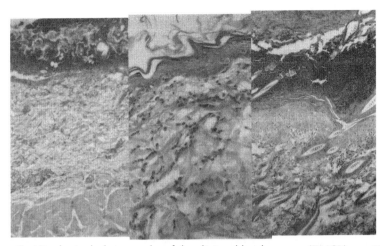

Figure 2. Histological photographs of the dinitrochlorobenzene (DNCB) reaction. Treatment of hypophysectomized (Hypox) rats with prolactin (PRL) restores immunocompetence in Hypox rats. Normal animals react with mononuclear cell infiltration of the challenge site, Hypox animals have no such infiltration. In Hypox animals treated with PRL, the inflammatory response is fully restored.[17] (In color in *Annals* online.)

tissue showed a direct correlation with immunocompetence.[20] This finding is in full accord with the requirement of cell proliferation for adaptive immune reactions. Tissue PRL was demonstrated in the thymus and the spleen of normal but not in Hypox rats.[21] It was also observed that long-surviving Hypox rats have trace amounts of PRL in their serum, which will increase up to 50% of normal by day 63 after surgery. Such animals showed normal bone marrow and immune function. If this residual PRL was neutralized with specific antibodies, the animals lost their immunocompetence, severe anemia developed, and all such animals died within 42 days after the commencement of antibody treatment.[22] Other experiments revealed that the tumor necrosis factor (TNF) response to bacterial lipopolysaccharide (LPS) endotoxin is controlled by the HPA axis. In adrenalectomized mice TNF blood levels rose 60 times over control levels within 30 min and the lethal dose of LPS was reduced 500 times in such animals. TNF levels were moderated and the sensitivity to endotoxin was decreased by dexamethasone (Dex) treatment.[23]

Mice with knockout genes for PRL or its receptor are immunocompetent.[24,25] This could be expected as such animals do have GHs, which are able to maintain immune function, as indicated by our experiments and those of others.[3,4,13–18]

The Regulation of Adaptive Immunity by Suppressor/Regulatory T Cells

During our original studies we observed that replacement doses of GLH stimulated and similar doses of ACTH suppressed adaptive immunity in Hypox rats. It was concluded from these observations that GLH maintains adaptive immune function in higher animals and that the HPA axis acts antagonistically by suppressing adaptive immunity. Thus GLH and HPA axis hormones were considered to be *immunoregulatory* because they were obligatory for normal immune function. Other hormones, (e.g., steroid, thyroid) were classified as *immunomodulators* as they played an optional role in immunoregulation.[26,27] Initially it was assumed that the HPA axis suppresses the thymus and T cell function via GC-induced apoptosis.[28]

Although this assumption may be correct in part, dead cells cannot be regulated. The idea of having suppressor cells for inhibition is much more compelling. Therefore, the gradually emerging concept of Tsr has been generally accepted. Suppressor T cells are heterogeneous; some of them work via cell-to-cell contact and others secrete inhibitory cytokines, such as interleukin (IL)-10 or transforming growth factor-beta (TGF-β).[29,30]

It is becoming increasingly apparent that GC and CAT stimulate the growth and differentiation of Tsr and of other suppressor cells. These observations demonstrate that GC and CAT have the capacity of suppressing adaptive immunity by tilting the balance in favor of Tsr.[31–40] It is also very important that, at the same time, GC and CAT enhance the production of APPs in the liver and in general play a key role in the amplification of natural immune mechanisms during APR, as is discussed below.

Acute Illness

The first review paper on the neuroendocrine changes of acute illness was published by Hans Selye. He proposed that "nocuous" stimuli (stressors) induce a stress response. Selye recognized that stressed organisms develop a defense reaction (general adaptation syndrome) against the insults encountered.[41] Today the response to various noxious insults is known as the APR.[7,42,43]

Clinically, APR is characterized by fever, loss of appetite, inactivity, and sleepiness. Changes in sleep are hallmarks of the APR to infectious challenge. The regulation of these responses involves a cytokine cascade within the brain, including IL-1 and TNF, and several other substances, such as GH-releasing hormone, PRL, nitric oxide (NO), and nuclear factor (NF)-κB. These substances are also involved in the regulation of normal spontaneous sleep.[44,45]

Endotoxin, infectious disease, and various forms of injury all elicit a systemic elevation of IL-1β, TNF-α, and IL-6, which are secreted by cells of the innate immune system, primarily by monocyte/macrophages.[42] Much attention has been paid recently to *colony-stimulating factors (CSF)*, which are cytokines originally described to stimulate bone marrow cells.[46] The bone marrow is recognized today as a fundamental organ in natural immunity as it provides the leukocytes that fulfill this function. The bone marrow is activated during APR, which results in the generation of *leukocytosis*.[47] Recent studies provided evidence that granulocyte macrophage CSF (GM-CSF), macrophage CSF, and granulocyte CSF are involved in the maintenance of host resistance to infectious disease,[48–52] parasitic infestation,[53] and cancer.[54,55] At least some of the CSFs show elevated levels in response to infectious disease.[56] GM-CSF has been proposed as a physiological regulator as it did increase host defense without causing or aggravating inflammation, which may lead to complications.[57] In addition GM-CSF stimulates adaptive immune reactions[58] and immunological tolerance.[59,60] GM-CSF influences dendritic cells, which present antigen to T lymphocytes, and invariant NK T cells that produce cytokines having important functions in inflammation, host defense, and immunoregulation.[61,62] GM-CSF is produced in the bone marrow, by mucosal epithelial cells in the lung, and also in the brain. Receptors are also present in the brain for this cytokine.[63,64] Macrophages play important roles in host defense and also regulate body metabolism.[65] GM-CSF is used currently for immunotherapy and for the production of recombinant vaccines.[66,67]

In turn the cytokines stimulate the hypothalamus, the bone marrow, liver, and the leukocytes directly or indirectly, thus eliciting an APR.[42,47,68] Profound changes occur in serum hormone levels, the HPA axis is activated, and there is also a *sympathetic outflow*, which raises serum CAT levels. GC exert a powerful suppressive effect on the adaptive immune system and also control the level of inflammatory cytokines. Through the activation of this axis and of the sympathetic nervous system, adaptive immune reactions are profoundly suppressed. APPs are induced in the liver, and natural antibody production is dramatically increased by a specific subset of B lymphocytes. Therefore, the conversion of the immune system from the adaptive mode of reactivity to the amplification of natural immunity takes place.[47,69–72] PRL and GH stimulate the adaptive immune system and usually become elevated within the first hour after endotoxin injection, which is followed by a decline and the level may become low normal to subnormal in serious cases of endotoxin shock. Luteinizing hormone (LH), follicle-stimulating hormone, estrogens, androgens, progesterone, and thyroid hormones all decline during infection and endotoxin shock, as a rule. Insulin, glucagon, α-melanocyte-stimulating hormone, endorphin, leptin, corticotropin-releasing hormone (CRH), and arginine VP are increased during endotoxemia.[23,42,47,68] It is clear that dynamic and diurnal changes of hormones should be kept in mind when hormonal alterations are taken into consideration during APR. Much remains to be elucidated about the nature and significance of APR.

A subset of bone marrow–derived macrophages in the brain, termed *perivascular cells*, synthesize prostaglandins after systemic cytokine or endotoxin challenges and play a critical role in the IL-1-induced HPA axis activation.[73] It has also been established that peptidergic sensory nerves present in the vagus and elsewhere provide feedback signals to the brain about the sites of local inflammation.[74]

Acute Phase Proteins

Protein synthesis is profoundly altered in the liver, which is most characteristic for APR. The synthesis of APPs is dramatically enhanced, whereas the production of some normal serum constituents, such as albumin and transferrin, is significantly decreased. In patients with acute illness, C-reactive protein (CRP) and serum amyloid A may increase over 1000-fold within 24–48 h; fibrinogen, "1-antitrypsin, and certain complement and properdin components

(e.g., factor B and C3) show a more moderate increase.[68]

CRP binds to C-type pneumococcal cell walls in the presence of Ca^{2+}. It is present in multiple species, from mammals to fish and crab. It consists of five identical subunits, which form a ring-shaped molecule named *pentraxin*, which also stands for a protein family. Serum amyloid P also belongs to this family.[74] CRP recognizes *homotopes*, which are frequently present on the surface of bacteria, fungi, parasites, and damaged cells and tissues. After combination with the specific homotope, CRP activates complement by the classical pathway, which leads to the induction of chemotaxis, of enhanced phagocytosis by neutrophil, leukocytes, and monocytes, and of tumoricidal activity in macrophages. CRP stimulates the synthesis of IL-1 and TNF-α and potentiates the cytotoxic activity of T lymphocytes, NK cells, and platelets. CRP localizes *in vivo* at sites of inflammation; it binds platelet-activating factor and blocks its activity. The clinical determination of CRP is diagnostic for the presence of infectious and inflammatory disease.[75–78] Denaturation takes place after attachment onto polystyrol plates, and free-CRP subunits attain a third conformation, referred to as *neoCRP*, which is a membrane protein on NK cells and macrophages and functions as a galactose-specific receptor. It also accumulates at injured sites of tissue. Monocyte/macrophages express a specific CRP receptor. Proteolytic fragments of CRP activate macrophages and neutrophils.[75] Human CRP protects mice from an otherwise lethal *Streptococcus pneumoniae* infection.[78]

Lipopolysaccharide-binding protein (LBP) shows a 100-fold increase (from 0.5–50 μg/mL) in the serum during an APR. It is capable of opsonizing LPS-bearing particles and may be required for the activation of complement by LPS through the alternate pathway. LBP–LPS complexes are also potent stimulators of cytokines from monocytes and macrophages after combining with CD14 and toll-like receptor 4 on the surface of these cells.[79,80] In humans, high-dose LBP suppressed the binding of both R-type and S-type LPS to CD14 and inhibited LPS-induced nuclear translocation of NF-κB. This inhibitory effect of serum could be mimicked by purified high-density lipoprotein (HDL) in serum-free medium, indicating an LBP-mediated transfer of S-type LPS to plasma lipoproteins, such as HDL.[81]

Haptoglobin (HG) is an APP that binds hemoglobin, thus preventing iron loss and renal damage. It is an antioxidant, has antibacterial activity, and plays a role in modulating many aspects of APR.[82,83] HG selectively suppressed *in vitro* the production of TNF-α, IL-10, and IL-12 by LPS-stimulated monocytes but failed to inhibit the production of IL-6, IL-8, and IL-1 receptor antagonist. HG knockout mice were more sensitive to LPS than were their wild-type counterparts.[84]

The APP α(1)-acid glycoprotein and α(1)-antitrypsin exert anti-apoptotic and anti-inflammatory effects and contribute to delayed type protection associated with ischemic preconditioning in the kidney and in other sites.[84]

Mannose-binding lectin (MBL) is an APP. It binds to the repeating sugar arrays on many microbial surfaces through multiple lectin domains. After binding, MBL is able to activate the complement system via an associated serum protease, MASP-2. There is an increased incidence of infections in individuals with mutations of MBL and an association with autoimmune disorders, such as systemic lupus erythematosus and rheumatoid arthritis.[85] The serum concentration of MBL is subject to large individual differences. GH regulates MBL levels.[86]

Other APPs are *proteinase inhibitors*, such as α2-macroglobulin, α1-acid glycoprotein, antithrombin III, α1-acute-phase globulin, and α1-proteinase inhibitor, which are abundant in the rat. Kupffer cells stimulate α2-macroglobulin synthesis by hepatocytes *in vitro* in the presence of 10^{-9} mol/L Dex. *Fibrinogen* is also an APP with an important role in blood coagulation and healing. α-Macrofetoprotein (α-MFP) is a strong inhibitor of inflammatory mediators, such as histamine (HA), bradykinin, serotonin, and prostaglandin E2, and inhibits polymorphonuclear chemotaxis.[87]

Metabolic Effect of Acute Phase Response

Pro-inflammatory cytokines, especially TNF, induce hyperleptinemia. This is an integral part of APR and is necessary for an integrated communication network to coordinate the energy status of the animal with the ability to fight pathogens.[88] Hyperglycemia and lipolysis are characteristic of APR, and catabolism prevails.[89,90]

In patients with APR the GH–insulin-like growth factor (IGF)-I axis is suppressed and catabolism prevails. Such patients were treated with GH in a controlled trial. GH treatment increased mortality. Deaths attributed to "septic shock or uncontrolled infection" occurred nearly four times more commonly in GH-treated patients compared to placebo-receiving patients. Although no data were given regarding immune parameters, the authors suggested that alterations in immune functions may have contributed to these fatalities.[91]

The APR is a massive neuroimmune and metabolic response that catabolizes the resources and tissues of the body in the interest of host defense and survival. The findings of Takala and co-workers[91] strongly suggest that the suppression of the GH–IGF-I axis in APR is required for intense catabolism to take place. A rapid release of nutrients and of energy is necessary under these conditions in order to maximally support the defense system of the body, which includes the HPA axis, sympathetic nervous system, bone marrow, $CD5^{+}$ B lymphocytes, leukocytes, and the liver.[27,47,68,92] Recent observations showed that GH inhibits the production of APPs in rats with burn injury and in human hepatocytes.[93,94] These findings strongly support the above hypothesis.

One may argue that the most efficient way to fuel the intensive systemic effort for survival in APR is by the rapid breakdown of bodily tissues. GH is a powerful anabolic hormone, which supports the T lymphocyte–dependent immune system, and acts as an antagonist of the HPA axis that promotes APR.[13–15,92–95] The results of this controlled trial support the hypothesis that the inhibition of the HPA axis and of catabolism by GH treatment in APR hampers the body's defense mechanisms, which may have fatal consequences.

The Regulation of Acute Phase Proteins

GC and *CAT* induce α-MFP synergistically in normal rats.[96] Near basal concentrations of GC exerted a stimulatory effect on hepatic APR, on the pro-inflammatory macrophage migration inhibition factor secretion, and on the expression of cytokine/chemokine receptors.[97] Adrenalin induces a high level of IL-6 in rats, which can be antagonized by propranolol. When IL-6 release is blocked, the fast reacting APP, α2-macroglobulin, and cysteine protease inhibitor are strongly depressed. Isoprenalin, a β2-adrenergic receptor agonist, also causes very high levels of IL-6, indicating that β2 receptors are involved.[98]

IL-6 is a major inducer of APP synthesis. Interferon (IFN)-γ, leukemia inhibitory factor, TGF-β, and oncostatin M also induce APP from the liver. IL-6 activates the genes of APP through the DNA binding protein called *NF-IL-6*. NF-IL-6 is a pleiotropic mediator of many inducible genes involved in the acute, immune, and inflammatory responses, similarly to NF-κB. Both NF-IL-6 and NF-κB binding sites are present in the inducible genes, such as IL-6, IL-8, and several acute phase genes.[99] In humans, IL-6 exerted a hyperglycemic effect, whereas IL-2 had an opposite effect.[100]

Immunoconversion in Acute Phase Response

During APR, the HPA axis and CAT are activated. This activation results in the suppression of the T cell–dependent adaptive immune response, which is supported further by the suppression of the hormones that are essential for the maintenance of the thymus and of T lymphocytes (e.g., PRL, GH, IGF-I). CAT and GC, which are released in large quantities during

APR, induce apoptosis in the thymus with a striking efficiency. The elevated level of TNF-α and zinc deficiency, which develops during APR, also contributes to thymic involution and to the suppression of the adaptive immune system.[7,27]

Healing

Febrile illness develops on numerous occasions during a lifetime. Most of these febrile episodes are followed by healing, return to health, and to normal immunocompetence. By now we understand much about APR, how it develops, and what it is doing. However, we know little about the recovery phase. Recent observations suggest that *VP* is the central hypothalamic coordinator during healing, which also leads to normal immune function (*immunoreversion*).[7] VP is primarily a neurohypophysial hormone produced in magnocellular neurons of the hypothalamic paraventricular and supraoptic nuclei, but parvocellular CRH neurons also co-express VP. VP acts as a second "releasing factor" for ACTH along with CRH. Aminergic, cholinergic, GABAergic, glutamatergic, and a number of peptidergic inputs have all been implicated in the regulation of CRH/VP neurons. VP is also expressed within the immune system.[7,101,102]

Vasopressin and Stress

Both CRH and VP are released during stress by the elevated levels of epinephrine (EP) and norepinephrine, and seconds later the secretion ACTH is induced, which elicits the secretion of GC by the adrenal cortex. CRH coordinates the endocrine, autonomic, behavioral, and immune responses to stress and also acts as a neurotransmitter or neuromodulator in the amygdala, dorsal raphe nucleus, hippocampus, and locus coeruleus. VP, 5-hydroxytryptamine, CAT, substance P, vasoactive intestinal polypeptide, neuropeptide Y, and cholecystokinin are produced in these loci. Cytokines, such as IL-1, stimulate CRH and VP gene expression and are implicated in immune–neuroendocrine regulation. Expression profiles of the CRH and VP genes are not uniform after stress exposure, and the VP gene appears to be more sensitive to GC suppression.[101–103] Cytokine-induced CRF and VP synthesis and/or release is modulated by CAT, prostaglandins, and NO.[104]

Compared to Wistar rats, Lewis rats exhibited low VP but identical CRH, and IL-1 priming significantly increased VP without affecting CRH stores. This is consistent with a shift to VP-dominated control of ACTH secretion, as described in Wistar rats under conditions of HPA hyper(re)activity. IL-1 priming of Lewis rats attenuated the ACTH responses to an IL-1 challenge 11 days later. There was no effect on immune reactivity.[105]

Immunoreactive CRH was significantly decreased in splenic extracts from arthritic rats. Low levels of VP were found in immune tissues, which significantly increased in spleens from arthritic animals, but thymic contents of VP were not altered.[106] Elevated plasma VP levels were noted in seven patients with status asthmaticus during the acute attack. These values returned to normal with resolution of the acute phase.[107]

Thirteen multiple sclerosis (MS) patients were studied at baseline and with provocative tests of HPA axis function (ovine CRH, VP, and ACTH stimulation). Compared to matched controls, patients with MS had significantly higher plasma cortisol levels at baseline but showed normal, rather than blunted, plasma ACTH responses to ovine CRH. Patients had blunted ACTH responses to VP stimulation and normal cortisol responses to high- and low-dose ACTH stimulation.[108]

Vasopressin in Chronic Inflammation

During chronic inflammatory diseases, such as adjuvant-induced arthritis of rats, CRH does not act as the major ACTH-releasing factor. This is also the case for EAE, eosinophilia-myalgia syndrome, systemic lupus erythemato-sus, and leishmaniasis. During chronic inflammation VP takes over as the major regulator of the HPA axis.[109]

Chronic intermittent exposure to immobilization, insulin-induced hypoglycemia, or psychological stress stimuli increased the number of CRH cells containing VP and the ratio of VP to CRH within the zona externa of the median eminence.[110–113] In chronically restrained rats exogenous VP but not CRH was found to increase plasma levels of both ACTH and corticosterone.[114] Chronic inflammation is associated with a much larger stimulation of VP than other stress models. Activation of CRH does not appear to play a role under these conditions. However, only CRH can stimulate proopiomelanocortin (POMC) transcription, not VP.[94,115] VP has been less potent than CRH in producing ACTH release from rat pituitaries. The effect of VP on CRF-mediated ACTH release is either synergistic or additive.[116,117]

Vasopressin and Cytokines

IL-1β significantly potentiated the acetylcholine-induced VP release. This effect was completely blocked by neutralizing antibodies to IL-1β, atropine, or mecamylamine.[118] In IL-1β-treated rats, the change in body temperature and VP release from the ventral septal area were negatively correlated.[119] In male rats the ACTH response to IL-1β was significantly reduced by both anti-CRH and anti-VP antisera compared to the levels after normal rabbit serum.[120] Similarly in rats, the *IL-6*-induced ACTH response was significantly suppressed by both anti-CRH and anti-VP antibodies. The TNF-α-induced ACTH response was not significantly affected by anti-VP antibody, although anti-CRH antibody suppressed the response.[121] IL-6 potentiated acetylcholine-induced VP release in rats.[122]

A single injection of recombinant mouse *IL-2* caused a significant increase in VP and oxytocin (OT) mRNA levels in the hypothalamus of nude mice. This effect was specific to the nude mouse.[123] IL-2 released VP from the hypothalamus and amygdala of rats *in vitro*. The IL-2- and acetylcholine-induced VP release was antagonized by Ng-methyl-L-arginine, which indicates a role for NO in this VP release.[124] IL-2 caused a dose-dependent stimulation of VP, but not CRH, secretion from both the intact rat hypothalamus *in vitro* and hypothalamic cell cultures.[125]

Centrally administered *leukemia inhibitory factor* significantly increased the plasma VP concentration from 5 to 60 min after the injection.[125]

The Role of Vasopressin in the Acute Phase Response

VP attenuated significantly the febrile response of rabbits to bacterial pyrogen.[126] Endotoxin may stimulate the generation of NO, which inhibits CRH and generates carbon monoxide, which modulates the release of VP. These are potential counter-regulatory controls of HPA activation.[127]

An inhibitor of central EP synthesis (SKF 64139) enhanced basal medial hypothalamus (BMH) and basal median eminence (BME) VP contents in adult male rats. LPS administration significantly decreased BMH VP in control and peripheral EP inhibitor (SKF 29661)-pretreated rats and diminished BME VP in all groups.[128]

In rats, CRH gene transcription was upregulated in the PVN 3–4 h following LPS injection. Transcripts of CRH receptor type A were present in the hypothalamus 6 h after endotoxin treatment. No alterations in cytoplasmic VP mRNA levels were noted in rats treated with LPS. ACTH secretion was stimulated within 30 min. These results suggest that systemic LPS acts first within the median eminence where it stimulates peptidic nerve terminals.[129]

LPS potently stimulated CRH and VP secretion into pituitary portal blood in alert normally behaving ewes and stimulated cortisol and progesterone secretion into peripheral blood. Both CRH and VP rose and fell simultaneously, although the peak of the VP response was approximately 10-fold greater than that of CRH. There was a significant suppression of gonadotropin-releasing hormone and LH pulsatile secretion in these same ewes and fever developed.[130]

In Holstein steers LPS induced fever, increased plasma ACTH, and cortisol. Pituitary VP receptor V3 mRNA was decreased at 2, 4, and 12 h following LPS administration and returned to basal by 24 h. A similar temporal regulation of pituitary CRH receptor (R)1 mRNA, but not pituitary POMC mRNA, was observed. Downregulation of CRHR1 mRNA was not observed in other brain regions following LPS administration (e.g., cerebellum, hypothalamus).[131]

Regulation of Pituitary Hormones by Vasopressin

The ACTH response to exogenous administration of VP was impaired in V1bR$^{-/-}$ mice, while CRH-stimulated ACTH release was not significantly different from that in the V1bR$^{+/+}$ mice. The increase in ACTH after a forced swim stress was significantly suppressed in V1bR$^{-/-}$ mice.[132]

In conscious male rats intracerebroventricular (i.c.v.) infusion of HA induced PRL secretion, which was inhibited by pretreatment with a specific antiserum to VP. A VP antagonist also inhibited the PRL response to HA and inhibited the PRL response to restraint stress. Pretreatment with a specific OT antagonist had no effect on the HA- or stress-induced PRL release.[133] VP antiserum (VP-Ab) was administered i.v. to lactating rats 15 min before permitting their previously isolated pups to suckle or to continuously suckled rats. The suckling-induced rise in plasma PRL levels was significantly less in VP-Ab-treated mothers when compared to rats receiving a similar amount of normal rabbit serum.[134] Anterior pituitary cells derived from juvenile female turkeys were incubated with posterior pituitary extracts or test substances for 3 h. Posterior pituitary extracts contained potent substance(s) which stimulated

PRL release in a concentration-dependent manner. Antisera to VP and vasoactive intestinal peptide (1:500) completely abolished the PRL-releasing activities.[135]

CRH or VP released ACTH and immunoreative β-endorphin (β-END) in response to HA and restraint stress. Pretreatment with CRH antiserum abolished the ACTH response to stress and inhibited the β-END response by 60%. Immunoneutralization with VP antiserum had only half the inhibitory effect of that seen with CRH antiserum. CRH (100 pmol i.v.) increased the plasma levels of ACTH and β-END. This effect was abolished by pretreatment with CRH antiserum, whereas pretreatment with VP antiserum prevented the CRH-induced ACTH release and inhibited the β-END response by 50%. VP (24–800 pmol i.v.) stimulated ACTH and β-END in a dose-dependent manner. CRH and VP antisera each prevented the effect of VP on ACTH secretion, whereas the β-END response to VP was only inhibited by about 60% by the antisera.[133]

Endogenous OT contributes to the control of basal GH release probably by stimulating somatostatin secretion and/or inhibiting GH-releasing hormone secretion or by both actions. Endogenous VP and OT play a physiologically significant stimulatory role in the control of basal ACTH release.[136]

The novel high-affinity nonpeptide CRHR1 antagonist R121919 attenuates the stress-induced release of corticosterone, PRL, and OT. The decrease in plasma *testosterone* following exposure to stress is abolished by R121919.[137]

In rats with paraventricular nucleus lesions, LPS was able to activate the hypophysial–adrenal system in the absence of hypophysiotrophic neuropeptides of paraventricular origin.[138]

Vasopressin and the Immune Response

Brattleboro diabetes insipidus (DI) rats were derived from Long–Evans (LE) rats and are homozygous for DI and lack VP. In DI rats there was a permanent decrease in the number of blood lymphocytes, increase in neutrophil count, reduced activity of macrophages, early involution of the thymus and spleen, and suppression of antibody production.[139] In DI rats, NK cell activity was significantly higher than in LE rats. VP replacement normalized water intake in DI rats but had no significant effect on NK cell activity. DI rats exhibited lower plasma corticosterone levels, which were not elevated by VP replacement.[140]

In mice with the disruption of VP receptor 1a (VPR1a) gene a shift was observed from IgM(high)/IgD(high) to the more mature IgM(low)/IgD(high) B cells. Splenic B-cell proliferation was significantly greater after anti-IgM stimulation, and enhanced IgG1 and IgG2b production occurred in response to immune challenge with T-dependent antigen. B-1 cells were increased in VPR1a$^{(-/-)}$ mice. T cell differentiation and activation were normal in VPR1a$^{(-/-)}$ mice.[141]

The VP-binding nonapeptide has the sequence Thr-Met-Lys-Val-Leu-Thr-Gly-Ser-Pro (binding peptide). VP and its six-amino acid N-terminal, cyclic ring pressinoic acid (PA) are both capable of replacing the IL-2 requirement for IFN-γ production by mouse splenic lymphocytes. The VP-binding peptide specifically and reversibly blocked VP help in IFN-γ production but failed to block the helper signal of PA. Thus the intact VP molecule and not just the N-terminal cyclic ring is important for interaction with the binding peptide.[142,143]

VP enhanced the autologous mixed lymphocyte response. Enhanced proliferation appeared to be specific for the arginine residues in position 8 of VP.[144]

In rats the i.c.v. administration of VP suppressed the proliferative response of splenic T cells and NK cytotoxicity in an adrenal-independent manner. These effects were completely reversed by i.c.v. pre-administration of the VPR1 receptor antagonist.[145]

VPR1 agonist induced a complex intracellular Ca^{2+}-signaling cascade in cortical

TABLE 1. The Neuroendocrine and Immune Effects of Neurointermediate Hypophysectomy and of Desmopressin Treatment[a]

	Control	Sham	Sham+DP	Hypox	Hypox+DP	NIL[c]	NIL+DP	NIL+TX
Adrenal weight		≠	↑↑↑	↓↓↓	↓	↑	↑↑	↑↑
Thymus weight		≠	≠	↓	↑ compared to Hypox	↓	≠	↓↓↓
Spleen weight		≠	↑↓	↓	↑ compared to Hypox	↑↓	≠↓	
Serum SRBC antibody		≠		↓↓		↓↓		
Serum SRBC C' fixing antibody	↑↑	↑↑		↓↓		↓↓		
Serum IgG, IgM, anti-SRBC	↑↑	↑↑		↓		↓		
Arthus reaction (SRBC)	↑↑	↑↑		↓		↓		
Serum IgG, IgM; intestinal IgA, anti- *Salmonella typhi**	↑↑	↑↑		↓↓		↓		
Serum IgG, IgM; intestinal IgA, anti- *Salmonella typhi**	↑↑	↑↑		↓↓		↓		
Contact sensitivity to DNCB	↑↑	↑↑		↓		↓		
EAE: clinical score	↑↑	↑↑	↓	↑	↑↑↑	↓↓	↑↑	
EAE: plasma ACTH and corticosterone		↑	↑	↓↓↓↓	↓↓↓↓	≠		
Adenohypophyseal cell counts		≠				GH[b] ↓ LH ↓		TSH ↑↑↑↑ GH ↓↓↓↓ PRL ↓↓↓

[a]Please see the text for a detailed explanation and for most abbreviations. Sham = sham-operated group of animals; Hypox = hypophysectomized animals; DP = desmopressin; NIL = neurointermediate pituitary lobectomy; TX = thyroidectomy; SRBC = sheep red blood cells; C' = serum complement; Ig = immunoglobulin (-G; -M; -A); DNCB = dinitrochlorobenzene; EAE = experimental autoimmune encephalitis; ACTH = adrenocorticotropin; GH = growth hormone; TSH = thyroid-stimulating hormone; LH = luteinizing hormone; PRL = prolactin; ↑, increase compared to intact control or sham operated control; ↓, decrease in relation to controls; ≠, no change with respect to the control; ↑↓, variable response.

[b]GH-, PRL-, TSH-, and LH-producing cell types were detected by immunocytochemistry.

[c]In long-surviving NIL rats (8 months), adrenal weight increased 30% whereas thymus weight decreased 50% when compared to the intact control. *Oral infection was used in the experiments with *Salmonella typhimurium*. Modified from Ref. 7.

astrocytes. It dramatically decreased the mRNA level of five cytokines, including IL-1β and TNF-α.[146]

Our Observations

Membrane VP receptors are present in several immune cell types.[142,147,148] We investigated the effect of neurointermediate pituitary lobectomy (NIL) on immune function of rats. NIL rats have low plasma levels of VP and OT.[149] The adrenal glands are enlarged, whereas the thymuses and spleens decreased in size in some experiments but not in others.[150,151] If thyroidectomy was also performed in NIL animals, the increase in adrenal size and decrease in thymus and spleen weights were exaggerated. NIL inhibited immune function, which included the IgG and IgM responses to sheep red blood cells,[152] plasma IgG, IgM,

TABLE 2. Hypothalamic Immunoregulation[a]

Parameter	CRH	VP
Pituitary adrenal axis	↑↑↑	↑↑
POMC	↑↑↑	0
Prolactin	↓↓	↑↑
Cytokines	Il-1, -6, TNF-α	Il-1,-2,-6, LIF
Adaptive Im.	↓↓↓	↑↑↑
Autoimmunity	↓↓↓	↑ permissive
Chronic inflam.	↓↓↓	↑↑
Nat. Imm., APR	↑↑↑	↑↑↑
LPS response	↑↑↑	↑↑↑

[a]Symbols are as for Table 1. 0, not influenced; CRH = corticotropin-releasing hormone; VP = vasopressin; POMC = proopiomelanocortin; Il = interleukin (-1; -2; -6); TNF = tumor necrosis factor; LIF = leukemia inhibitory factor; APR = acute phase response; LPS = lipoplisaccharide.

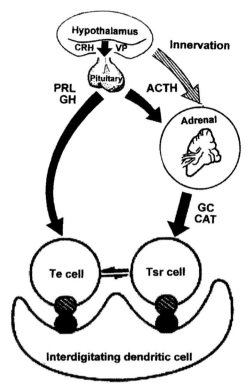

Figure 3. Hypothalamic regulation of immuno-competence. During health the hypothalamic neuropepetide vasopressin (VP) stimulates the secretion of prolactin (PRL), growth hormone (GH), and also adrenocorticotropic hormone (ACTH) by the pituitary gland. PRL and GH stimulate effector T cells (Te), and glucocorticoids (GC) and catecholamines (CAT) stimulate suppressor/regulatory T cells (Tsr). Thus VP maintains normal well-balanced (homeostatic) hormone levels, which lead to normal immune function. Corticotropin-releasing hormone (CRH) is a powerful stimulant of the pituitary–adrenal axis during acute illness and stress. Under these conditions GC and CAT levels rise and grossly elevate Tsr levels. The Te/Tsr balance tilts toward Tsr, which leads to the suppression of adaptive immune function and to the amplification of natural immunity (see Fig. 4).

and intestinal secretion of IgA to *Salmonella typhimurium*[153] and delayed type-cell-mediated immunity to DNCB and the Arthus reaction.[154] Decreased incidence and severity of EAE[19] and failure to develop inflammation in adjuvant-induced arthritis were also observed in NIL animals.[155]

Using the EAE model in NIL rats, we examined the effects of *desmopressin (DP)*, a synthetic analog of VP, on the immune/inflammatory responses and on HPA axis activity. The results showed that NIL induces a decreased incidence and severity of the EAE with no increase in HPA activity and DP treatment restored the susceptibility of the NIL animals to EAE, which was accompanied with high ACTH and corticosterone plasma levels (Tables 1 and 2; Fig. 3).[156]

Conclusions

This overview indicates that VP participates in immunoregulation, both by regulating pituitary hormones and by direct effect on immunocytes. It seems certain that VP is required for the maintenance of adaptive immunocompetence. GLH are responsible for the maintenance of thymus func-

tion and of the T cell–regulated adaptive immune system in a competent state. It is clear that VP has the capacity to stimulate both the HPA axis and PRL in a balanced fashion. This is in contrast with CRH, which stimulates the HPA axis exclusively. In APR, CRH is dominant because of its resistance to GC inhibition, whereas VP is in the background. However, as it has been established,

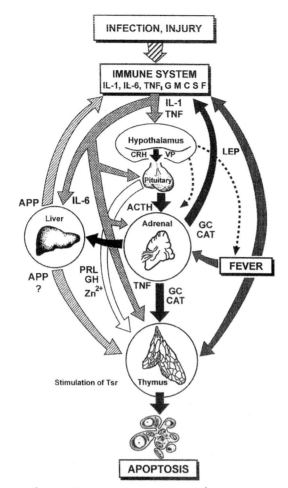

Figure 4. Immunoconversion and immunoreversion during the acute phase response (APR). The APR is a systemic inflammatory reaction to infectious agents and to other forms of injury. Fever is a hallmark of the APR, so it is commonly known as febrile illness. Immune-derived cytokines [primarily interleukin (IL)-1, IL-6, tumor necrosis factor (TNF)-α, and granulocyte macrophage colony-stimulating factors (GM-CSF)] are released by the immune system and act either on nerve terminals or on the brain and on leukocytes. The cytokines stimulate the hypothalamus, and a powerful neuroendocrine and metabolic response to the infection/injury is initiated. CSF activate the bone marrow-derived leukocytes. From the hypothalamus, CRH and VP are secreted during APR. Both of these peptides stimulate the hypothalamus–pituitary–adrenal (HPA) axis. In addition VP stimulates PRL secretion. Initially CRH has a dominant role during APR, and the activation of the HPA axis prevails. This is coupled with "sympathetic outflow" from the adrenal gland. The increased level of GC and CAT, together with TNF-α, are of prime importance for inducing

during chronic inflammatory disease VP will take over the regulation of the HPA axis. Moreover, VP has the capacity to stimulate PRL synthesis, which is suppressed during APR. PRL is an important immunostimulator, and is capable of restoring adaptive immunocompetence, which sets the stage for recovery and healing. At the same time VP also maintains the HPA function at physiological levels, which maintains

thymus involution (e.g., by inducing apoptosis of $CD8^+4^+$ thymocytes) and for inhibiting the T cell–dependent adaptive immune system. Other factors that contribute to thymic suppression are the downregulation of GH and PRL synthesis and zinc deficiency.[7,28] Under these conditions, suppressor/regulatory T-lymphocyte (Tsr) numbers are grossly elevated in response to GC and CAT and suppress adaptive immunity systemically. During APR the synthesis of acute phase proteins (APPs) is amplified in the liver by IL-6, GC, and CAT. Serum C-reactive protein (CRP) will rise as much as 1000 times the basal level within 24–48 h. CRP is capable of recognizing pathogenic organisms and activating complement and leukocytes for phagocytosis and cytotoxicity. Other serum proteins with similar biology are lipopolysaccharide-binding protein (LBP) and mannan-binding protein (MBP). Additional APP are fibrinogen and a number of anti-inflammatory and enzyme inhibitory proteins, which also rise in the serum during APR. Natural antibodies that are polyspecific, similar to CRP, LBP, and MBP, are also stimulated during APR and serve to identify pathogenic agents, which is followed by immune activation. Therefore the essence of febrile illness is to switch the immune system over from the adaptive (T cell–dependent) mode of reactivity to the activation of innate/natural immune mechanisms. This process has been coined as *immunoconversion.*[7] During the chronic phase of inflammatory disease, CRH will subside and VP will take over the regulation of the HPA axis. Because VP also stimulates PRL secretion, it is hypothesized that VP alters the *neuroendocrine milieu* to favor the restoration of adaptive immunocompetence. During healing, immune reactivity returns to normal physiological levels, which is named *immunoreversion.* VP maintains normal immune reactivity in healthy animals. It is the primary activator of the HPA axis during chronic inflammatory disease and also contributes to APR. We propose that VP is the hypothalamic coordinator of the healing process from acute illness. (Modified from Ref. 157.)

innate immunity by acting synergistically with catecholamines. These observations promise a better understanding of illness and recovery and are expected to significantly aid patient management. Additional studies are required to unravel in more detail the control of immune function by the hypothalamus via the pituitary gland (Fig. 4).

Acknowledgments

Supported by Univesidad Autonoma de Aguascalientes (UAA) PIFF08-1 and Consejo Nacional de Ciencia y Tecnología (CONACYT)-62317, Mexico.

Conflicts of Interest

The authors declare no conflicts of interest.

References

1. Berczi, I. & A. Szentivanyi. 2003. Growth and lactogenic hormones, insulin-like growth factor and insulin. In *Neuroimmune Biology, Volume 3: The Immune-Neuroendocrine Circuitry. History and Progress.* I. Berczi & A. Szentivanyi, Eds.: 129–153. Elsevier. Amsterdam.
2. O'Connor, J.C. *et al.* 2008. Regulation of IGF-I function by proinflammatory cytokines: at the interface of immunology and endocrinology. *Cell Immunol.* **252:** 91–110.
3. Savino, W. 2007. Neuroendocrine control of T cell development in mammals: role of growth hormone in modulating thymocyte migration. *Exp. Physiol.* **92:** 813–817.
4. Kelley, K.W. *et al.* 2007. Protein hormones and immunity. *Brain Behav. Immun.* **21:** 384–392.
5. Venkatesh, J. *et al.* 2006. Cutting edge: hormonal milieu, not antigenic specificity, determines the mature fenotype of autoreactive B cells. *J. Immun.* **176:** 3311–3314.
6. Bertok, L. & D.A. Chow, Eds. 2005. *Natural Immunity.* I. Berczi & A. Szentivanyi, Series Eds. Elsevier. Amsterdam.
7. Berczi, I. *et al.* 2006. Chapter 14. Immunoconversion in the acute phase response. In *Cytokines, Stress and Immunity.* N.P. Plotnikoff *et al.* Eds.: 215–254. CRC Press, Taylor & Francis Group. Boca Raton, FL.
8. Straub, R.H. & E. Mocchegiani, Eds. 2004. *Neuroimmune Biology Volume 4. The Neuroendocrine Immune Network in Ageing.* I. Berczi, A. Szentivanyi, Series Eds. Elsevier. Amsterdam.
9. Janeway, C.A. Jr. *et al.* Ed. 2005. *Immunobiology,* 6th ed. Garland Science Publishing. New York.
10. Berczi, I. *et al.* 1993. Hormones in self tolerance and autoimmunity: a role in the pathogenesis of rheumatoid arthritis? *Autoimmunity* **16:** 45–56.
11. Berczi, I. & A. Szentivanyi. 2003. The immune-neuroendocrine circuitry. In *Neuroimmune Biology, Volume 3: The Immune-Neuroendocrine Circuitry. History and Progress.* I. Berczi & A. Szentivanyi, Eds.: 561–592. Elsevier. Amsterdam.
12. Nagy, E. & I. Berczi. 1978 Immunodeficiency in hypophysectomized rats. *Acta. Endocrinol.* **89:** 530–537.
13. Berczi, I. *et al.* 1981. Regulation of humoral immunity in rats by pituitary hormones. *Acta. Endocrinol.* **98:** 506–513.
14. Nagy, E. *et al.* 1983. Regulation of immunity in rats by lactogenic and growth hormones. *Acta. Endocrinol.* **102:** 351–357.
15. Nagy, E. *et al.* 1983. Immunomodulation by bromocriptine. *Immunopharmacology* **6:** 231–243.
16. Berczi, I. *et al.* 1984. The influence of pituitary hormones on adjuvant arthritis. *Arthritis Rheum.* **27:** 682–688.
17. Berczi, I. *et al.* 1983. Pituitary hormones and contact sensitivity in rats. *Allergy* **38:** 325–330.
18. Nagy, E. & I. Berczi. 1989. Pituitary dependence of bone marrow function. *Br. J. Haematol.* **71:** 457–462.
19. Quintanar-Stephano, A. *et al.* 2005. Neurointermediate pituitary lobectomy decreases the incidence and severity of experimental autoimmune encephalomyelitis in Lewis rats. *J. Endocrinol.* **184:** 51–58.
20. Berczi, I. *et al.* 1991. Pituitary hormones regulate c-myc and DNA synthesis in lymphoid tissue. *J. Immunol.* **146:** 2201–2206.
21. Berczi I. Neuroimmune biology: an introduction. In *Neuroimmune Biology Volume 1: New Foundation of Biology.* I. Berczi & R. Gorczynski, Eds.: 3–45. Elsevier. Amsterdam.
22. Nagy, E. & I. Berczi. 1991. Hypophysectomized rats depend on residual prolactin for survival. *Endocrinology* **128:** 2776–2784.
23. Ramachandra, R.N. *et al.* 1992. Neuro-hormonal host defence in endotoxin shock. *Brain Behav. Immun.* **6:** 157–169.
24. Horseman, N.D. *et al.* 1997. Defective mammopoiesis, but normal hematopoiesis, in mice with a targeted disruption of the prolactin gene. *EMBO J.* **16:** 6926–6935.

25. Bouchard, B. *et al.* 1999. Immune system development and function in prolactin receptor-deficient mice. *J. Immunol.* **163:** 576–582.

26. Beczi, I. 1986. Immunoregulation by the pituitary gland. In *Pituitary Function and Immunity*. I. Berczi, Ed.: 227–240. CRC Press, Inc. Boca Raton, FL.

27. del Rey, A. *et al.* Eds. 2008. *Neuroimmune Biology Volume 7: The Hypothalamus-Pituitary-Adrenal Axis*. I. Berczi & A. Szentivanyi, Series Eds.: Elsevier. Amsterdam.

28. Haeryfar, S.M.M. & I. Berczi. 2001. The thymus and the acute phase response. *Cell. Mol. Biol.* **47:** 145–156.

29. Schwartz, A. & R.K. Gershon. 1984. Regulation of in vitro cytotoxic T lymphocyte generation. III. Interactions or regulatory T cell subsets in suppressor and target populations. *J. Mol. Cell. Immunol.* **1:** 237–252.

30. Shevach, E.M. 2008. Special regulatory T cell review: how I became a T suppressor/regulatory cell maven. *Immunology* **123:** 3–5.

31. Peek, E.J. *et al.* 2005. Interleukin-10-secreting "regulatory" T cells induced by glucocorticoids and by beta-2-agonists. *Am. J. Respir. Cell. Mol. Biol.* **33:** 105–111.

32. Negrini, S. *et al.* 2006. Endocrine regulation of suppressor lymphocytes: role of the glucocorticoid-induced TNF-like receptor. *Ann. N. Y. Acad. Sci.* **1069:** 377–385.

33. Kizaki, T. *et al.* 1996. Glucocorticoid-mediated generation of suppressor macrophages with high density Fc gamma RII during acute cold stress. *Endocrinology* **137:** 4260–4267.

34. Ikeda, T. *et al.* 1989. In vitro effect of prednisolone on peripheral blood suppressor T cell activity in patients with alcoholic hepatitis. *Clin. Immunol. Immunopathol.* **53**(2 Pt 1):225–232.

35. Nouri-Aria, K.T. *et al.* 1982. Effect of corticosteroids on suppressor-cell activity in "autoimmune" and viral chronic active hepatitis. *N. Engl. J. Med.* **307:** 1301–1304.

36. Szentivanyi, A. 1968. The beta adrenergic theory of the atopic abnormality in bronchial asthma. *J. Allergy* **42:** 203–232.

37. Li, X. *et al.* 2004. The induction of splenic suppressor T cells through an immune-privileged site requires an intact sympathetic nervous system. *J. Neuroimmunol.* **153:** 40–49.

38. Karaszewski, J.W. *et al.* 1991. Increased lymphocyte beta-adrenergic receptor density in progressive multiple sclerosis is specific for the CD8+, CD28− suppressor cell. *Ann. Neurol.* **30:** 42–47.

39. Van Tits, L.J. *et al.* 1990. Catecholamines increase lymphocyte beta 2-adrenergic receptors via a beta 2-adrenergic, spleen-dependent process. *Am. J. Physiol.* **258**(1 Pt 1):E191–E202.

40. Karpus, W.J. *et al.* 1988. Central catecholamine neurotoxin administration. 1. Immunological changes associated with the suppression of experimental autoimmune encephalomyelitis. *J. Neuroimmunol.* **18:** 61–73.

41. Selye, H. 1946. The general adaptation syndrome and the diseases of adaptation. *J. Clin. Endocrinol.* **6:** 117–230.

42. Berczi, I. 1998. Neuroendocrine response to endotoxin. *Ann. N. Y. Acad. Sci.* **851:** 411–415.

43. Paltrinieri, S. 2008. The feline acute phase reaction. *Vet. J.* **177:** 26–35.

44. Krueger, J.M. *et al.* 2003. Sleep in host defense. *Brain Behav. Immun.* **17**(Suppl 1): S41.

45. Krueger, J.M. *et al.* 2008. Cytokines and sleep. In *Neuroimmune Biology, Volume 6: Cytokines and the Brain*. C. Phelps & E.A. Korneva, Eds.: 214–240. I. Berczi & A. Szentivanyi, Series Eds. Elsevier. Amsterdam.

46. Metcalf, D. 2008. Hematopoietic cytokines. *Blood* **111:** 485–491.

47. Berczi, I. & A. Szentivanyi. 2003. The acute phase response. In *Neuroimmune Biology, Volume 3: The Immune-Neuroendocrine Circuitry. History and Progress*. I. Berczi & A. Szentivanyi, Eds.: 463–494. Elsevier. Amsterdam.

48. O'Mahony, D.S. *et al.* 2008. Differential constitutive and cytokine-modulated expression of human Toll-like receptors in primary neutrophils, monocytes, and macrophages. *Int. J. Med. Sci.* **5:** 1–8.

49. Spight, D. *et al.* 2008. Granulocyte-macrophage-colony-stimulating factor dependent peritoneal macrophage responses determined by survival in experimentally induced peritonitis and sepsis in mice. *Shock* **30:** 434–442.

50. Heit, B. *et al.* 2006. HIV and other lentiviral infections cause defects in neutrophil chemotaxis, recruitment, and cell structure: immunorestorative effects of granulocyte-macrophage colony-stimulating factor. *J. Immunol.* **177:** 6405–6414.

51. Ballinger, M.N. 2006. Role of granulocyte macrophage colony-stimulating factor during gram-negative lung infection with Pseudomonas aeruginosa. *Am. J. Respir. Cell. Mol. Biol.* **34:** 766–774.

52. Kobayashi, S.D. *et al.* 2005. Spontaneous neutrophil apoptosis and regulation of cell survival by granulocyte macrophage-colony stimulating factor. *J. Leukoc. Biol.* **78:** 1408–1418.

53. Kaur, A. 2004. Bioimmunotherapy of rodent malaria: co-treatment with recombinant mouse granulocyte-macrophage colony-stimulating factor and an enkephalin fragment peptide Tyr-Gly-Gly. *Acta. Trop.* **91:** 27–41.

54. Everly, J.J. & S. Lonial. 2005. Immunomodulatory effects of human recombinant granulocyte-macrophage colony-stimulating factor (rhuGM-CSF): evidence of antitumour activity. *Expert Opin. Biol. Ther.* **5:** 293–311.

55. Ezaki, K. & M. Tsuzuki. 1997. Cytokine therapy for hematological malignancies. *Gan To Kagaku Ryoho. Suppl.* **1:** 182–194.

56. Selig, C. & W. Nothdurft. Cytokines and progenitor cells of granulocytopoiesis in peripheral blood of patients with bacterial infections. *Infect. Immun.* **63:** 104–109.

57. Presneill, J.J. 2002. A randomized phase II trial of granulocyte-macrophage colony-stimulating factor therapy in severe sepsis with respiratory dysfunction. *Am. J. Respir. Crit. Care Med.* **166:** 129–130.

58. Mels, A.K. *et al.* 2001. Immune-stimulating effects of low-dose perioperative recombinant granulocyte-macrophage colony-stimulating factor in patients operated on for primary colorectal carcinoma. *Br. J. Surg.* **88:** 539–544.

59. Ganguly, D. *et al.* 2007. Granulocyte-macrophage colony-stimulating factor drives monocytes to CD14low CD83+ DCSIGN- interleukin-10-producing myeloid cells with differential effects on T-cell subsets. *Immunology* **121:** 499–507.

60. Jinushi, M. *et al.* 2007. MFG-E8-mediated uptake of apoptotic cells by APCs links the pro- and anti-inflammatory activities of GM-CSF. *J. Clin. Invest.* **117:** 1902–1913.

61. Han, S. *et al.* 2005. Macrophage-colony stimulating factor enhances MHC-restricted presentation of exogenous antigen in dendritic cells. *Cytokine* **32:** 187–193.

62. Bezbradica, J.S. 2006. Granulocyte-macrophage colony-stimulating factor regulates effector differentiation of invariant natural killer T cells during thymic ontogeny. *Immunity* **25:** 487–497.

63. Baleeiro, C.E., P.J. Christensen, S.B. Morris, *et al.* 2006. GM-CSF and the impaired pulmonary innate immune response following hyperoxic stress. *Am. J. Physiol. Lung Cell. Mol. Physiol.* **291:** L1246–L1255.

64. Franzen, R. *et al.* 2004. Nervous system injury: focus on the inflammatory cytokine 'granulocyte-macrophage colony stimulating factor'. *Neurosci. Lett.* **361:** 76–78.

65. Naito, M. 2008. Macrophage differentiation and function in health and disease. *Pathol. Int.* **58:** 143–155.

66. Encke, J. *et al.* 2006. Genetic vaccination with Flt3-L and GM-CSF as adjuvants: enhancement of cellular and humoral immune responses that results in protective immunity in a murine model of hepatitis C virus infection. *World J. Gastroenterol.* **12:** 7118–7125.

67. McCormick, S. *et al.* 2006. Manipulation of dendritic cells for host defence against intracellular infections. *Biochem. Soc. Trans.* **34**(Pt 2): 283–286.

68. Berczi, I. & E. Nagy. 1994. Neurohormonal control of cytokines during injury. In *Brain Control of Responses to Trauma.* N.J. Rothwell & F. Berkenbosch, Eds.: 32–107. Cambridge University Press. Cambridge, UK.

69. Wexler, B.C. *et al.* 1957. Effects of bacterial polysaccharide (Piromen) on the pituitary-adrenal axis: adrenal ascorbic acid, cholesterol and histological alterations. *Endocrinology* **61:** 300–308.

70. Wilder, R.L. 1995. Neuroendocrine-immune system interactions and autoimmunity. *Annu. Rev. Immunol.* **13:** 307–338.

71. Torpy, D.J. & G.P. Chrousos. 1996. The three way interaction between the hypothalamic–pituitary–adrenal and gonadal axes and the immune system. *Rheumatol. London: Bailliere Tindall* **10:** 181–198.

72. Berczi, I. *et al.* 1996. The immune effects of neuropeptides. *Rheumatol, London: Bailliere Tindall* **10:** 227–257.

73. Schiltz, J.C. & P.E. Sawchenko. 2003. Signaling the brain in systemic inflammation: the role of perivascular cells. *Front. Biosci.* **8:** S1321–S1329.

74. Jancso, G. Ed. 2008. Neurogenic inflammation in health and disease. In *Neuroimmune Biology,* Volume 8. I. Berczi & A. Szentivanyi, Series Eds. Elsevier. Amsterdam.

75. Kolb-Bachofen, V. 1991. A review on the biological properties of C-reactive protein. *Immunobiology* **183:** 133–445.

76. Ballou, S.P. & I. Kushner. 1992. C-reactive protein and the acute phase response. *Adv. Intern. Med.* **37:** 313–336.

77. Young, B. *et al.* 1991. C-reactive protein: a critical review. *Pathology* **23:** 118–124.

78. Mold, C. *et al.* 1981. C-reactive protein is protective against Streptococcus pneumoniae infection in mice. *J. Exp. Med.* **154:** 1703–1708.

79. Raetz, C.R.H. *et al.* 1991. Gram-negative endotoxin: an extraordinary lipid with profound effects on eukaryotic signal transduction. *FASEB J.* **5:** 2652–2660.

80. Flo, T.H. & A. Aderem. 2005. Pathogen recognition by Toll-like receptors. In *Neuroimmune Biology, Volume 5: Natural Immunity.* L. Bertok & D.A. Chow, Eds.: 167–182. I. Berczi & A. Szetivanyi, Series Eds. Elsevier. Amsterdam.

81. Hamann, L. *et al.* 2005. Acute-phase concentrations of lipopolysaccharide (LPS)-binding protein inhibit innate immune cell activation by different LPS chemotypes via different mechanisms. *Infect. Immun.* **73:** 193–200.

82. Wassell, J. 2000. Haptoglobin: function and polymorphism. *Clin. Lab.* **46:** 547–552.

83. Arredouani, M.S. *et al.* 2005. Haptoglobin dampens endotoxin-induced inflammatory effects both in vitro and in vivo. *Immunology* **114:** 263–271.

84. Daemen, M.A. *et al.* 2000. Functional protection by acute phase proteins alpha(1)-acid glycoprotein and alpha(1)-antitrypsin against ischemia/reperfusion injury by preventing apoptosis and inflammation. *Circulation* **102:** 1420–1426.

85. Liu, H. *et al.* 2001. Characterization and quantification of mouse mannan-binding lectins (MBL-A and MBL-C) and study of acute phase responses. *Scand. J. Immunol.* **53:** 489–497.

86. Hansen, T.K. *et al.* 2003. Intensive insulin therapy exerts antiinflammatory effects in critically ill patients and counteracts the adverse effect of low mannose-binding lectin levels. *J. Clin. Endocrinol. Metab.* **88:** 1082–1088.

87. Bauer, J. *et al.* 1984. Induction of rat alpha2-macroglobulin in vivo and in heaptocyte primary cultures: synergistic action of glucocorticoids and a Kupffer cell derived factor. *FEBS Lett.* **177:** 89–94.

88. Finck, B.N. & R.W. Johnson. 2000. Tumor necrosis factor-alpha regulates secretion of the adipocyte-derived cytokine, leptin. *Microsc. Res. Tech.* **50:** 209–215.

89. Hsieh, Y.C. *et al.* 2007. Metabolic modulators following trauma sepsis: sex hormones. *Crit. Care Med.* **35**(9 Suppl): S621–S629.

90. Collier, B. *et al.* 2008. Glucose control and the inflammatory response. *Nutr. Clin. Pract.* **23:** 3–15.

91. Takala, J. *et al.* 1999. Increased mortality associated with growth hormone treatment in critically ill adults. *N. Engl. J. Med.* **341:** 785–792.

92. Berczi, I. *et al.* 2001. Natural immunity and neuroimmune host defence. *Ann. N. Y. Acad. Sci.* **917:** 248–257.

93. Jeschke, M.G. *et al.* 1999. Recombinant human growth hormone alters acute phase reactant proteins, cytokine expression, and liver morphology in burned rats. *J. Surg. Res.* **83:** 122–129.

94. Derfalvi, B. *et al.* 2000. Interleukin-6-induced production of type II acute phase proteins and expression of junB gene are downregulated by human recombinant growth hormone in vitro. *Cell. Biol. Int.* **24:** 109–114.

95. Berczi, I. 1986. The influence of pituitary-adrenal axis on the immune system. In *Pituitary Function and Immunity.* I. Berczi, Ed.: 49–132. CRC Press. Boca Raton, FL.

96. van Gool, J. *et al.* 1984. Glucocorticoids and catecholamines as mediators of acute-phase proteins, especially rat alpha-macrofoetoprotein. *Biochem. J.* **220:** 125–152.

97. Yeager, M.P. *et al.* 2004. Glucocorticoid regulation of the inflammatory response to injury. *Acta. Anaesthesiol. Scand.* **48:** 799–813.

98. Van Gool, J. *et al.* 1990. The relation among stress, adrenalin, interleukin 6, and acute phase proteins in the rat. *Clin. Immunol. Immunopathol.* **57:** 200–210.

99. Akira, S. & T. Kishimoto. 1992. IL-6 and NF-IL6 in acute-phase response and viral infection. *Immunol. Rev.* **127:** 26–50.

100. Harnish, M.J. *et al.* 2005. Differential regulation of human blood glucose level by interleukin-2 and -6. *Exp. Clin. Endocrinol. Diabetes* **113:** 43–48.

101. Ekman, R. *et al.* 2001. Arginine vasopressin in the cytoplasm and nuclear fraction of lymphocytes from healthy donors and patients with depression or schizophrenia. *Peptides* **22:** 67–72.

102. Itoi, K. *et al.* 2004. Regulatory mechanisms of corticotropin-releasing hormone and vasopressin gene expression in the hypothalamus. *J. Neuroendocrinol.* **16:** 348–355.

103. Carrasco, G.A. & L.D. Van de Kar. Neuroendocrine pharmacology of stress. *Eur. J. Pharmacol.* **463:** 235–272.

104. Turnbull, A.V. *et al.* 1998. Mechanisms of hypothalamic-pituitary-adrenal axis stimulation by immune signals in the adult rat. *Ann. N. Y. Acad. Sci.* **840:** 434–443.

105. Huitinga, I. *et al.* 2000. Priming with interleukin-1beta suppresses experimental allergic encephalomyelitis in the Lewis rat. *J. Neuroendocrinol.* **12:** 1186–1193.

106. Chowdrey, H.S. *et al.* 1995. Evidence for arginine vasopressin as the primary activator of the HPA axis during adjuvant-induced arthritis. *Br. J. Pharmacol.* **116:** 2417–2424.

107. Baker, J.W. *et al.* 1976. Elevated plasma antidiuretic hormone levels in status asthmaticus. *Mayo Clin. Proc.* **51:** 31–34.

108. Michelson, D. *et al.* 1994. Multiple sclerosis is associated with alterations in hypothalamic-pituitary-adrenal axis function. *J. Clin. Endocrinol. Metab.* **79:** 848–853.

109. Harbuz, M.S. *et al.* 2003. Hypothalamo-pituitary-adrenal axis and chronic immune activation. *Ann. N. Y. Acad. Sci.* **992:** 99–106.

110. DeGoeij, D. *et al.* 1991. Repeated stress activation of corticotropin releasing factor neurons enhances vasopressin stores and colocalization with corticotropin-releasing factor in the median eminence of rats. *Neuroendocrinology* **53:** 150–159.

111. DeGoeij, D. *et al.* 1992. Chronic intermittent stress enhances vasopressin but not corticotropin releasing factor secretion during hypoglycemia. *Am. J. Physiol.* **263:** E394–E399.

112. DeGoeij, D. *et al.* 1992. Chronic psychological stress enhances vasopressin but not corticotropin releasing

factor, in the external zone of the median eminence of male rats: relationship to subordinate status. *Endocinology* **131:** 847–853.

113. DeGoeij, D. *et al.* 1992. Repeated stress enhances vasopressin synthesis in corticotropin releasing factor neurons in the paraventricular nucleus. *Brain Res.* **577:** 165–168.

114. Hashimoto, K. *et al.* 1988. Corticotropin-releasing hormones and pituitary-adrenocortical response in chronically stressed rats. *Regul. Pept.* **23:** 117–126.

115. Levin, N. *et al.* 1989. Modulation of basal and corticotropin-releasing factor-stimulated proopiomelanocortin gene expression by vasopressin in rat anterior pituitary. *Endocinology* **125:** 2957–2966.

116. Antoni, F.A. 1986. Hypothalamic control of adrenocorticotropin secretion: advances since the discovery of 41-residue corticotropin releasing factor. *Endocrinol. Rev.* **7:** 351–378.

117. Gilles, G. *et al.* 1982. Corticotropin releasing activity of the new CRF is potentiated several times by vasopressin. *Nature* **299:** 355–357.

118. Raber, J. *et al.* 1994. IL-1 beta potentiates the acetylcholine-induced release of vasopressin from the hypothalamus in vitro, but not from the amygdala. *Neuroendocrinology* **59:** 208–217.

119. Wilkinson, M.F. *et al.* 1994. Central interleukin-1 beta stimulation of vasopressin release into the rat brain: activation of an antipyretic pathway. *J. Physiol.* **481**(Pt 3): 641–646.

120. Sasaki, S. *et al.* 1995. The role of arginine vasopressin in interleukin-1 beta-induced adrenocorticotropin secretion in the rat. *Neuroimmunomodulation* **2:** 134–136.

121. Kageyama, K. *et al.* 1995. In vivo evidence that arginine vasopressin is involved in the adrenocorticotropin response induced by interleukin-6 but not by tumor necrosis factor-alpha in the rat. *Neuroimmunomodulation* **2:** 137–140.

122. Raber, J. & F.E. Bloom. 1994. IL-2 induces vasopressin release from the hypothalamus and the amygdala: role of nitric oxide-mediated signaling. *J. Neurosci.* **14:** 6187–6195.

123. Pardy, K. *et al.* 1993. The influence of interleukin-2 on vasopressin and oxytocin gene expression in the rodent hypothalamus. *J. Neuroimmunol.* **42:** 131–138.

124. Hillhouse, E.W. 1994. Interleukin-2 stimulates the secretion of arginine vasopressin but not corticotropin-releasing hormone from rat hypothalamic cells in vitro. *Brain Res.* **650:** 323–325.

125. Ishizaki, S. *et al.* 2004. Leukemia inhibitory factor stimulates vasopressin release in rats. *Neurosci. Lett.* **359:** 77–80.

126. Malkinson, T.J. *et al.* 1987. Perfusion of the septum of the rabbit with vasopressin antiserum enhances endotoxin fever. *Peptides* **8:** 385–389.

127. Kostoglou-Athanassiou, I. *et al.* 1998. Endotoxin stimulates an endogenous pathway regulating corticotropin-releasing hormone and vasopressin release involving the generation of nitric oxide and carbon monoxide. *J. Neuroimmunol.* **86:** 104–109.

128. Giovambattista, A. *et al.* 2000. Modulatory role of the epinergic system in the neuroendocrine-immune system function. *Neuroimmunomodulation* **8:** 98–106.

129. Lee, S. *et al.* 1995. Systemic endotoxin increases steady-state gene expression of hypothalamic nitric oxide synthase: comparison with corticotropin-releasing factor and vasopressin gene transcripts. *Brain Res.* **705:** 136–148.

130. Battaglia, D.F. *et al.* 1998. Systemic challenge with endotoxin stimulates corticotropin-releasing hormone and arginine vasopressin secretion into hypophyseal portal blood: coincidence with gonadotropin-releasing hormone suppression. *Endocrinology* **139:** 4175–4181.

131. Qahwash, I.M. *et al.* 2002. Bacterial lipopolysaccharide-induced coordinate down-regulation of arginine vasopressin receptor V3 and corticotropin-releasing factor receptor 1 messenger ribonucleic acids in the anterior pituitary of endotoxemic steers. *Endocrine* **18:** 13–20.

132. Tanoue, A. *et al.* 2004. The vasopressin V1b receptor critically regulates hypothalamic-pituitary-adrenal axis activity under both stress and resting conditions. *J. Clin. Invest.* **113:** 302–309.

133. Kjaer, A. *et al.* 1992. Histamine- and stress-induced secretion of ACTH and beta-endorphin: involvement of corticotropin-releasing hormone and vasopressin. *Neuroendocrinology* **56:** 419–428.

134. Nagy, G.M. *et al.* 1991. Attenuation of the suckling-induced prolactin release and the high afternoon oscillations of plasma prolactin secretion of lactating rats by antiserum to vasopressin. *Neuroendocrinology* **54:** 566–570.

135. el Halawani, M.E. *et al.* 1992. Evidence of a role for the turkey posterior pituitary in prolactin release. *Gen. Comp. Endocrinol.* **87:** 436–442.

136. Franci, C.R. *et al.* 1993. Actions of endogenous vasopressin and oxytocin on anterior pituitary hormone secretion. *Neuroendocrinology* **57:** 693–699.

137. Keck, M.E. *et al.* 2003. The high-affinity nonpeptide CRH1 receptor antagonist R121919 attenuates stress-induced alterations in plasma oxytocin, prolactin, and testosterone secretion in rats. *Pharmacopsychiatry* **36:** 27–31.

138. Elenkov, I.J. *et al.* 1992. Lipopolysaccharide is able to bypass corticotrophin-releasing factor in affecting plasma ACTH and corticosterone levels: evidence from rats with lesions of the paraventricular nucleus. *J. Endocrinol.* **133:** 231–236.

139. Khegai, I.I. *et al.* 2003. Immune system in vasopressin-deficient rats during ontogeny. *Bull. Exp. Biol. Med.* **136:** 448–450.

140. Yirmiya, R. *et al.* 1989. Natural killer cell activity in vasopressin-deficient rats (Brattleboro strain). *Brain Res.* **479:** 16–22.

141. Hu, S.B. *et al.* 2003. Vasopressin receptor 1a-mediated negative regulation of B cell receptor signaling. *J. Neuroimmunol.* **135:** 72–81.

142. Johnson, H.M. & B.A. Torres. A novel arginine vasopressin-binding peptide that blocks arginine vasopressin modulation of immune function. *J. Immunol.* **141:** 2420–2423.

143. Torres, B.A. & H.M. Johnson. Arginine vasopressin-binding peptides derived from the bovine and rat genomes differ in their abilities to block arginine vasopressin modulation of murine immune function. *J. Neuroimmunol.* **27:** 191–199.

144. Bell, J. *et al.* 1993. Identification and characterization of [125I]arginine vasopressin binding sites on human peripheral blood mononuclear cells. *Life Sci.* **52:** 95–105.

145. Shibasaki, T. *et al.* 1998. Brain vasopressin is involved in stress-induced suppression of immune function in the rat. *Brain Res.* **808:** 84–92.

146. Zhao, L. & R.D. Brinton. 2004. Suppression of proinflammatory cytokines interleukin-1beta and tumor necrosis factor-alpha in astrocytes by a V1 vasopressin receptor agonist: a cAMP response element-binding protein-dependent mechanism. *J. Neurosci.* **24:** 2226–2235.

147. Elands, J. *et al.* 1990. Neurohypophyseal hormone receptors in the thymus, spleen, and lymphocytes. *Endocrinology* **126:** 2703–2710.

148. Bell, J. *et al.* 1993. Identification and characterization of [125] arginine vasopressin binding sites on human peripheral blood mononuclear cells. *Life Sci.* **52:** 95–105.

149. Moll, J. & D. De Wied. 1962. Observations on the hypothalamo-posthypophyseal system of the posterior lobectomized rat. *Gen. Comp. Endocrinol.* **2:** 215–228.

150. Miller, R.E. *et al.* 1974. Anterior hypophysial function in the posterior-hypophysectomised rat: normal regulation of the adrenal system. *Neuroendocrinology* **14:** 233–250.

151. Organista-Esparza, A. *et al.* 2003. Efectos de la lobectomía neurointermedia hipofisiaria y la hipofisectomía sobre la respuesta inmune humoral en la rata Wistar. In *Proc. XLVI National Congress of Physiological Sciences.* Aguascalientes, Mexico.

152. Quintanar, A. *et al.* 2007. Increased IgM and decreased IgG response to rabbit red blood cell immunization in protracted hypophysectomized and neurointermediate pituitary lobectomized rats. *FASEB J.* Abstract No. 962.2.

153. Campos-Rodríguez, R. *et al.* 2006. Hypophysectomy and neurointermediate pituitary lobectomy reduce serum immunoglobulin M (IgM) and IgG and intestinal IgA responses to Salmonella enterica serovar Thyphimurium infection in rats. *Infect. Immun.* **74:** 1883–1889.

154. Quintanar-Stephano, A. *et al.* 2004. Effects of neurointermedate pituitary lobectomy on humoral and cell-mediated immune responses in the rat. *Neuroimmunomodulation* **11:** 233.

155. Quintanar-Stephano, A. *et al.* 2005. Protection Against Adjuvant-induced Arthritis (AIA) by the Excision of the Neuro-intermediate Pituitary Lobe (NIL) in Lewis Rats. *FASEB J.* Abstract No 7407.

156. Quintanar-Stephano, A. 2004. Effects of neurointermediate pituitary lobectomy and desmopressin on experimental autoimmune encephalomyelitis in rats. *FASEB J.* Abstract No. 833.13.

157. Berczi, I. 2007. Integration and regulation of higher organisms by the neuroimmune supersystem. *Int. J. Integrative Biol.* **1:** 216–231.

The Role of Neuroimmunomodulation in Alzheimer's Disease

Ricardo B. Maccioni,[a,b,c] Leonel E. Rojo,[b,c,d]
Jorge A. Fernández,[a,c] and Rodrigo O. Kuljis[a,e]

[a]International Center for Biomedicine, [b]Laboratory of Cellular and Molecular
Neurosciences, Faculty of Sciences, University of Chile, Santiago, Chile

[c]Mind and Brain Institute, International Center for Biomedicine, Santiago, Chile

[d]Department of Pharmaceutical Sciences, Arturo Prat University,
Iquique, Chile

[e]University of Miami School of Medicine, Miami, Florida, USA

The idea that alterations in the brain immunomodulation are critical for Alzheimer's disease (AD) pathogenesis provides the most integrative view on this cognitive disorder, considering that converging research lines have revealed the involvement of inflammatory processes in AD. We have proposed the damage signal hypothesis as a unifying scheme in that release of endogenous damage/alarm signals, in response to accumulated cell distress (dyslipidemia, vascular insults, head injury, oxidative stress, iron overload, folate deficiency), is the earliest triggering event in AD, leading to activation of innate immunity and the inflammatory cascade. Inflammatory cytokines play a dual role, either promoting neurodegeneration or neuroprotection. This equilibrium is shifted toward the neurodegenerative phenotype upon the action of several risk factors that trigger innate damage signals that activate microglia and the release of tumor necrosis factor-α, interleukin-6, and some trophic factors. In this neuroimmunomodulatory hypothesis we integrate different risk factors with microaglial activation and the resulting neuronal alterations and hyperphosphorylations of tau protein. The progression of AD, with slowly increasing damage in brain parenchyma preceding the onset of symptoms, suggests that tissue distress triggering damage signals drives neuroinflammation. These signals via toll-like receptors, receptors for highly glycosylated end products, or other glial receptors activate sensors of the native immune system, inducing the anomalous release of cytokines and promoting the neurodegenerative cascade, a hallmark of brain damage that correlates with cognitive decline.

Key words: Alzheimer's disease; immunomodulation hypothesis; neuroinflammation; innate immunity; cytokines; glial cells; neurons; tau protein; hyperphosphorylations; neuronal degeneration

Introduction

Alzheimer's disease (AD) is the principal cause of dementia throughout the world and the fourth cause of death in developed economies after cancer, cardiovascular diseases, and vascular stroke. However, the set of disorders that cause cognitive impairment and that include vascular brain disorders, stroke, and brain trauma, accounts for one of the largest factors of morbidity and mortality.[1,2] In the United States approximately 5 million people are affected by AD, and mortality from this disease is near 100,000 per year, with a cost to the economy of over $100 bn.

Address for correspondence: Dr. Ricardo B. Maccioni, The Mind and Brain Institute, International Center for Biomedicine (ICC), Avda. Providencia 455, Dept. 303, Santiago, Chile. Voice: +562 878 7228. rmaccion@manquehue.net

Neuroimmunomodulation: Ann. N.Y. Acad. Sci. 1153: 240–246 (2009).
doi: 10.1111/j.1749-6632.2008.03972.x © 2009 New York Academy of Sciences.

Considering that AD accounts for the largest number of dementia cases, including dementia from Lewy bodies, frontotemporal dementia (FTD-17), and vascular dementia, and that age is the main risk factor, the prevalence of these pathologies in an aging society is presently a major medical puzzle and a major challenge for science.

Among many postulates for the pathogenesis of AD, the more plausible explanation is based on the findings that tau hyperphosphorylations constitute a common final pathway of altered signaling mechanisms in degenerating neurons. However, this does not account for all the sequence of events after the early triggering factors that lead to neuronal degeneration. AD is a multifactorial disease. Several risk factors as well as the contribution of genetic vulnerability and polymorphisms among certain groups of subjects are involved in its pathogenesis. Strong evidence has been cumulated on the role of neuroinflammation in AD pathogenesis. Neuropathological studies in human brains demonstrating the activation of glial cells[3] has been corroborated by *in vitro* studies in which amyloid Aβ-exposed and activated glial cells overproduce pro-inflammatory cytokines, which in turn trigger a neurodegenerative cascade in living neurons.[4-6] Studies with transgenic animal models of AD have also demonstrated that brain inflammation appears to be a key component of AD pathogenesis.[7] Moreover, epidemiological data show that individuals consuming nonsteroidal anti-inflammatory drugs (NSAIDs) have a lower risk of AD.[8] In fact, inflammation is associated with brain lesions in AD while a sparing effect of NSAIDs has been shown; these NSAIDs are also protective in animal models of AD.[7] In fact, patients receiving systemic NSAIDs developed significantly less AD manifestations, suggesting that ameliorating inflammation in the brain helps to prevent or slow down the onset of AD.[3,9] However, this effect may not apply to all NSAIDs equally; a more recent study failed to demonstrate such an effect for certain drugs, such as naproxen and celecoxib.[10]

How Does Neuroinflammation Participate in AD Pathogenesis?

Neuroinflammation is characterized by the generation of a set of pro-inflammatory mediators locally produced by host cells, indicating the engagement of the innate immune system. In this context, AD can be considered an autotoxic disease in which an innate immune system uses local phagocytes, such as microglia, as an effector. Activated complement fragments and inflammatory cytokines have been identified in lesions (Figs. 1 and 2). AD exhibits marked inflammatory phenomena from the inherent toxicity of aggregates of Aβ oligomers (much earlier than the other lesion, the senile plaques) and small aggregates of the hyperphosphorylated tau protein. Thus, the AD phenotype is a result of the convergence of multiple risk factors that activate one or more danger/alarm signal detectors, with microglial activation, production of nuclear factor (NF)-κB, and inducing multiple degeneration-promoting signals, such as tumor necrosis factor (TNF)-α, interleukin (IL)-1β, and IL-6, that converge to produce an abnormal processing of tau protein (Fig. 2). These anomalous signals lead to an overactivation of some cell cycle enzymes, such as cdk5 and the neuronal glycogen synthase kinase, with the consequent tau hyperphosphorylations.[11,12] Increasing evidence has accumulated on the substantial toxicity of abnormally phosphorylated tau variants contributing to the neurodegenerative cascade.[13-15] Once this pathway is triggered, the expression of clinicopathological disorders cannot be stopped.

Several lines of evidence indicate that under certain experimental conditions, damage/alarm signals, such as oxidative stress, exposure to toxins, hypoxia, oxidized low-density lipoproteins, or mechanical damage promote neuronal degeneration.[16-18] The resulting inflammatory cytokines in all of these situations can play a dual role either promoting neurodegeneration or assisting neuroprotection.[5,6,9] Thus, if pro-inflammatory mediators were simply protective, one should expect that

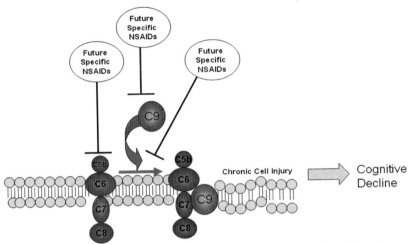

Figure 1. Formation of the membrane attack complex (MAC) on the surface of brain cells as a result of the activation of the complement system and potential targets for future specific nonsteroidal anti-inflammatory drugs NSAIDs against Alzheimer's disease (AD) during early stages of brain damage. (In color in *Annals* online.)

individuals receiving NSAIDs would be at a higher risk of AD, which appears not to be the case.[3,9] In fact, the evidence indicates that only a few pro-inflammatory molecules, such as TNF-α,[6] exert neuroprotective effects.

Innate Immunity in Alzheimers's Disease

Neuronal damage in AD occurs long before the clinical onset of the disease, a decade or even longer time intervals,[1] as a consequence of the permanent action for years of the various exogenous or endogenous risk factors. Among the major risk factors are chronic stress, blood lipid disorders,[17,19–22] repeated mechanical head trauma, oxidative stress,[23,24] brain iron overload,[25] folic acid deficiency, K$^+$ efflux, and several others, such as genetic polymorphisms.[26] All these conditions, or the convergence of several of these, are sufficient to trigger danger/alarm signals[27] that, through activation of innate immunity, modify the normal activity of microglial cell receptors, such as toll-like receptors (TLRs), receptors for highly glycosylated end products (RAGEs), and other sensitive receptors on the glial cell surface. Thus, activated glial cells respond with an

overproduction of pro-inflammatory cytokines, such as TNF-α, IL-1β, and IL-6, which are found to be considerable increased in AD.[9,28–30] In this context, we have proposed a novel unifying hypothesis that the release of endogenous damage/alarm signals,[16] in response to converging and accumulated cell distress (e.g., dyslipidemia, vascular insults, head injury, oxidative stress, folate deficiency), is the earliest triggering event in AD pathogenesis, which then leads to the activation of innate immunity[3,9] and, subsequently, an inflammatory cascade (Figs. 1 and 2). In this hypothesis we consider the risk factors that have been analyzed separately and in different contexts, with microglial activation, tau hyperphosphorylation in the affected neurons, and the resulting neuronal damage. The protracted progression of the disease, with slowly increasing damage in brain parenchyma preceding the onset of symptoms, suggests that moderate tissue distress triggering damage/alarm signals drives an escalating inflammatory process until tissue damage causes progressive eventually irreversible pathology. This hypothesis is based on known facts about AD and experimental models of AD as well as our own reviews of these complex sets of factors.[5,9,14,16]

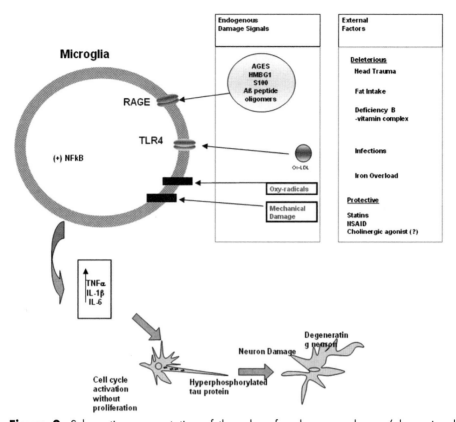

Figure 2. Schematic representation of the roles of endogenous danger/alarm signals in the innate immune system at the early stages of Alzheimer's disease (AD) pathogenesis. Danger signals include advanced glycation end products (AGES), HMBG1 (high-mobility box group 1), S-100 proteins, and amyloid -β (Aβ) peptide oligomers (but not β-pleated fibrillar aggregates). These activate microglia through the AGES or receptors for highly glycosylated end products (RAGE), shown here as a transmembrane protein. Oxidized low-density lipoproteins (oxLDL) activate toll-like receptors (TLRs), particularly TLR4. Additional danger signals are trauma and oxyradical damage, possibly acting on separate receptors (black boxes inserted in the membrane) as well as by inducing the production of additional Aβ peptide oligomers, AGES, and S-100 protein that contribute to this process. These danger signals trigger innate immune system alarm mechanisms resulting in long-term overproduction of tumor necrosis factor alpha (TNF-α), interleukin 1-beta (IL-1β), and IL-6. These signals would then mediate neuronal damage that is reflected in alterations, such as tau hyperphosphorylation, which eventually result in neuronal degeneration and progressively more severe clinical manifestations of cognitive and behavioral decline unrelated to the amyloid aggregation process. (In color in *Annals* online.)

Future Avenues for Rational Development of New Anti-inflammatory Agents against AD

Activated complement fragments as well as inflammatory cytokines have been identified in association with the histologically evident lesions in the brain of patients affected with AD.[31,32] The activation of the complement system induces formation of the membrane attack complex (MAC) on the surface of brain cells[33] (Fig. 1). Thus, a slow, chronic, asymptomatic, and autotoxic process leads to progressive neurodegeneration stages and to cognitive impairment in Alzheimer patients. From the point of view of an integrated analysis of this evidence, we propose potential targets for future specific NSAIDs against early stages of brain damage. Considering that Aβ extracellular deposits and neurofibrillary tangles are present during early preclinical stages of AD until the terminal stages, their ability to strongly activate complement system provides a mechanism for initiating and sustaining chronic, low-level, inflammatory responses that may accumulate over the disease course.[34] This supports the idea that the complement system cascade intervention can be a pharmacological approach to AD in the near future. Besides Aβ effects on the complement system, amyloid oligomers also signal through RAGE receptors, resulting in the sustained production of NF-kB, which is involved in the inflammatory cascade (Fig. 2).

Innate Immunity in AD and Other Degenerative Diseases

The notion that endogenous signals of damage trigger the earliest events of AD pathogenesis finds further support in the natural history of the inherited forms of early onset AD in which mutations in the affected genes are expressed as an increased production of pro-inflammatory Aβ peptide oligomers; this needs decades to cause pathology and correlates with a more precocious onset of the familial forms of this disease compared to the most prevalent sporadic forms of the disease. Along the same line of evidence, persons with Down's syndrome, a condition associated with a high risk of AD, exhibit increased serum levels of Aβ in childhood and adolescence and rapidly accumulating senile plaques and neurofibrillary tangles thereafter. Intriguingly, plasma Aβ levels in these subjects correlate inversely with age,[35] a key observation that contradicts the highly prevalent amyloid hypothesis. In summary, we propose that the disease phenotype/neurological condition that has so far been called "Alzheimer's disease" is not a result of a single "cause" but to the convergence of multiple risk factors that

coalesce in the activation of one or more damage/danger signal detectors (Fig. 1). The long-term effect of these triggering factors results in microglial activation and the protracted production of NF-κB, inducing multiple predominantly degeneration-promoting signals, such as the inflammatory cytokines. All of these converge to produce abnormal processing of tau protein, which acts as a final common pathway.[1,16] Recent reports describe the roles of IL-6 and TNF-α on AD pathogenesis. We reported that IL-6 induces tau hyperphosphorylation and neuronal cell death, both mediated by deregulation of the cdk5/p35 complex.[4] We have also reported that TNF-α can decrease cdk5 activity and prevent hippocampal neuron death induced by Aβ$_{1-42}$ peptide *in vitro*.[6] Once this pathway has been triggered by multiple mediators of inflammation, the full expression of the clinicopathological disorder probably cannot be stopped. In this hypothetical scheme, interstitial amyloid deposits, senile plaques, neurofibrillary tangles, neuronal degeneration, and, of course, clinical manifestations occur subsequently. The key element of this proposal, which is experimentally testable, is that the danger/alarm signals must activate the sensors of the innate immune system in the brain. It remains to be determined precisely how this hypothetical chain of events is unique to what we conceptualize today as "Alzheimer's disease," as there are phenotypically distinct disorders that are also associated with inflammatory phenomena but that do not result in the clinical and histopathological manifestations considered to define AD. Among the possible explanations for this conundrum, we propose that the location where these phenomena are triggered (e.g., medial aspect of the temporal lobe in AD versus lateral aspect of the temporal and/or frontal lobe in the so-called frontotemporal atrophies versus midbrain and diencephalon in progressive supranuclear palsy) may alter the time course, topographic distribution, lesion array, and, ultimately, clinical manifestations of the ensuing disorder. As a complementary (and not necessarily mutually exclusive) explanation, there is also an emerging molecular basis for the phenotypic diversity among neurodegenerative disorders that exhibit inflammatory phenomena. For example, there is a differential activation of TLRs in animal models of AD versus models of other disorders. In fact, TLR2 is activated in models of AD but not in models of other degenerative disorders. Furthermore, it is plausible that other mediators of innate immunity may also be expressed differentially in distinct neurodegenerative disorders, which is another important avenue for further experimental assessment.

Acknowledgments

This research has been supported by grants from the Fondo Nacional de Desarrollo Científico y Tecnológico (1080254), the International Center for Biomedicine (ICC), and Neuroinnovation Ltd. We thank the helpful contribution of the psychologist Alejandra Sekler.

Conflicts of Interest

The authors declare no conflicts of interest.

References

1. Maccioni, R.B., L. Barbeito & J.P. Muñoz. 2001. The molecular bases of Alzheimer's disease and other neurodegenerative disorders. *Arch. Med. Res.* **32:** 367–381.
2. Terry, R.D. 2000. Where in the brain does Alzheimer's disease begin? *Ann. Neurol.* **47:** 421.
3. McGeer, P.L., M. Schulzer & E.G. McGeer. 1996. Artritis and anti-inflammatory agents as possible protective factors for Alzheimer's disease: a review of 17 epidemiologic studies. *Neurology* **47:** 425–432.
4. Quintanilla, R.A., D.I. Orellana, C. González-Billault & R.B. Maccioni. 2004. Interleukin-6 induces Alzheimer-type phosphorylation of tau protein by deregulating the cdk5/p35 pathway. *Exp. Cell Res.* **295:** 245–257.
5. Orellana, D.I., R.A. Quintanilla, C. Gonzalez-Billault & R.B. Maccioni. 2005. Role of the JAKs/STATs pathway in the intracellular calcium changes induced by interleukin-6 in hippocampal neurons. *Neurotox. Res.* **8:** 295–304.
6. Orellana, D.I., R.A. Quintanilla & R.B. Maccioni. 2007. Neuroprotective effect of TNFalpha against the beta-amyloid neurotoxicity mediated by CDK5 kinase. *Biochim. Biophys. Acta* **1773:** 254–263.
7. Yan, Q., J. Zhang, H. Liu, *et al.* 2003. Anti-inflammatory drug therapy alters beta-amyloid processing and deposition in an animal model of Alzheimer's disease. *J. Neurosci.* **23:** 7504–7509.
8. McGeer, P.L., J. Rogers & E.G. McGeer. 2006. Inflammation, antiinflammatory agents and Alzheimer disease: the last 12 years. *J. Alzheimer's Dis.* **9**(3 Suppl): 271–276.
9. Rojo, L.E., J.A. Fernández, A.A. Maccioni, *et al.* 2008. Neuro-inflammation: implications for the pathogenesis and molecular diagnosis of Alzheimer's disease. *Arch. Med. Res.* **39:** 1–16.
10. Lyketsos, C.G. *et al.* 2007. Naproxen and celecoxib do not prevent AD in early results from a randomized controlled trial. *Neurology* **68:** 1800–1808.
11. Alvarez, A., R. Toro, A. Caceres & R.B. Maccioni. 1999. Inhibition of tau phosphorylating protein kinase cdk5 prevents beta-amyloid-induced neuronal death. *FEBS Lett.* **459:** 421–426.
12. Alvarez, A., J.P. Muñoz & R.B. Maccioni. 2001. A cdk5/p35 stable complex is involved in the beta-amyloid induced deregulation of Cdk5 activity in hippocampal neurons. *Exp. Cell Res.* **264:** 266–275.
13. Lavados, M., G. Farias, F. Rothhammer, *et al.* 2005. ApoE alleles and tau markers in patients with different levels of cognitive impairment. *Arch. Med. Res.* **36:** 474–479.
14. Maccioni, R.B., M. Lavados, C.B. Maccioni & A. Mendoza. 2004. Biological markers of Alzheimer's disease and mild cognitive impairment. *Curr. Alzheimer Res.* **1:** 307–314.
15. Maccioni, R.B., M. Lavados, C.B. Maccioni, *et al.* 2006. Anomalously phosphorylated tau protein and Abeta fragments in the CSF of Alzheimer's and MCI subjects. *Neurobiol. Aging* **27:** 237–244.
16. Fernandez, J., L. Rojo, R.O. Kuljis & R.B. Maccioni. 2008. The damage signals hypothesis of Alzheimer's disease pathogenesis. *J. Alz. Dis.* **14:** 329–333.
17. Wolozin, B., W. Kellman, P. Ruosseau, *et al.* 2000. Decreased prevalence of Alzheimer disease associated with 3-hydroxy-3-methylglutaryl coenzyme A reductase inhibitors. *Arch. Neurol.* **57:** 1439–1443.
18. Rojo, L., M.K. Sjöberg, P. Hernández, *et al.* 2006. Roles of cholesterol and lipids in the etiopathogenesis of Alzheimer's disease. *J. Biomed. Biotechnol.* 73976.
19. Yaffe, K. 2007. Metabolic syndrome and cognitive decline. *Curr. Alzheimer Res.* **2:** 123–126. Review.

20. Sekler, M.A., J.M. Jiménez, L.E. Rojo, *et al.* 2008. Cognitive impairment associated with Alzheimer's disease: links with oxidative stress and cholesterol metabolism. *J. Neuropsychiatr. Dis. Treat.* **4:** 1–8.

21. Reid, P.C., Y. Urano, T. Kodama & T. Hamakubo. 2007. Alzheimer's disease: cholesterol, membrane rafts, isoprenoids and statins. *J. Cell Mol. Med.* **11:** 383–392. Review.

22. Reitz, C., M.X. Tang, J. Manly, *et al.* 2008. Plasma lipid levels in the elderly are not associated with the risk of mild cognitive impairment. *Dement. Geriatr. Cogn. Disord.* **25:** 232–237.

23. Köseoglu, E. & Y. Karaman. 2007. Relations between homocysteine, folate and vitamine B12 in vascular dementia and Alzheimer disease. *Clin. Biochem.* **40:** 859–863.

24. Zambrano, C.A., J.T. Egaña, M.T. Núñez, *et al.* 2004. Oxidative stress promotes tau dephosphorylation in neuronal cells: the roles of cdk5 and PP1. *Free Rad. Biol. Med.* **36:** 1393–1402.

25. Lavados, M., M. Guillon, M.C. Mujica, *et al.* 2008. Mild cognitive impairment and Alzheimer patients display different levels of Redox-active CSF iron. *J. Alz. Dis.* **13:** 225–232.

26. Lio, D., G. Annoni, F. Licastro, *et al.* 2006. Tumor Necrosis factorα-308A/G polymorphism is associated with age at onset of Alzheimer's disease. *Mech. Ageing Dev.* **127:** 567–571.

27. Seong, S.Y. & P. Matzinger. 2004. Hydrophobicity: an ancient damage-associated molecular pattern that initiates innate immune responses. *Nat. Rev. Immunol.* **4:** 469–478.

28. Braida, D., P. Sacerdote, A.E. Panerai, *et al.* 2004. Cognitive function in young and adult IL (interleukin)-6 deficient mice. *Behav. Brain Res.* **153:** 423–429.

29. Dik, M.G., C. Jonker, C.E. Hack, *et al.* 2005. Serum inflammatory proteins and cognitive decline in older persons. *Neurology* **64:** 1371–1377.

30. Lanzrein, A.S., C.M. Johnston, V.H. Perry, *et al.* 1998. Longitudinal study of inflammatory factors in serum, cerebrospinal fluid, and brain tissue in Alzheimer disease: IL-1beta, IL-6, IL-1 receptor antagonist, TNF-alpha, the soluble TNF receptors I and II, and alpha1- antichymotrypsin. *Alzheimer Dis. Assoc. Disord.* **12:** 215–227.

31. Itagaki, S., H. Akiyama, H. Saito & P.L. McGeer. 1994. Ultrastructural localization of complement membrane attack complex (MAC)-like immunoreactivity in brains of patients with Alzheimer's disease. *Brain Res.* **645:** 78–84.

32. Bonifati, D.M. & U. Kishore. 2007. Role of complement in neurodegeneration and neuroinflammation. *Mol. Immunol.* **44:** 999–1010.

33. Webster, S., L.F. Lue, L. Brachova, *et al.* 1997. Molecular and cellular characterization of the membrane attack complex, C5b-9, in Alzheimer's disease. *Neurobiol. Aging* **18:** 415–421.

34. Shen, Y., L. Lue, L. Yang, *et al.* 2001. Complement activation by neurofibrillary tangles in Alzheimer's disease. *Neurosci. Lett.* **305:** 165–168.

35. Metha, P.D., G. Capone, A. Jewell & R.L. Freeland. 2007. Increase in amyloid beta protein levels in children and adolescents with Down syndrome. *J. Neurol. Sci.* **254:** 22–27.

The Adrenal Steroid Response during Tuberculosis and Its Effects on the Mycobacterial-driven IFN-γ Production of Patients and Their Household Contacts

Veronica Bozza,[a] **Luciano D'Attilio,**[a] **Griselda Didoli,**[a]
Natalia Santucci,[a] **Luis Nannini,**[b] **Cristina Bogue,**[c]
Adriana Del Rey,[d] **Hugo Besedovsky,**[d] **Maria Luisa Bay,**[a]
and Oscar Bottasso[a]

[a]*Institute of Immunology, School of Medical Sciences, Rosario, Argentina*

[b]*Eva Peron School Hospital, Granadero Baigorria, Santa Fe, Argentina*

[c]*Carrasco Hospital, Rosario, Santa Fe, Argentina*

[d]*Institut für Physiologie und Pathophysiologie, Marburg, Germany*

Earlier studies revealed that patients with tuberculosis (TB) have imbalanced immunoendocrine responses and that adrenal steroids [cortisol and dehydroepiandrosterone (DHEA)] can modify their specific cell-mediated immune response. Because most household contacts (HHCs) of contagious TB patients develop a subclinical and self-controlled process (latent TB), we studied some features of their immune and endocrine responses, particularly those related to the hypothalamic–pituitary–adrenal axis. Nineteen HHCs, 24 untreated TB patients (15 moderate, 9 advanced), and 18 healthy controls of similar age were studied. Patients had increased and reduced levels of cortisol and DHEA, respectively. DHEA levels were also reduced in HHCs. Stimulation of peripheral blood mononuclear cells (PBMC) with *Mycobacterium tuberculosis* sonicate resulted in increased *in vitro* lymphoproliferation in HHCs, while advanced patients showed the lowest response. Significantly higher amounts of interferon (IFN)-γ were detected in supernatants from stimulated PBMC of HHCs when compared to controls and TB patients. Addition of cortisol to the cultures inhibited mycobacterial antigen-driven IFN-γ production in all groups, although HHC supernatant contained significantly higher concentrations. In contrast, addition of DHEA to cultures of cells from HHCs resulted in increased IFN-γ levels. These results suggest the existence of a particular immunoendocrine relation assuring a preserved IFN-γ production in healthy housemates of TB patients.

Key words: tuberculosis; household contacts; interferon-γ; cortisol; dehydroepiandrosterone; immunoendocrine interactions

Introduction

An estimated one-third of the world population is believed to be infected with *Mycobacterium tuberculosis*, the etiologic agent of tuberculosis (TB), with 3 million deaths per year attributable to this disease.[1] The infection occurs in the lungs, but the microorganism can seed any organ via hematogenous spread. Epidemiological data suggest that only about 10% of the individuals infected with *M. tuberculosis* have a lifetime risk of developing TB.[2,3] This group presumably lacks the ability to control

Address for correspondence: Oscar Bottasso, Institute of Immunology, School of Medical Sciences, National University of Rosario, Santa Fe 3100, Rosario, Argentina. Voice: +54 341 4804559; fax: +54 341 34804569.
bottasso@uolsinectis.com.ar

Neuroimmunomodulation: Ann. N.Y. Acad. Sci. 1153: 247–255 (2009).
doi: 10.1111/j.1749-6632.2008.03976.x © 2009 New York Academy of Sciences.

the infection by failing to develop a protective response in time to prevent disease. Conversely, it is generally thought that the majority of people infected with *M. tuberculosis* have a clinically latent infection. It takes place in immunocompetent individuals in whom the infection remains dormant or latent through mechanisms that prevent bacillary proliferation, limiting its dissemination. Although these individuals may continue to be persistently infected with *M. tuberculosis* and remain latent carriers of the organism, they do not present clinical symptoms and are not contagious to others.[2,3]

The immune response against *M. tuberculosis* is complex, and the immunological events involved in protection have not been fully elucidated. Cytokine-mediated immune responses to *M. tuberculosis* infection are important determinants for development of clinical disease/latent infection. There is consensus that Th1 cells, via production of interferon-γ (IFN-γ), are associated with a protective response resulting from the activation of macrophages and subsequent destruction of intracellular bacilli, whereas Th2 cytokines seem to be detrimental. According to the Th1/Th2 paradigm, failure to resolve the infection in susceptible individuals is a consequence of the downregulation of Th1-mediated immunity.[4,5]

Because immunological and endocrine responses are closely connected and work in conjunction to shape the type of the defensive reaction against a pathogenic insult, endocrine factors are likely to contribute to the control or establishment of TB infection. The hypothalamus–pituitary–adrenal (HPA) axis and the ultimate production of the steroids cortisol and dehydroepiandrosterone (DHEA) in particular are well known for their immunoregulatory effects during normal and pathological conditions.[6–9] Our *in vitro* studies with *M. tuberculosis*-stimulated peripheral mononuclear cells (PBMC) from patients with pulmonary TB indicate that cortisol, within a range of physiological concentrations, decreases mycobacterial antigen-driven proliferation and IFN-γ production, with more pro-

nounced effects in severely ill patients.[10] TB patients showed a modest increase of circulating cortisol with profoundly decreased levels of DHEA, resulting in an increased cortisol/DHEA ratio.[11]

Latent tuberculosis infection (LTBI) can be viewed as an equilibrium between the host and the bacillus in which a robust defensive response ensures the formation of a granulomatous lesion that apparently restrains the infection and prevents active disease from occurring.[12] Hence, understanding LTBI is crucial for understanding the mechanisms underlying disease control. Since healthy household contacts (HHCs) of contagious TB patients constitute a suitable group of persons with LTBI, we studied some features of their immune and endocrine responses, in particular those related to the HPA axis.

Materials and Methods

Study Groups

Patients (six females and 18 males) with newly diagnosed lung TB and no HIV co-infection were recruited for these studies. Diagnosis was based on clinical and radiological data together with the identification of TB bacilli in sputum. The age of the patients ranged from 18 to 71 years (mean ± SD, 40.7 ± 16.9 years). Disease severity was determined according to the radiological pattern and was classified into moderate ($n = 15$) or advanced ($n = 9$). A group of 19 HIV-1 seronegative HHCs were selected from first-grade contacts of acid-fast bacilli-positive TB patients. Each HHC shared the same house or room with an index patient for at least 3 months before the patient's TB diagnosis. The control population was composed of 18 healthy volunteers without any known prior contact with TB patients. HHCs and controls had similar age and sex distribution, and none had clinical or radiological evidence of active pulmonary TB or of any other respiratory disease or acute, chronic, or immunocompromising diseases or therapies.

Blood samples were obtained from all donors at entry into the study; TB patients were sampled before initiation of antituberculous treatment. Samples were obtained at 8:00 AM to avoid differences caused by circadian variations. Additional exclusion criteria included disease states that affect the adrenal glands, the HPA, or hypothalamus–pituitary–gonadal axes or requiring corticosteroid treatment, pregnancy, and age below 18 years. This work was approved by the Ethical Committee of the Facultad de Ciencias Medicas, Universidad Nacional de Rosario, Argentina. Participants were enrolled provided informed consent had been obtained.

Mononuclear Cell Isolation and *in Vitro* Stimulation

PBMC were obtained from fresh EDTA-treated blood. After centrifugation the buffy coat was separated and diluted 1:1 in RPMI 1640 (PAA Laboratories GmbH, Linz, Austria) containing standard concentrations of L-glutamin, penicillin, and streptomycin [culture medium (CM)]. The cell suspension was layered over a Ficoll-Triyosom gradient (density 1.077; Amersham Biosciences, Piscataway, NJ) and centrifuged at 400 g for 30 min at room temperature (19–22°C). PBMC recovered from the interface were washed three times with CM and resuspended in CM containing 10% heat-inactivated, pooled, normal AB human sera (CMS; PAA Laboratories). Cells were cultured in quadruplicate in flat-bottomed microtiter plates (2×10^5 cells/well in 200 μL) with or without addition of antigen obtained by sonication of heat-killed H37Rv *M. tuberculosis* (whole sonicated antigen from *M. tuberculosis* (WSA); 8 μg/mL, kindly provided by Dr. J.L. Stanford, Free University College of London, London). The *M. tuberculosis* strain used to prepare the WSA had been isolated from a patient with open pulmonary TB fully sensitive to anti-TB drugs. Bacilli were cultured in Sauton's agar

and further suspended in borate-buffered physiological saline. The sonicate filtrate was diluted to 1 mg/mL with borate buffer. PBMC cultures were incubated for 5 days at 37°C in a 5% CO_2-humidified atmosphere and pulsed with ^{3}H-thymidine for 18 h before cell harvesting. Proliferative responses are expressed as the stimulation index (SI), calculated by dividing the count per minute of stimulated cultures by the count per minute of cells from the same individual without stimulation.

Cytokine Measurements

To evaluate cytokine production, 10^6 cells/mL were cultured with or without addition of 8 μg/mL of WSA. Since IFN-γ response peaked 96 h following stimulation,[9] culture supernatants were collected after 96 h and stored at −20°C until used for cytokine determinations. The concentration of IFN-γ in supernatants from stimulated or unstimulated cultures was determined by ELISA using commercially available kits (OptEIA Set; Pharmingen, San Diego, CA), and following the guidelines provided by the manufacturer. Samples were assayed in duplicate and results are expressed as the average of the two determinations. Cytokines were quantified with reference to standard curves generated using human recombinant cytokines.

Studies on the *in Vitro* Effects of Cortisol and DHEA

PBMC were cultured as described above with the addition of different physiological concentrations of cortisol (10^{-6} mol/L) and/or DHEA (10^{-7} mol/L, 10^{-8} mol/L, 10^{-9} mol/L). Inhibitory and stimulating doses of both compounds were determined in a pilot study using PBMC from healthy volunteers stimulated with WSA *in vitro*. The effect of the hormones on cytokine production by antigen-stimulated PBMC was studied in supernatants from 96-h cultures. Lymphoproliferation was analyzed as described above. Cultures exposed to the same final concentration of alcohol needed to dissolve the hormones were used as further controls. This alcohol concentration did not affect cell viability, cell proliferation, or cytokine production (data not shown). The following combinations were used: neither stimulation nor treatments (baseline); WSA-stimulation, with or without addition of DHEA and/or cortisol.

Hormone Determinations

Immediately after collection, Trasylol® (100 U/mL; Bayer, Leverkusen, Germany) was added to the plasma and samples were preserved at −20°C. Levels of cortisol, DHEA, and DHEA-sulfate (DHEAS) were measured in plasma with commercially available ELISA kits, according to the instructions of the manufacturer (DRG Systems, Marburg, Germany). The detection limits were 2.5 ng/mL for cortisol, 0.1 ng/mL for DHEA, and 0.044 μg/mL for DHEAS.

Statistical Analysis

Because of individual variations in cell proliferation and cytokine production in patients and control subjects, data are given as the median and 25–75 percentiles. Plasma levels of hormones are given as mean ± SE of the mean. Statistical comparisons were performed by the Kruskall–Wallis and Mann–Whitney U tests. Related samples were analyzed by the Wilcoxon and Friedman tests. Correlations between hormone levels and the *in vitro* mycobacterial-driven immune response (lymphoproliferation and cytokine production) were analyzed by parametric and nonparametric methods. A P-value < 0.05 was considered statistically significant.

Results

Results from adrenal steroid levels in plasma are depicted in Figure 1. Mean levels of corti-

sol in patients with advanced TB were significantly higher than in HHCs, controls, and patients with moderate TB ($P < 0.01$). Cases with moderate TB had a modest increase in cortisol levels, statistically different from those of HHCs ($P < 0.04$). While measurements of DHEAS revealed no between-group differences, DHEA concentration in plasma of TB patients was remarkably lower (60–65% decrease) than that of the controls ($P < 0.02$, Fig. 1). Levels of DHEA were also lower in HHCs, roughly 50% of those of the controls ($P < 0.02$, Fig. 1). The ratio cortisol/DHEA was significantly increased in both groups of TB patients compared to controls and HHCs ($P < 0.01$). Interestingly, the cortisol/DHEA ratio was also higher in HHCs compared to controls ($P < 0.04$, Fig. 1). The DHEAS/DHEA ratio was increased among advanced patients, nearly reaching statistical significance with respect to the other groups. There were no significant associations between age and hormone concentrations in plasma.

Data of the *in vitro* proliferation of PBMC from the different groups are presented in Table 1. PBMC from advanced TB patients had significantly lower median proliferative responses to WSA than the remaining groups ($P < 0.02$). Cells obtained from HHCs had a higher mycobacteria-driven proliferation than controls, but the trend did not reach statistical significance.

There was a negative correlation between cortisol/DHEA ratio and antigen-specific proliferation (r, -0.35; $n = 52$, $P < 0.01$).

Antigen-stimulated IFN-γ production was increased among HHCs and significantly different from all other groups ($P < 0.001$, Table 2). Patients with moderate disease also had a higher IFN-γ production, when compared to those of the advanced cases ($P < 0.05$, Table 2). Treatment with cortisol resulted in a significant reduction of IFN-γ in culture supernatants in all groups when compared to their untreated counterparts (Table 2). Comparisons among groups revealed higher IFN-γ concentrations in the group of HHCs ($P < 0.05$) than

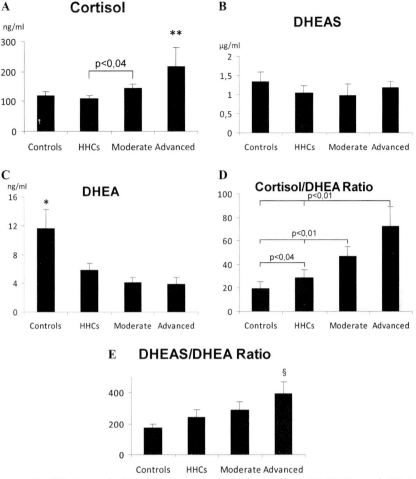

Figure 1. (**A**) Cortisol, (**B**) dehydroepiandrosterone-sulfate (DHEAS), and (**C**) DHEA plasma levels and (**D**) cortisol/DHEA and (**E**) DHEAS/DHEA ratios in controls, household contacts (HHCs), and tuberculosis patients with moderate or advanced disease. Data are given as means ± SE of the mean ng/mL, except for DHEAS, which is represented in μg/mL. DHEAS and DHEA concentrations employed for calculating the DHEAS/DHEA ratio were in ng/mL. *significantly different from the remaining groups, $P < 0.02$. **significantly different from the remaining groups, $P < 0.01$. §comparisons with the remaining groups, $P = 0.05$.

in all other groups. Reduced IFN-γ concentrations were observed in cultures treated with cortisol plus DHEA in any of the concentrations tested, but the supernatants from HHCs contained significantly higher levels than the other groups (Table 2).

Analysis of changes in cultures exposed to DHEA revealed a dissimilar pattern of group differences when compared to their respective unexposed cells. While all tested doses of DHEA significantly decreased IFN-γ levels in culture supernatants from patients with moder-

ate TB, concentrations of this cytokine were not significantly modified in DHEA-treated cultures of advanced patients (Table 2). Interestingly, IFN-γ production by cells from HHCs and controls was only decreased when treated with 10^{-7} mol/L or 10^{-8} mol/L DHEA, respectively. Furthermore, treatment of cells from HHCs with 10^{-8} mol/L and 10^{-9} mol/L DHEA resulted in increased amounts of IFN-γ (Table 2), which were the highest concentrations of the cytokine obtained under the experimental conditions tested here.

TABLE 1. Proliferative Responses of Peripheral Mononuclear Cells (PBMC) from Controls, Household Contacts (HHCs), and Patients with Moderate or Advanced Tuberculosis (TB) to Specific Antigen Stimulation

Groups	SI WSA
Controls ($n = 13$)	18.78 (11.9–40.9)
HHCs ($n = 19$)	28.6 (14.1–65.19)
Moderate ($n = 13$)	19.2 (14–30.17)
Advanced ($n = 8$)	7.26 (3.38–11.19)*

Cultures were stimulated for 5 days in the presence of whole sonicated antigen from *M. tuberculosis* (WSA). Values correspond to the stimulation index (SI) and are expressed as median (25–75 percentiles).

*Significantly different from all other groups, $P < 0.02$.

The relative change of IFN-γ concentrations was also calculated according to the formula: cytokine concentration in stimulated cultures/cytokine concentration in stimulated hormone-treated cultures × 100. The relative decrease in IFN-γ concentrations in cortisol-treated cultures revealed no differences among groups. In DHEA-treated cultures, in particular at the 10^{-9} mol/L concentration, cultures from HHCs revealed a hormone-dependent increment of IFN-γ levels, which was significantly different from the other groups ($P < 0.05$).

HHCs were next classified into two groups of similar age and sex distribution depending on their consanguinity ($n = 13$) or not ($n = 7$) with the TB patient. All supernatants from WSA-stimulated cultures and WSA-stimulated DHEA-treated (10^{-8}–10^{-9} mol/L) cultures of PBMC from consanguineous HHCs contained significantly higher amounts of IFN-γ than the non-consanguineous counterparts ($P < 0.03$ and $P < 0.015$, respectively).

Discussion

TB represents a chronic and complex interaction between the host and the pathogen, with protective and damaging responses existing throughout. Exposure to *M. tuberculosis* in most immunocompetent humans leads to the subsequent expansion of

TABLE 2. Levels of Interferon (IFN)-γ in 96-h Culture Supernatants from WSA-stimulated PBMCs of Controls, HCCs, and TB Patients in the Absence or Presence of Glucocorticoids and/or Dehydroepiandrosterone (DHEA)

| | Hormone treatment | | | Groups | | | |
| | Cortisol | DHEA | Controls ($n = 18$) | HCCs ($n = 13$) | Moderate ($n = 15$) | Advanced ($n = 8$) | Overall P-value |
Stimulation							
Baseline	—	—	4.5 (4.5–4.5)	8 (4.5–24.5)	4.5 (4.5–9)	4.5 (4.5–28)	ns
WSA	—	—	781.5 (416–1227)	2670 (1313–6206)	1202 (656–2764)	807 (287–957)^a	<0.001
WSA	10^{-6} mol/L	—	264 (97–483)§	630 (146–1743)‡	234 (57–812)§	62.5 (9.5–331.2)†	<0.05
WSA		10^{-7} mol/L	804 (311–1115)	1966 (896–5716)*	1111 (448–1677)*	722 (268–941)	<0.025
WSA		10^{-8} mol/L	654 (250–1061)**	3439 (1404–5303)	893 (496–1878)*	648 (192–924)	<0.005
WSA		10^{-9} mol/L	718 (338–1295)	3978 (1687–5950)	1070 (585–1912)*	623 (136–956)	<0.001
WSA	10^{-6} mol/L	10^{-7} mol/L	238 (69–451.7)§	588 (215–2715)**	209 (79–427)§	34 (9–303)†	<0.01
WSA	10^{-6} mol/L	10^{-8} mol/L	226 (82–502)§	525 (206.5–2200)‡	145 (72–524)§	48 (9–251)‡	<0.01
WSA	10^{-6} mol/L	10^{-9} mol/L	199 (82–523)§	467 (93.5–3475)‡	354 (97–599)§	45 (9–289.5)†	=0.05

Data represent median and (25–75) percentiles (pg/mL).
Comparisons between groups: overall P values or ^{a} significantly different from moderate patients, $P < 0.05$.
Comparisons within groups are referred to differences in relation to their respective WSA-stimulated cultures without hormones.
*$P < 0.02$, **$P < 0.01$, †$P < 0.005$, ‡$P < 0.002$, §$P < 0.001$.

mycobacteria-specific T lymphocyte populations that result in granuloma formation where the infection is contained but not eradicated. This condition of persisting infection at a subclinical level is termed *LTBI*.[12] Studies in healthy humans who are likely infected with *M. tuberculosis* are important for developing a better understanding of the process by which infection is controlled, at least in its beginning. The robust antigen-dependent production of IFN-γ detected in HHCs may be involved in this process. This cytokine, which is mainly produced by specific CD4[+] T lymphocytes upon recognition of mycobacterial epitopes, enhances the capacity of macrophages to suppress replication of, or possibly kill, the phagosome-resident organisms.[4,5] Studies in human macrophages showed that IFN-γ stimulates the production of tumor necrosis factor and 1,25 dihydroxycholecalciferol, both of which facilitate mycobacterial inhibition, probably from the generation of reactive oxygen and nitrogen intermediates, as well as control intracellular iron levels.[13,14]

Treatment with cortisol revealed no differential effect of this hormone on cells obtained either from controls, HHCs, or TB patients because decreased amounts of IFN-γ were observed in all groups, although IFN-γ levels continued to be comparatively higher in HHCs. This is in line with our previous studies[10] and reports in the literature showing that glucocorticoids can inhibit Th1 cells.[15–17] While in most cases the IFN-γ response was modestly decreased or unchanged by DHEA, IFN-γ production was even increased in cell cultures from HHCs treated with the lower concentrations of DHEA. This result confirms the facilitating effects of DHEA on Th1 responses[9] and adds novel evidence of a differential effect related to the host status, at least during infection with *M. tuberculosis*.

GCs exert anti-inflammatory effects and favor an immune response inefficient in eliminating intracellular pathogens,[6–8] whereas DHEA counteracts this Th2-promoting effect of GCs, although it also exerts potent anti-inflammatory effects.[9] The increased cortisol/DHEA ratio detected in TB patients may be detrimental for the development of an appropriate cell-mediated immune response, and the inverse correlation between the cortisol/DHEA ratio and *in vitro* specific lymphoproliferation supports this assumption.

A different situation seems to be present in HHCs as they displayed the highest IFN-γ production in the presence of a slightly augmented cortisol/DHEA ratio and they also had a DHEA-dependent increment of IFN-γ levels.

We have previously shown that exposure of a human adrenal cell line to products released by antigen-stimulated lymphoid cells obtained from TB patients results in a marked reduction in the concentration of DHEA, which is the biologically active hormone, in the supernatant of the adrenal cell cultures.[11] On the other hand, it has been shown that bacterial products and pro-inflammatory cytokines can inhibit the activity of DHEAS sulfatase in macrophages, which reduces the transformation of the sulfatated mediator into DHEA.[18] Thus, it is possible that inhibition of DHEA synthesis by the adrenal gland and the conversion of DHEAS into DHEA at the site of inflammation could result in the reduced levels of DHEA that we have detected. The fact that such reduction does not only occur in TB patients but also in HHCs indicates that this effect is determined by immune mechanisms activated by the infection with *M. tuberculosis* rather than being a consequence of the overt expression of the disease.

A question to be answered with respect to LTBI is the difference in IFN-γ production when HHCs were classified according to consanguinity. One possibility for the increased IFN-γ production among consanguineous HHCs is that they may share some genetic background rendering them more susceptible to be infected upon exposure.

Studies carried out in Ethiopia showed that healthy individuals who control a latent infection with *M. tuberculosis* express higher levels of IFN-γ than healthy individuals and more IFN-γ gene expression than TB patients.[19] In a 2-year follow-up study, it was shown that infected individuals who remained healthy had an increased production of IFN-γ when PBMC were stimulated with purified mycobacteria protein derivate but lower production when stimulated with the early secretory antigenic 6-kDa protein, an *M. tuberculosis*-specific antigen.[20] In our studies, none of the HHCs had clinical or radiological signs of disease and they produced more IFN-γ in response to WSA stimulation than controls and TB patients, warranting follow-up studies of this population.

Partly because IFN-γ is necessary for host immunity against TB and partly from the lack of a gold standard for a true correlate of protective immunity, measurement of IFN-γ production is being widely used. Nevertheless, additional factors should act in concert to confer sufficient protection. Studies in different infectious diseases indicate that CD4 T cells secreting only IFN-γ predominate in infections with an acute or persistently high antigen load, like acute, untreated, HIV-1 infection or untreated TB.[21–23] In contrast, a polyfunctional response of CD4 T cells secreting IFN-γ only, IFN-γ and IL-2, or IL-2 only, is characteristic of infections with a persistently low antigen load, for example during latent asymptomatic cytomegalovirus infection[21]; whereas CD4 T cells secreting only IL-2 are associated with cleared or treated infections.[21,23,24]

The defense of an organism against infection requires a series of coordinated neural, endocrine, and immunological reactions that allow pathogen clearance and recovery of the injured tissue. In conclusion, although the protective mechanisms accounting for the different resistance showed by TB patients and HHCs are not fully identified, the present results suggest the existence of a particular immunoendocrine relation assuring a preserved IFN-γ production in healthy contacts of contagious TB patients.

Acknowledgments

The present study received financial support from a Fondo para la Investigación Científica y Tecnológica (FONCYT) research grant (BID 1728/OC-AR 5-25462).

Conflicts of Interest

The authors declare no conflicts of interest.

References

1. World Health. Organization Global tuberculosis control: surveillance, planning, financing. WHO report 2006. www.who.int/entity/tb/publications/global_report/2006/pdf/full_report_correctedversion.pdf
2. Bloom, B.R. & C.J. Murray. 1992. Tuberculosis: commentary on a re-emergent killer. *Science* **257:** 1055–1064.
3. Comstock, G.W. 1982. Epidemiology of tuberculosis. *Am. Rev. Respir. Dis.* **125:** 8–15.
4. Flynn, J.L. 2004. Immunology of tuberculosis and implications in vaccine development. *Tuberculosis* **84:** 93–101.
5. Bottasso, O., M.L. Bay, H. Besedovsky, *et al*. 2007. The immuno-endocrine component in the pathogenesis of tuberculosis. *Scand. J. Immunol.* **66:** 166–175.
6. Besedovsky, H. & A. del Rey. 1996. Immune-neuroendocrine interactions: facts and hypothesis. *Endocr. Rev.* **17:** 64–95.
7. Turnbull, A.V. & C.L. Rivier. 1999. Regulation of the hypothalamic-pituitary-adrenal axis by cytokines: actions and mechanisms of action. *Physiological Rev.* **79:** 1–71.
8. Elenkov, I.J. & G.P. Chrousos. 1999. Stress hormones, Th1/Th2 patterns, pro/anti-inflammatory cytokines and susceptibility to disease. *Trends Endocrinol. Metab.* **10:** 359–368.
9. Dillon, J. 2005. dehydroepiandrosterone, dehydroepiandrosterone sulfate and related steroids: their role in inflammatory, allergic and immunological disorders. *Curr. Drug Targets Inflamm. Allergy* **4:** 377–385.
10. Mahuad, C., M.L. Bay, M.A. Farroni, *et al*. 2004. Cortisol and dehydroepiandrosterone affect the response of peripheral blood mononuclear cells to mycobacterial antigens during tuberculosis. *Scand. J. Immunol.* **60:** 639–646.
11. del Rey, A., C.V. Mahuad, V.V. Bozza, *et al*. 2007. Endocrine and cytokine responses in humans with pulmonary tuberculosis. *Brain Behav. Immun.* **21:** 171–179.
12. Morrison, J., M. Pai & P.C. Hopewell. 2008. Tuberculosis and latent tuberculosis infection in close contacts of people with pulmonary tuberculosis in low-income

and middle-income countries: a systematic review and meta-analysis. *Lancet Infec. Dis.* **8:** 359–368.

13. Rook, G.A., J. Steele, L. Fraher, *et al.* 1986. Vitamin D₃, gamma interferon, and control of proliferation of *Mycobacterium tuberculosis* by human monocytes. *Immunology* **57:** 159–163.

14. Denis, M. 1991. Killing of *Mycobacterium tuberculosis* within human monocytes: activation by cytokines and calcitriol. *Clin. Exp. Immunol.* **84:** 200–208.

15. Miyaura, H. & M. Iwata. 2002. Direct and indirect inhibition of Th1 development by progesterone and glucocorticoids. *J. Immunol.* **168:**1087–1094.

16. Ramirez, F., D.J. Fowell, M. Puklavec, *et al.* 1996. Glucocorticoids promote a Th2 cytokine response by CD4+ T cells in vitro. *J. Immunol.* **156:** 2406–2412.

17. Padgett, D.A., J.F. Sheridan, R. Loria. 1995. Steroid hormone regulation of a polyclonal Th2 immune response. *Ann. N. Y. Acad. Sci.* **774:** 323–325.

18. Hennebold J.D. & R.A. Daynes. 1994. Regulation of macrophage dehydroepiandrosterone sulfate metabolism by inflammatory cytokines. *Endocrinology* **135:** 67–75.

19. Demissie, A., M. Abebe, A. Aseffa, *et al.* 2004. Healthy individuals that control a latent infection with *Mycobacterium tuberculosis* express high levels of Th1 cytokines and the IL-4 antagonist IL-4δ2. *J. Immunol.* **172:** 6938–6943.

20. Doherty, T.M., A. Demissie, J. Olob, *et al.* 2002. Immune responses to the *Mycobacterium tuberculosis*-specific antigen ESAT-6 signal subclinical infection among contacts of tuberculosis patients. *J. Clin. Microbiol.* **40:** 704–706.

21. Harari, A., F. Vallelian, P.R. Meylan, *et al.* 2005. Functional heterogeneity of memory CD4 T cell responses in different conditions of antigen exposure and persistence. *J. Immunol.* **174:** 1037–1045.

22. Younes, S.A., B. Yassine-Diab, A.R. Dumont, *et al.* 2003. HIV-1 viremia prevents the establishment of interleukin 2–producing HIV-specific memory CD4+ T cells endowed with proliferative capacity. *J. Exp. Med.* **198:** 1909–1922.

23. Millington, K.A., J.A. Innes, S. Hackforth, *et al.* 2007. Dynamic relationship between IFN-γ and IL-2 profile of *Mycobacterium tuberculosis*–specific T cells and antigen load. *J. Immunol.* **178:** 5217–5226.

24. Correa, R., A. Harari, F. Vallelian, *et al.* 2007. Functional patterns of HIV-1-specific CD4 T-cell responses in children are influenced by the extent of virus suppression and exposure. *AIDS* **21:** 23–30.

The Chemokine CCL5 Is Essential for Leukocyte Recruitment in a Model of Severe *Herpes simplex* Encephalitis

Márcia Carvalho Vilela,[a] Daniel Santos Mansur,[b] Norinne Lacerda-Queiroz,[c] David Henrique Rodrigues,[c] Graciela Kunrath Lima,[b] Rosa Maria Esteves Arantes,[d] Erna Geessien Kroon,[b] Marco Antônio da Silva Campos,[e] Mauro Martins Teixeira,[c] and Antônio Lúcio Teixeira[a]

[a]Departamento de Clínica Médica, Faculdade de Medicina, [b]Departamento de Microbiologia, Instituto de Ciências Biológicas, [c]Departamento de Bioquímica e Imunologia, Instituto de Ciências Biológicas, and [d]Departamento de Patologia Geral, Instituto de Ciências Biológicas, Universidade Federal de Minas Gerais, Belo Horizonte, Brazil [e]Centro de Pesquisas René Rachou, Fiocruz, Belo Horizonte, Brazil

The *Herpes simplex virus*-1 (HSV-1) is responsible for several clinical manifestations in humans, including encephalitis. To induce encephalitis, C57BL/6 mice were inoculated with 10^4 plaque-forming cells of HSV-1 by the intracranial route. Met-RANTES (regulated upon activation, normal T cell expressed and presumably secreted) ($10\,\mu g$/mouse), a CC chemokine family receptor (CCR)1 and CCR5 antagonist, was given subcutaneously the day before, immediately after, and at days 1, 2, and 3 after infection. Treatment with Met-RANTES had no effect on the viral titers. In contrast, intravital microscopy revealed that treatment with Met-RANTES decreased the number of leukocytes adherent to the pial microvasculature at days 1 and 3 after infection. The levels of the chemokines CCL3, CCL5, CXCL1, and CXCL9 increased after infection and were enhanced further by the treatment with Met-RANTES. Treatment with a polyclonal anti-CCL5 antibody 2 h before the intravital microscopy decreased leukocyte adhesion in the microcirculation of infected mice. In conclusion, CCL5, a chemokine that binds to CCR1 and CCR5, is essential for leukocyte adhesion during HSV-1 encephalitis. However, blocking of CCR1 and CCR5 did not affect HSV-1 replication, suggesting that other immune mechanisms are involved in the process of infection control.

Key words: CCL5; Met-RANTES; *Herpes* virus; encephalitis; intravital microscopy

Introduction

The chemokine family is responsible for the trafficking of leukocytes and plays a major role in the functioning of the immune system.[1,2] Chemokines are small (8–10 kDa) basic polypeptides and they can be subdivided into four main families based on the number and the mutual placement of the cysteine residues in the N-terminal region of the peptide.[3,4] The effects of chemokines are mediated by cell surface receptors that belong to the family of G protein-coupled receptors. CCL5, previously known as RANTES (regulated upon activation, normal T cell expressed and presumably secreted), is a member of the CC chemokine family and recruits monocytes, T cells, basophils, and eosinophils via the chemokine receptors CCR1, CCR3, and CCR5.[5]

Address for correspondence: Antônio Lúcio Teixeira, Departamento de Clínica Médica, Faculdade de Medicina, UFMG, Av. Alfredo Balena, 190. Santa Efigênia, Belo Horizonte, Brazil 30130-100. Voice/fax: 55-31-34092651. altexr@gmail.com

Neuroimmunomodulation: Ann. N.Y. Acad. Sci. 1153: 256–263 (2009).
doi: 10.1111/j.1749-6632.2008.03959.x © 2009 New York Academy of Sciences.

The discovery that human immunodeficiency virus-1 (HIV-1) uses CCR5 as a cofactor for cellular entry stimulated the research in this field aimed at the development of potent, well-tolerated, small-molecule antagonists of chemokine receptors. Modifications of the amino-terminal region of chemokines have led to receptor antagonists, including Met-RANTES (CCL5 with the N terminus methionine) and AOP-RANTES (aminooxipentane RANTES), which also block infection by HIV-1. Met-RANTES was obtained when RANTES/CCL5 was expressed in *Escherichia coli* and the initiating methionine was retained.[6]

There are several lines of evidence implicating CCL5 in neuroinflammatory processes. For example, CCL5 may play an important role in multiple sclerosis (MS) by recruiting T cells expressing the cognate chemokine receptor, CCR5, to the central nervous system (CNS).[7,8] Anti-CCL5 antibodies diminished leukocyte infiltration into the CNS and reduced neurological symptoms in a viral model of MS.[9] In other experimental models, such as rheumatoid arthritis and colitis, mice treated with Met-RANTES had less severe clinical symptoms and reduced inflammatory parameters.[10,11]

Herpes simplex virus-1 (HSV-1) is an alphaherpervirus able to infect most cell types and establishes latent infections in neurons. HSV-1 is the major cause of sporadic acute focal encephalitis in humans.[12] Despite the progress in antiviral therapy, HSV-1 encephalitis is still one of the most devastating infectious diseases of the CNS, with a mortality of up to 20% and neurological sequel in over 50% of the survivors.[13] Recently our group demonstrated that a severe model of encephalitis caused by HSV-1 was followed by increased CNS levels of CCL5 and other chemokines, including CCL2, CCL3, CXCL1, and CXCL9. Moreover, we performed intravital microscopy and observed an increase in the levels of rolling and adhered leukocytes in meningeal vessels of infected mice.[14]

In the present study we aimed to explore the possible involvement of CCL5 in the trafficking of leukocytes into the CNS by using intravital microscopy of mice infected with an intracerebral inoculum of HSV-1.

Experimental Procedures

Mouse Strains

Male (age 6–9 weeks) C57BL/6 mice were obtained from Animal Care Facilities of the Institute of Biological Sciences, Federal University of Minas Gerais, Belo Horizonte, Brazil. The local ethics committee for animal research approved all the experimental procedures described here.

Virus

HSV-1 strain EK[15] was allowed to multiply in Vero cells and was maintained with minimal essential medium (GIBCO, Grand Island, NY) containing 5% fetal bovine serum (FBS) (GIBCO) and 25 $\mu g/\mu L$ of ciprofloxacin (Cellofarm, Carapina, ES, Brazil) at 37°C in 5% CO_2. Virus was purified in sucrose gradient and the titers determined in Vero cells as previously described.[16,17] The virus titers obtained were 1.1×10^8 plaque-forming cells (PFU)/mL for HSV-1.

Vero Cells

Vero cells were maintained in minimal essential medium (GIBCO) supplemented with 5% heat-inactivated FBS and antibiotics in 5% CO_2 at 37°C. These cells were used for virus multiplication.

Infection with HSV-1

Mice were anesthetized by intraperitoneal injection of a mixture of ketamine (150 mg/kg) and xylazine (10 mg/kg), and a 10^4-PFU inoculum of the purified HSV-1 resuspended in 10 μL of phosphate-buffered saline (PBS) was injected intracranially in the right side of a sagittal suture at the level of the eyes. Control mice received PBS.

Treatment of HSV-1–infected Mice with Met-RANTES or Anti-RANTES

Met-RANTES was injected daily with 0.1 mL and 10 μg/mouse. Treatment was given subcutaneously the day before, immediately after, and at days 1, 2, and 3 after HSV-1 infection.[18] Met-RANTES was a kind gift from Dr. Amanda Proudfoot (Merck-Serono Pharmaceutical Research Institute, Geneva, Switzerland). To evaluate the role of CCL5 on leukocyte adhesion, another group of animals was treated with an intraperitoneal injection of 300 μL/mouse of anti-murine CCL5 antibody 2 h before the intravital microscopy.[19] Control animals received nonimmune rabbit sera.

Intravital Microscopy

Intravital microscopy of the mouse brain microvasculature was performed as previously described.[20,21] Briefly, mice were anesthetized by intraperitoneal injection of a mixture of ketamine (150 mg/kg) and xylazine (10 mg/kg), and the tail vein was cannulated for administration of fluorescent dyes. A craniotomy was performed using a high-speed drill (Beltec, Araraquara, SP, Brazil), and the dura mater was removed to expose the underlying pial vasculature. Throughout the experiment, mice were maintained at 37°C with a heating pad and the exposed brain was continuously superfused with artificial cerebrospinal fluid buffer, an ionic composition in mmol/L: NaCl 132, KCl 1.95, $CaCl_2$ 1.71, $MgCl_2$ 0.64, $NaHCO_3$ 24.6, dextrose 3.71, and urea 6.7, pH 7.4, at 37°C.

Leukocytes were fluorescently labeled by intravenous administration of rhodamine 6G (Sigma, St. Louis, MO) (0.5 mg/kg body weight) and were observed by using a microscope (Olympus B201 (Tokyo, Japan), X20 objective lens, corresponding to 100 μm of

area) outfitted with a fluorescent light source (epi-illumination at 510–560 nm, using a 590-nm emission filter). A silicon-intensified camera mounted on the microscope projected the image onto a monitor. The number of rolling and adherent leukocytes was determined offline during video playback analysis. Leukocytes were considered adherent to the venular endothelium if they remained stationary for a minimum of 30 s. Rolling leukocytes were defined as white cells moving at a velocity lower than that of erythrocytes within a given vessel. Pial vessels with diameters ranging from 50 to 120 μm were used, as most adhesion occurred in vessels of these sizes. Because of the greater variability in size of these vessels, we expressed leukocyte adhesion as number of cells/100 μm.

ELISA of the Proteins in the CNS

Brain tissue extracts were obtained from control and infected mice after intravital microscopy, and the left hemisphere was stored at −20°C. Thereafter, the brain was homogenized in extraction solution (100 mg of tissue per 1 mL) containing: 0.4 mol/L NaCl, 0.05% Tween 20, 0.5% BSA, 0.1 mmol/L Phenyl methyl sulfonil fluoride, 0.1 mmol/L benzethonium chloride, 10 mmol/L EDTA and 20 KI aprotinin, using Ultra-Turrax (Fisher Scientific, Pittsburgh, PA). Brain homogenate was centrifuged at 3000 g for 10 min at 4°C, and the supernatants were collected and stored at −20°C. The concentration of chemokines CXCL1, CXCL9, CCL2, CCL3, and CCL5 was determined using ELISA.

The supernatants of brain tissue were assayed in an ELISA setup using commercially available antibodies, according to the procedures provided by the manufacturer (R&D Systems, Minneapolis, MN).

Statistical Analysis

Data are shown as mean ± SEM. A one-way ANOVA with Tukey's correction was used for

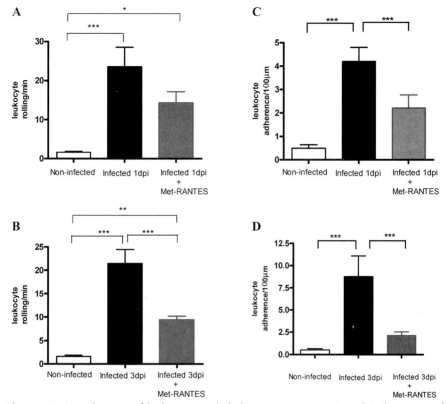

Figure 1. Visualization of leukocyte–endothelium interaction at 1 and 3 days post infection (d.p.i.) with *Herpes simplex virus* (HSV)-1. Mice were inoculated with 10^4 plaque-forming cells (PFU) of HSV-1 by the intracranial route. Groups are: noninfected mice (*n* = 6), infected mice (*n* = 6), and Met-RANTES (regulated upon activation, normal T cell expressed and presumably secreted) treatment in infected mice (*n* = 5) from 1 day before the infection to 3 d.p.i. Intravital microscopy was used to assess rolling (**A, B**) and adhesion (**C, D**) of leukocytes in the brain microvasculature. Data indicate mean ± SEM of cells per minute (**A, B**) or per 100 μm (**C, D**). Statistically significant results were indicated by ***$P < 0.001$, **$P < 0.01$, and *$P < 0.05$. Statistical analysis used was one-way ANOVA with Tukey's correction.

multiple comparisons. Statistical significance was set at $P < 0.05$.

Results

Treatment with Met-RANTES Decreased Rolling and Adherence of Leukocytes to Meningeal Vessels of HSV-1–infected Mice

C57Bl/6 mice developed encephalitis after intracranial infection with 10^4 PFU of HSV-1. These animals died from days 3 to 6 after infection. Intravital microscopy showed an increase in rolling and adhesion of leukocytes in meningeal vessels of infected mice at days 1 and 3 after infection (Fig. 1). The procedure was not performed later because of the excessive lethality rates. Treatment with Met-RANTES before and during the infection significantly decreased both leukocyte rolling and adhesion (Fig. 1).

Treatment with Met-RANTES Was Associated with Higher Chemokine Levels in the Brain Tissue of HSV-1–infected Mice

HSV-1–infected mice had increased levels of the chemokines CXCL1, CXCL9, CCL2,

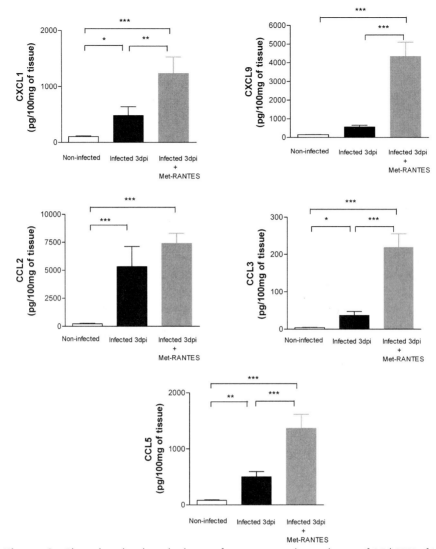

Figure 2. Chemokine levels in the brain after intracranial inoculation of 10^4 PFU of HSV-1. Groups are: noninfected mice ($n = 8$), infected mice ($n = 8$), and Met-RANTES treatment in infected mice ($n = 6$) from 1 day before to 3 days after infection. The concentration of the chemokines CXCL1, CXCL9, CCL2, CCL3, and CCL5 at 3 d.p.i. was measured in brain extracts by ELISA. Data indicate mean $\pm$ SEM. Statistically significant results were indicated by ***$P < 0.001$, **$P < 0.01$, and *$P < 0.05$. Statistical analysis used was one-way ANOVA with Tukey's correction.

CCL3, and CCL5 in the brain at days 1 and 3 after infection. Despite the decreased leukocyte rolling and adhesion, treatment with Met-RANTES significantly enhanced the levels of chemokines in the brain of infected mice at day 3 (Fig. 2) but not at day 1 (data not shown) after infection.

Treatment with Met-RANTES Did Not Modify HSV-1 Viral Load in the Brain

Treatment with Met-RANTES did not alter virus titers in brain at day 1 (untreated mice, log $10^{5.022}$ PFU; Met-RANTES treatment, log $10^{5.573}$ PFU per mg of tissue; P value $= 0.15$)

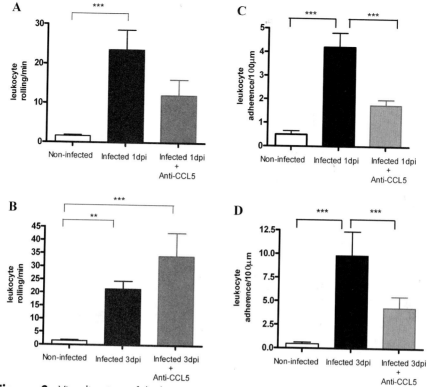

Figure 3. Visualization of leukocyte–endothelium interaction at 1 and 3 d.p.i. with HSV-1. Mice were intracranially inoculated with 10^4 PFU of HSV-1. Groups are: noninfected mice ($n = 6$), infected mice ($n = 6$), and anti-CCL5 treatment in infected mice ($n = 6$) 2 h before intravital microscopy. Intravital microscopy was used to assess rolling (**A, B**) and adhesion (**C, D**) of leukocytes in the brain microvasculature. Data indicate mean ± SEM of cells per minute (**A, B**) or per 100 μm (**C, D**). Statistically significant results were indicated by ***$P < 0.001$, **$P < 0.01$, and *$P < 0.05$. Statistical analysis used was one-way ANOVA with Tukey's correction.

and day 3 (untreated mice, log $10^{5.653}$ PFU; Met-RANTES treatment, log $10^{5.213}$ PFU per mg of tissue; P value = 0.18) after infection.

Treatment with Anti-CCL5 Antibody Reduced Leukocyte Adherence to the Meningeal Vessels of HSV-1–infected Mice

A series of experiments were performed to confirm that CCL5 was indeed relevant for the adhesion of leukocytes to meningeal vessels. To this end, infected animals were treated with a polyclonal anti-CCL5 antibody 2 h before intravital microscopy. As seen in Figure 3, acute treatment with the antibody greatly decreased the adherence of leukocytes to meningeal ves-

sels at days 1 and 3 after infection. In contrast, leukocyte rolling was not significantly affected by the treatment (Fig. 3).

Discussion

The present study investigated the role of the chemokine CCL5 and its receptors for leukocyte/endothelial cell interaction in a model of HSV-1–induced encephalitis in mice. We showed that CCL5 plays a relevant role in the recruitment of leukocytes into the brain of HSV-1–infected mice. This result was demonstrated using two different tools, Met-RANTES, an antagonist for CCR1 and CCR5, and an anti-CCL5 antibody.

The recruitment of leukocytes is composed of a series of events dependent on multiple protein interactions.[22,23] Intravital microscopy studies allow the visualization of leukocyte/endothelial cell interaction in vessels *in vivo* and have revealed that leukocytes must first tether and roll along the venular wall before they can attach firmly and emigrate from the vasculature.[24] Chemokines act mainly on the adhesion step of this highly regulated process.[25,26]

Both strategies used in the present study to antagonize the action of CCL5 significantly reduced the adherence of leukocytes to the meningeal endothelium. In a previous study of our group, we showed that anti-CCL5 antibody decreased leukocyte adhesion but not rolling in an MOG (myelin oligodendrocyte glycoprotein)-induced, experimental, autoimmune encephalomyelitis.[21] Unexpectedly, the rolling of leukocytes was also reduced by treatment with Met-RANTES but not the antibody. It is of note that whereas the antibody was given just prior to the intravital microscopy, Met-RANTES was given daily from the day before the infection. So, it is possible that daily treatment with Met-RANTES may have modified the expression of mediators relevant for the expression of adhesion molecules for leukocyte rolling.

Met-RANTES treatment was also followed by a significant increase in CCL3, CCL5, CXCL1, and CXCL9 levels. Blocking the action of a determined chemokine may result in compensatory mechanisms leading to the overproduction of other chemokines. In line with this result, Thapa and colleagues showed recently that mice deficient in CCR5 ($CCR5^{-/-}$) expressed higher levels of TNF, CXCL1, CCL2, CCL3, and CCL5 in the brain after HSV-2 infection.[27]

In our work treatment with Met-RANTES was neither associated with a reduction nor with an increase of HSV-1 titers. Interestingly, administration of Met-RANTES during a generalized HSV-2 infection in mice led to impaired antiviral response with significantly higher viral load in the liver. This may suggest that CCR1 and/or CCR5 are important for both viral clearance and eventual control of the immune response in this model.[28] In our model, blockade of both CCR1 and CCR5 led no change in viral loads when a high inoculum was injected in the brain. However, further studies are necessary to fully define the involvement of CCL5 and its receptor on the control of HSV-1 replication when the virus is given at different sites and at low inoculum.

In summary, we showed that CCL5 plays an important role in the adhesion of leukocytes in the brain microcirculation in herpetic encephalitis.

Acknowledgments

This work was supported by Conselho Nacional de Desenvolvimento Científico e Tecnológico (CNPq) and Fundação de Amparo à Pesquisa do Estado de Minas Gerais (Fapemig), Brazil.

Conflicts of Interest

The authors declare no conflicts of interest.

References

1. Wells, T.N.C., C.A. Power & A.E.I. Proudfoot. 1998. Definition, function and pathophysiological significance of chemokine receptors Trends. *Pharmacol. Sci.* **19:** 376–380.

2. Luster, A.D. 1998. Chemokines-chemotactic cytokines that mediate inflammation. *N. Engl. J. Med.* **338:** 436–445.

3. Baggiolini, M. 2001. Chemokines in pathology and medicine. *J. Intern. Med.* **250:** 91–104.

4. Baggiolini, M. 1998. Chemokines and leukocyte traffic. *Nature* **392:** 565–568.

5. Schall, T.J., K. Bacon, K.J. Toy & D.V. Goeddel. 1990. Selective attraction of monocytes and T lymphocytes of the memory phenotype by cytokine RANTES. *Nature* **347:** 669–671.

6. Proudfoot, A.E. *et al.* 1996. Extension of recombinant human RANTES by the retention of the initiating

methionine produces a potent antagonist. *J. Biol. Chem.* **271:** 2599–2603.

7. Balashov, K.E. *et al.* 1999. CCR5(+) and CXCR3(+) T cells are increased in multiple sclerosis and their ligands MIP-1alpha and IP-10 are expressed in demyelinating brain lesions. *Proc. Natl. Acad. Sci. USA* **96:** 6873–6878.

8. Sørensen, T.L. *et al.* 1999. Expression of specific chemokines and chemokine receptors in the central nervous system of multiple sclerosis patients. *J. Clin. Invest.* **103:** 807–815.

9. Glass, W.G. *et al.* 2004. Antibody targeting of the CC chemokine ligand 5 results in diminished leukocyte infiltration into the central nervous system and reduced neurologic disease in a viral model of multiple sclerosis. *J. Immunol.* **172:** 4018–4025.

10. Morteau, O. *et al.* 2002. Genetic deficiency in the chemokine receptor CCR1 protects against acute Clostridium difficile toxin A enteritis in mice. *Gastroenterology* **122:** 725–733.

11. Plater-Zyberk, C. *et al.* 1997. Effect of a CC chemokine receptor antagonist on collagen induced arthritis in DBA/1 mice. *Immunol. Lett.* **57:** 117–120.

12. Whithey, R.J. & B. Roizman. 2001. Herpes simplex virus infections. *Lancet* **357:** 1513–1518.

13. Raschilas, F. *et al.* 2002. Outcome of and prognostic factors for herpes simplex encephalitis in adult patients: results of a multicenter study. *Clin. Infect. Dis.* **35:** 254–260.

14. Vilela, M.C. 2008. Investigação do recrutamento celular em camundongos selvagens e TNFR1$^{-/-}$ no modelo experimental de encefalite herpética grave. Master thesis, Universidade Federal de Minas Gerais, Belo Horizonte, Brazil.

15. Nogueira, M.L. *et al.* 2001. Detection of herpesvirus DNA by the polymerase chain reaction (PCR) in the vitreos samples from patients with necrotizing retinitis. *J. Clin. Pathol.* **54:** 103–106.

16. Joklik, W.K. 1962. The purification of four strains of poxvirus. *Virology* **18:** 9–18.

17. Campos, M.A. & E.G. Kroon. 1993. Critical period of irreversible block of vaccinia virus replication. *Rev. Microbiol.* **24:** 104–110.

18. Matsui, M. *et al.* 2002. Treatment of experimental autoimmune encephalomyelitis with the chemokine receptor antagonist Met-RANTES. *J. Neuroimmunol.* **128:** 16–22.

19. Coelho, P.S. *et al.* 2002. Glycosylphosphatidylinositol -anchored mucin-like glycoproteins isolated from Trypanosoma cruzi trypomastigotes induce in vivo leukocyte recruitment dependent on MCP-1 production by IFN-gamma-primed-macrophages. *J. Leukoc. Biol.* **71:** 837–844.

20. Carvalho-Tavares, J. *et al.* 2000. A role for platelets and endothelial selectins in tumor necrosis factor- induced leukocyte recruitment in the brain microvasculature. *Circ. Res.* **87:** 1141–1148.

21. dos Santos, A.C. *et al.* 2005. CCL2 and CCL5 mediate leukocyte adhesion in experimental autoimmune encephalomyelitis—an intravital microscopy study. *J. Neuroimmunol.* **162:** 122–129.

22. Ley, K. 1996. Molecular mechanisms of leukocyte recruitment in the inflammatory process. *Cardiovasc. Res.* **32:** 733–742.

23. Kubes, P. & P.A. Ward. 2000. Leukocyte recruitment and the acute inflammatory response. *Brain Pathol.* **10:** 127–135.

24. Kerfoot, S.M. & P. Kubes. 2002. Overlapping roles of P-selectin and alpha 4 integrin to recruit leukocytes to the central nervous system in experimental autoimmune encephalomyelitis. *J. Immunol.* **69:** 1000–1006.

25. Mogensen, T.H. & S.R. Paludan. 2001. Molecular pathways in virus-induced cytokine production. *Microbiol. Mol. Biol. Rev.* **65:** 131–150.

26. Kennedy, P.G. & A. Chaudhuri. 2002. Herpes simplex encephalitis. *J. Neurol. Neurosurg. Psychiatry* **73:** 237–278.

27. Thapa, M., W.A. Kuziel & D.J. Carr. 2007. Susceptibility of CCR5-deficient mice to genital herpes simplex virus type 2 is linked to NK cell mobilization. *J. Virol.* **81:** 3704–3713.

28. Sørensen, L.N. & S.R. Paludan. 2004. Blocking CC chemokine receptor (CCR) 1 and CCR5 during herpes simplex virus type 2 infection in vivo impairs host defence and perturbs the cytokine response. *Scand. J. Immunol.* **59:** 321–333.

Neuroendocrine-immunology of Experimental Chagas' Disease

Eduardo Roggero,[a] **Ana R. Pérez,**[a] **Oscar A. Bottasso,**[a] **Hugo O. Besedovsky,**[b] **and Adriana del Rey**[b]

[a]*Instituto de Inmunología, Facultad de Ciencias Médicas, Universidad Nacional de Rosario, Rosario, Argentina*

[b]*Department of Immunophysiology, Institute of Physiology and Pathophysiology, Medical Faculty, Philipps University, Marburg, Germany*

The cytokine-mediated stimulation of the hypothalamus–pituitary–adrenal (HPA) axis is relevant for immunoregulation and survival during bacterial endotoxemia and certain viral infections. However, only limited information is available regarding the effect of endogenous glucocorticoids on parasitic diseases. Here, we discuss evidence that the increased levels of corticosterone that occur following *Trypanosoma cruzi* infection in mice is an endocrine response that protects the host by impeding an excessive production of pro-inflammatory cytokines. Comparative studies between susceptible C57Bl/6J and resistant Balb/c mice indicate that the predisposition to the disease depends on the appropriate timing and magnitude of the activation of the HPA axis. However, this endocrine response also results in thymus atrophy and depletion of CD4$^+$CD8$^+$ by apoptosis. On the other hand, using tumor necrosis factor (TNF)-receptor knockout mice, we found that TNF-α plays a complex role during this disease; it is involved in the mediation of cardiac tissue damage but it also contributes to prolonged survival. Taken together, this evidence indicates that a subtle balance between endocrine responses and cytokine production is necessary for an efficient defense against *T. cruzi* infection.

Key words: *Trypanosoma cruzi* infection; endogenous glucocorticoids; cytokines; tumor necrosis factor; thymus; apoptosis; Chagas' disease

Introduction

One of the most frequent parasitic diseases in Latin American countries is Chagas' disease (also known as American trypanosomiasis). Approximately 18 million people in Central and South America are infected with the intracellular parasite *Trypanosoma cruzi*, and more than 100 million people are at risk of infection. The parasite is transmitted to humans and other mammals mostly by hematophagous insects. The human disease occurs in two stages: an acute stage shortly after the infection and a chronic stage that may develop over 20–40 years. Chronic infections result in various neurological disorders, damage of the heart muscle (cardiomyopathy is the most serious manifestation), and sometimes dilation of the digestive tract (megacolon and megaesophagus). Chagas' disease can be fatal, in most cases as a result of the cardiac sequelae.[1,2]

In the following paragraphs we describe the relevance of cytokine and hypothalamus–pituitary–adrenal (HPA) axis interactions for the course of acute *T. cruzi* infection and the thymus atrophy that infected mice develop in parallel. Furthermore, we discuss results illustrating the relevance of tumor necrosis factor (TNF)-α for the activation of the HPA axis and the course of the infection in mice genetically deficient in the receptors for this cytokine. More

Address for correspondence: Adriana del Rey, Department of Immunophysiology, Institute of Physiology and Pathophysiology, Medical Faculty, Deutschhausstrasse 2, 35037 Marburg, Germany. Voice: +49 6421 2862175; fax: +49 6421 2868925. delrey@mailer.uni-marburg.de

Neuroimmunomodulation: Ann. N.Y. Acad. Sci. 1153: 264–271 (2009).
doi: 10.1111/j.1749-6632.2008.03982.x © 2009 New York Academy of Sciences.

details about the methodology used and the results can be found in recent publications from our group.[3–6]

T. cruzi Infection in Mice

Balb/c and C57Bl/6J mice are useful models for studying the immune response to intracellular pathogens because these strains display a different sensitivity to the infection and mount a different type of immune response.[7–10] We have previously shown that inoculation of *T. cruzi* into C57Bl/6J mice leads to a progressive and lethal disease with profound thymic atrophy and loss of $CD4^+CD8^+$ thymocytes, while more than 50% of the Balb/c mice recover.[3] It seems that the increased morbidity of C57Bl/6J mice does not result from an aggravated infection because parasitemia, myocardial parasite nests, and the number of amastigotes in peritoneal macrophages are comparable in both strains. The main differences between infected C57Bl/6J and Balb/c mice are observed in cytokine levels.[3] Although blood levels of TNF-α, interferon (IFN)-γ, interleukin (IL)-1β, and IL-10 are increased in both strains of mice, C57Bl/6J mice display higher TNF-α and lower IL-10 and IL-1β levels than Balb/c mice. Interestingly, peritoneal macrophages from C57Bl/6J mice also produce more TNF-α than those from Balb/c mice when exposed to the parasite *in vitro*. These results suggest that the fatal outcome in C57Bl/6J mice may be linked to an unbalanced relation between cytokines, a proposal that agrees with the report that the cachexia associated with *T. cruzi* infection in mice is attenuated by antibodies to TNF-α.[11] However, it is known that pro-inflammatory cytokines also elicit neuroendocrine responses that can affect the course of inflammatory, infectious, and autoimmune diseases.[12] Therefore, we studied whether alterations in immune–neuroendocrine interactions could also contribute to the different sensitivity to *T. cruzi* infection in these mouse strains.

Changes in Endogenous Corticosterone Levels and the Fate of Thymic Cells during T. cruzi Infection

In the past two decades, several studies have dealt with the immunopathogenesis of *T. cruzi* infection, but there are few reports on the role that neuroendocrine mechanisms may play in the development of the disease.[13–15] We have chosen to study the significance of endogenous glucocorticoid levels for the course of *T. cruzi* infection because the cytokine pattern and the thymic alterations described during this disease are compatible with the hypothesis that the HPA axis might be activated in the mouse model of Chagas' disease used in our studies. Indeed, TNF-α, IL-1β, IL-6, and IFN-γ, which can stimulate the HPA axis (for review, see Refs. 16, 17), are among the cytokines released during *T. cruzi* infection.[3,18] To study the relevance of interactions between cytokines and the HPA axis for the susceptibility and course of *T. cruzi* infection, we have performed comparative studies on possible changes in the release of corticosterone, the main glucocorticoid in mice, in C57Bl/6J and Balb/c mice following inoculation of the parasite.

Basal corticosterone levels in blood are significantly lower in C57Bl/6J mice than in the Balb/c counterparts. While no major changes were detected in glucocorticoid blood levels in C57Bl/6J mice during the first week after inoculation of *T. cruzi* trypomastigotes, Balb/c mice showed a progressive increase in the levels of this hormone following injection of the parasite. Two weeks after infection, increased levels of corticosterone were detected in both mouse strains. Analysis of the increase in glucocorticoid blood levels relative to the mean levels of control mice showed that during the early phase of infection the HPA axis of Balb/c mice was, in contrast to C57Bl/6J mice, already stimulated. For example, on day 5 after *T. cruzi* injection there was no significant increase in corticosterone blood levels in C57Bl/6J mice

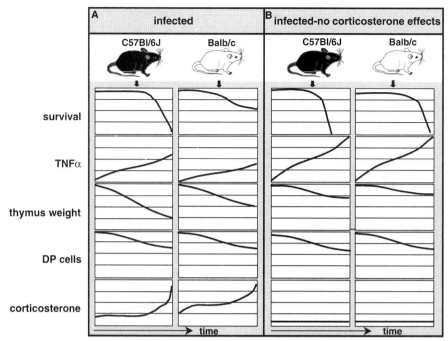

Figure 1. Schematic representation of changes in different parameters during *T cruzi* infection. Comparative effects in survival, tumor necrosis factor (TNF)-α plasma levels, thymus weight, CD4+CD8+ double positive (DP) cells, and corticosterone blood levels between susceptible C57Bl/6J and resistant Balb/c mice during *T. cruzi* infection in intact mice (**A**) and following adrenalectomy and treatment with the glucocorticoid receptor blocker RU486 (**B**). Interference with effects of increased levels of endogenous corticosterone causes increased lethality and TNF-α production but reduces thymus atrophy and apoptosis of DP thymic cells.

relative to the corresponding controls, whereas the levels increased about twofold in infected Balb/c mice. However, 18 days after infection, the relative increase in glucocorticoid levels was twofold higher in C57Bl/6J than in Balb/c mice. These results are schematically represented in Figure 1A.

Severe thymic atrophy during *T. cruzi* infection was observed in C57Bl/6J mice.[3] The progressive diminution in the absolute and relative weight of the gland during the course of the infection was paralleled by a loss of immature double positive (DP) thymic cells, an increase in the percentage of apoptotic cells, and a considerable rise in glucocorticoid levels in plasma. Eighteen days after infection, the reduction in the weight of the thymus was more marked in C57Bl/6J mice (about 70%) than in Balb/c mice (about 36%). A similar difference between the two strains was observed

in the reduction of DP thymocytes. The findings described above prompted us to analyze whether a blockade of glucocorticoid receptors or adrenalectomy affects survival, thymus involution, and cytokine production during *T. cruzi* infection.

Increase in Endogenous Glucocorticoid Levels Prolongs Survival of *T. cruzi*–infected Mice

As mentioned, infection of C57Bl/6J mice with *T. cruzi* is lethal, even with an inoculation of a low number of parasites. Daily treatment with the glucocorticoid receptor blocker RU486 decreased significantly the mean survival time of these mice.[5] The Balb/c strain is more resistant to infection because more than half of the animals that received the same number of parasites as the C57Bl/6J mice survived. Only 40% of the infected Balb/c mice died from *T. cruzi* infection.[3] However, treatment with the blocker RU486 not only significantly shortened the survival time but also resulted in death of all infected Balb/c mice. Interestingly, Balb/c mice treated with the blocker from day 2 after infection died earlier than those in which the blockade was delayed until day 10 post infection. In C57Bl/6J mice, the mortality was the same when the treatment started on day 2 or later (day 10). These results strongly indicate that the early increase in corticosterone blood levels induced by *T. cruzi* inoculation into Balb/c hosts contributes to protecting these animals. Adrenalectomy exerts effects similar to those of the blocker RU486 in *T. cruzi*-infected C57Bl/6J mice. These results are schematically shown in Figure 1A.

Interference with Glucocorticoid Actions Results in Increased Production of Pro-inflammatory Cytokines in *T. cruzi*–infected Mice

To study the influence of endogenous glucocorticoids on the immunoendocrine status during *T. cruzi* infection, systemic levels of pro-inflammatory cytokines and corticosterone were evaluated in adrenalectomized mice inoculated with the parasite or in which glucocorticoid levels were blocked by administration of RU486 at different times after infection. In some experiments, adrenalectomy was combined with administration of the blocker. Although these treatments did not result in complete depletion of glucocorticoids, the concentration of TNF-α, IL-1β, and IL-6 in blood of infected mice was significantly elevated in both C57Bl/6J and Balb/c mice when endogenous corticosterone levels were markedly decreased.[5] These results are schematically represented in Figure 1B.

Interference with Glucocorticoid Effects Reduces Thymic Atrophy and Thymocyte Apotosis in *T. cruzi*–infected Mice

Blockade of glucocorticoid effects and/or adrenalectomy results in thymic protection, as reflected by a markedly decreased thymic atrophy and decreased percentage of apoptotic cells in *T. cruzi*–infected mice. Histologically, the thymus showed preservation of the gland structure, with a cortical pattern and proportion of DP cells similar to that of normal mice. The protection exerted by the combination of adrenalectomy and glucocorticoid blockade was significantly higher than that of each treatment alone.[5] These results, schematically shown in Figure 1B, illustrate the relevance of increased glucocorticoid levels for thymic involution during *T. cruzi* infection.

TNF-α Does Not Mediate Thymus Involution in *T. cruzi*–infected Mice

One of the most marked consequences of the abrogation of glucocorticoid effects in infected mice observed in parallel to a marked reduction in thymic involution was a 4.5-fold increase in systemic TNF-α concentrations compared to those of untreated infected mice. These results already indicate that TNF-α is not directly involved in thymic atrophy. However TNF-α may also exert synergistic effects with endogenous glucocorticoids as it has been shown *in vitro* that TNF-α can induce apoptosis of immature T cells.[19] This possibility was studied using TNF-receptor 1 and TNF-receptor 2 knockout (R1KO, R2KO) mice and also mice that lack both types of receptors (double knockout (DKO)). A clear thymus involution was evident 15 days after *T. cruzi* inoculation in wild-type as well as in the three types of knockout mice. Surprisingly, thymus atrophy (as reflected by relative thymic weight, loss of DP cells, and apoptosis) was even more pronounced in DKO and R1KO mice compared to the corresponding infected wild-type control.[6] Two weeks after infection, the relative thymus weight in DKO and R1KO was half of that observed in their wild-type counterparts. The histology of the gland showed that the thymic cortex virtually disappeared in DKO mice. Similar results were obtained in R1KO mice. In line with the marked thymus weight loss and the histological pattern, the DP population was drastically depleted in DKO and R1KO mice. R2KO showed the smallest difference with respect to the wild-type control. Although basal apoptosis in non-infected DKO and R1KO mice was less than in the normal wild-type mice, the percentage of apoptotic cells in the thymus of infected knockout mice relative to the corresponding basal levels showed that thymocyte cell death was significantly more increased in DKO and R1KO mice than in the wild type. These studies indicate that, although basal TNF-α levels may mediate apoptotic effects, this cytokine might be anti-apoptotic when it is produced under conditions in which other immune or endocrine products are also released, such as during *T. cruzi* infection.

TNF-α Affects Survival, Cytokine Production, and the Response of the HPA Axis in *T. cruzi*–infected Mice

In wild-type mice, mortality caused by *T. cruzi* infection was 100%. No significant difference in the survival time of infected R2KO animals was observed, but the survival time of infected, DKO, and R1KO mice was significantly shortened and the number of blood and tissue parasites was higher when compared to infected wild-type mice.[6] However, in contrast to the severe injury observed in infected wild-type mice, no inflammatory infiltration or fiber destruction was observed in myocardial tissue of DKO mice, indicating the relevance of TNF-α for the development of the cardiac pathology. Thus, in line with other reports, our data indicate that TNF-α plays a complex role during

this disease; it is involved in the mediation of cardiac tissue damage but it also contributes to prolonged survival.

The possibility that cytokine production and HPA axis stimulation are altered in infected, TNF-α-receptor, knockout mice was also studied.[6] TNF-α, IL-1β, and IL-6 concentrations were increased to a greater extent in infected knockout animals than in the infected wild-type mice. Interestingly, TNF-α levels in infected DKO mice were significantly higher than those of the two single knockout mice. This marked release of TNF-α may reflect a feedback mechanism activated by the absence of signals conveyed by the cytokine. IL-1β levels were significantly higher in the three knockout mice than in wild-type mice, while IL-6 concentration was markedly augmented only in DKO mice. Such augmented levels may explain the more pronounced stimulation of the HPA axis observed in DKO and R1KO mice, which showed an 18- and 10-fold increase in corticosterone plasma levels, respectively, compared to the fourfold increase observed in infected wild-type mice. This marked stimulation of the HPA axis in DKO mice may be responsible for the deletion of most of the DP population. These results are schematically represented in Figure 2.

Overview: The Cytokine–HPA Axis Circuit in *T. cruzi*–infected Mice

The data discussed here provide further confirmation to our earlier proposal[20,21] that the immunoregulatory circuit integrated by cytokines and the HPA axis also operates during infection with a protozoan parasite. It has been shown that this circuit exerts protective functions during different experimental and human autoimmune, inflammatory, and viral and bacterial diseases (for review, see Refs. 12, 16). The results reported here show for the first time that blockade of the increase of endogenous corticosterone levels in a model of an intracellular parasite not only accelerates death of C57Bl/6J mice but also results in 100%

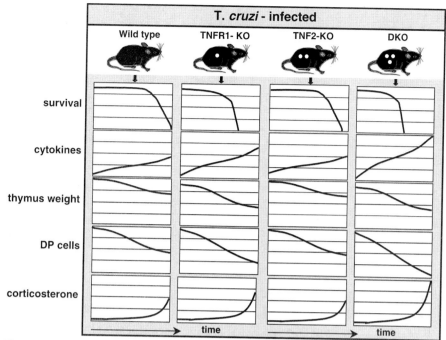

Figure 2. Schematic representation of effects of the lack of TNF-α signals in different parameters during *T. cruzi* infection. Survival, cytokine [TNF-α, IL-1, IL-6] plasma levels, thymus weight, CD4+CD8+ double positive (DP) thymic cells, and corticosterone blood levels in wild-type, TNF-receptor 1 and 2 knockout (R1KO, R2KO) mice, and TNF-receptor 1 and 2 double knockout (DKO) mice. The lack of TNF-α signaling in *T. cruzi*–infected R1KO and DKO mice results in advanced lethality and in a marked increase in IL-1 and corticosterone blood levels without interfering with thymus atrophy and apoptosis of DP thymic cells. However, *T. cruzi* infection causes less inflammatory damage in the heart of these knockout mice compared to wild-type mice (not shown in the figure).

mortality in the less susceptible strain Balb/c. A seemingly paradoxical result is that interference with the cytokine–HPA axis circuit, at the level of either glucocorticoid or TNF-α effects, aggravates the disease but is protective for the thymus. The absence of TNF-α signaling also accelerates the lethal course of the disease. Taken together, the data show that the operation of the cytokine–HPA axis circuit is highly beneficial in impeding the expression of the disease and in retarding its lethal course in susceptible animals. Our data also illustrate the complexity, redundancy, and limitations of the biological effect of this regulatory feedback mechanism. Glucocorticoids can limit the overshoot of inflammatory mechanisms by controlling cytokine production. However, when these hormones are released during a prolonged time,

the physiologic role of inflammatory process, innate immunity, and Th1 and Th17 mechanisms can be inhibited, thus favoring super infections. Furthermore, glucocorticoids can inhibit protein synthesis and affect glucose homeostasis, effects that can debilitate the organism during disease. There is a high redundancy in the capacity of cytokines to stimulate the HPA axis. The results obtained in TNF-α knockout mice show that, in the absence of the signals mediated by this cytokine, there is a clear hyperproduction of IL-1 (about 20-fold), an effect that in DKO mice was paralleled by increased IL-6 levels. IL-1 is considered the most potent of all these mediators in its capacity to stimulate the HPA axis. Thus, these cytokines may have induced the several-fold increase in corticosterone levels in the infected,

TNF receptor (TNFR), knockout mice over the already increased levels in infected wild-type mice. The amounts of corticosterone released in *T. cruzi*–infected TNFR-deficient mice are at the limit of the capacity of the adrenal gland to release these hormones, as observed, for example, during the Waterhouse–Friderichsen sepsis syndrome in humans in which an acute exhaustion of the adrenal cortex is observed. Such levels were clearly not enough for a balanced feedback inhibition of the production of IL-1 and other pro-inflammatory cytokines induced by the parasite. This pattern of cytokine and glucocorticoid production, together with deficient antiparasitic effects from the absence of TNF signals, are likely contributing factors to the accelerated death of infected, TNFR, DKO mice. In general, the effect of the mediators that integrate the immune–cytokine–HPA axis circuit follows a bell-shaped curve. Adaptive and regulatory effects that contribute to re-establish health are exerted within a defined range of concentrations, but hypoproduction or hyperproduction can result in deleterious interactions.

In conclusion, our results indicate that, as with all control systems, both the lack of activation and the hyperactivity of the cytokine–HPA axis circuit can aggravate the course of *T. cruzi* infection.

Acknowledgments

This work was partially supported by the Deutsche Forschungsgemeinschaft (DFG).

Conflicts of Interest

The authors declare no conflicts of interest.

References

1. Teixeira, A.R., N. Nitz, M.C. Guimaro, *et al.* 2006. Chagas disease. *Postgrad. Med. J.* **82:** 788–798.
2. Moncayo, A. & M.I. Ortiz Yanine. 2006. An update on Chagas disease (human American trypanosomiasis). *Ann. Trop. Med. Parasitol.* **100:** 663–677.
3. Roggero, E., A. Perez, M. Tamae-Kakazu, *et al.* 2002. Differential susceptibility to acute Trypanosoma cruzi infection in BALB/c and C57BL/6 mice is not associated with a distinct parasite load but cytokine abnormalities. *Clin. Exp. Immunol.* **128:** 421–428.
4. Roggero, E., I. Piazzon, I. Nepomnaschy, *et al.* 2004. Thymocyte depletion during acute Trypanosoma cruzi infection in C57Bl/6J mice is partly reverted by lipopolysaccharide pretreatment. *FEMS Immunol. Med. Microbiol.* **41:** 123–131.
5. Roggero, E., A.R. Perez, M. Tamae-Kakazu, *et al.* 2006. Endogenous glucocorticoids cause thymus atrophy but are protective during acute Trypanosoma cruzi infection. *J. Endocrinol.* **190:** 495–503.
6. Perez, A.R., E. Roggero, A. Nicora, *et al.* 2007. Thymus atrophy during Trypanosoma cruzi infection is caused by an immuno-endocrine imbalance. *Brain Behav. Immun.* **21:** 890–900.
7. Heinzel, F.P., R.M. Rerko & A.M. Hujer. 1998. Underproduction of interleukin-12 in susceptible mice during progressive leishmaniasis is due to decreased CD40 activity. *Cell Immunol.* **184:** 129–142.
8. Appelberg, R., A.G. Castro, J. Pedrosa, *et al.* 1994. Role of gamma interferon and tumor necrosis factor alpha during T-cell-independent and -dependent phases of Mycobacterium avium infection. *Infect. Immun.* **62:** 3962–3971.
9. Wrightsman, R., S. Krassner & J. Watson. 1982. Genetic control of responses to Trypanosoma cruzi in mice: multiple genes influencing parasitemia and survival. *Infect. Immun.* **36:** 637–644.
10. Andrade, V., M. Barral-Netto & S.G. Andrade. 1985. Patterns of resistance of inbred mice to Trypanosoma cruzi are determined by parasite strain. *Braz. J. Med. Biol. Res.* **18:** 499–506.
11. Truyens, C., F. Torrico, A. Angelo-Barrios, *et al.* 1995. The cachexia associated with Trypanosoma cruzi acute infection in mice is attenuated by anti-TNF-alpha, but not by anti-IL-6 or anti-IFN-gamma antibodies. *Parasite Immunol.* **17:** 561–568.
12. Besedovsky, H.O. & A. del Rey. 2006. Regulating inflammation by glucocorticoids. *Nat. Immunol.* **7:** 537.
13. Savino, W., M.C. Leite-de-Moraes, M. Hontebeyrie-Joskowicz & M. Dardenne. 1989. Studies on the thymus in Chagas' disease. I. Changes in the thymic microenvironment in mice acutely infected with Trypanosoma cruzi. *Eur. J. Immunol.* **19:** 1727–1733.
14. Leite de Moraes, M.C., M. Hontebeyrie-Joskowicz, F. Leboulenger, *et al.* 1991. Studies on the thymus in Chagas' disease. II. Thymocyte subset fluctuations

in Trypanosoma cruzi–infected mice: relationship to stress. *Scand. J. Immunol.* **33:** 267–275.

15. Correa-de-Santana, E., M. Paez-Pereda, M. Theodoropoulou, *et al.* 2006. Hypothalamus-pituitary-adrenal axis during Trypanosoma cruzi acute infection in mice. *J. Neuroimmunol.* **173:** 12–22.

16. Besedovsky, H.O. & A. del Rey. 1996. Immune-neuro-endocrine interactions: facts and hypotheses. *Endocr. Rev.* **17:** 64–102.

17. Turnbull, A.V. & C.L. Rivier. 1999. Regulation of the hypothalamic-pituitary-adrenal axis by cytokines: actions and mechanisms of action. *Physiol. Rev.* **79:** 1–71.

18. Gao, W. & M.A. Pereira. 2002. Interleukin-6 is required for parasite specific response and host resistance to Trypanosoma cruzi. *Int. J. Parasitol.* **32:** 167–170.

19. Hernandez-Caselles, T. & O. Stutman. 1993. Immune functions of tumor necrosis factor. I. Tumor necrosis factor induces apoptosis of mouse thymocytes and can also stimulate or inhibit IL-6-induced proliferation depending on the concentration of mitogenic costimulation. *J. Immunol.* **151:** 3999–4012.

20. Besedovsky, H.O., A.E. del Rey & E. Sorkin. 1985. Immune-neuroendocrine interactions. *J. Immunol.* **135:** 750s–754s.

21. Besedovsky, H., A. del Rey, E. Sorkin & C.A. Dinarello. 1986. Immunoregulatory feedback between interleukin-1 and glucocorticoid hormones. *Science* **233:** 652–654.

Index of Contributors